The Mind within the Net

The Mind within the Net
Models of Learning, Thinking, and Acting

Manfred Spitzer

A Bradford Book
The MIT Press
Cambridge, Massachusetts
London, England

© 1999 Massachusetts Institute of Technology

This work originally appeared in German under the title *Geist im Netz*.
All rights reserved. No part of this book may be reproduced in any form or by any electronic or mechanical means (including photocopying, recording, or information storage and retrieval) without permission in writing from the publisher.

This book was set in Sabon by Wellington Graphics and was printed and bound in the United States of America.

Library of Congress Cataloging-in-Publication Data

Spitzer, Manfred.
  [Geist im Netz. English]
  The mind within the net : models of learning, thinking, and acting / Manfred Spitzer.
    p.   cm.
  "A Bradford Book"
  Translation of: Geist im Netz.
  Includes bibliographical references and index.
  ISBN 0-262-19406-6 (hardcover : alk. paper)
  1. Neural networks (Neurobiology)   I. Title.
QP363.3.S55   1998
612.8'2—dc2   98-10911
                 CIP

For Ulla, Anja, Thomas, Stefan, and Markus

Contents

Preface

How does the brain work? How do billions of neurons bring about ideas, sensations, emotions, and actions? Why do children play, and why do they learn faster than elderly people? What can go wrong in perception, thinking, learning, and acting?

The 1990s are the decade of the brain. In the past ten years the field of neuroscience has yielded a wealth of knowledge that allows us to study these questions within a framework created by neurobiology and neural network theory. Neurophysiology has told us a great deal about how individual neurons work, and neural network theory is demonstrating how neurons work *together*. In the years ahead, we can expect to learn much more about the underlying principles of neural networks and how they produce the higher cognitive functions.

How do networks built out of neurons work? How do they produce higher and the highest cognitive functions? What are their underlying principles? The first part of this book provides an introduction to the basic structure of neural networks. In the second part I report on some of the most important discoveries that have been made by studying neural networks. In the third part I describe in some detail several applications of network models that throw new light on normal and abnormal states of mind. In my view, insights gained from these models will change the way we think about ourselves and about other people.

What is this book good for? And for whom is it written? It may be argued that a complex mathematical theory about a specific class of cells is much too complicated to yield understandings relevant to real life. Obviously, I do not agree, for several reasons. First, important discoveries in neuroscience have undoubtedly been made in the recent past. Secondly, these discoveries—because they concern such basic human activities as thinking and acting—are relevant not just to a few scientists but to the general public as well. Thirdly, as a psychiatrist, I am intrigued by the insights that have already resulted from several network models of mental disorder. In other words, computer models can help us understand what appear to be the most private if all human experiences. Neuroscience and neural network theory can also make us understand why a toddler should listen to childrens songs rather than to complex music and why some elderly people have trouble finding their way around in a new environment.

Some may find it hard to believe that a mathematical theory can fundamentally change the way in which we think about learning, creativity, thinking, and acting, or how we can apply it in such varied domains as kindergartens, schools, politics, television programming, and retirement homes. It may even help us understand individuals struggling with mental disorders like problems of concentration or delusions. It is just these possibilities that motivated me to write this book. In my view, what researchers have discovered is no longer just for the laboratory; it has become directly relevant to all of us. In this respect, then, this book is about *your* brain, *your* thoughts, skills, and actions, *your* children and *our* society.

Not only the layperson, but also the specialist has difficulty keeping track of the latest news from research and development. The more you know, the more you know what you do not know; you read one paper and you want to read ten more, and so on. Moreover, the relevant papers in neurobiology, neural network theory, psychology, and psychiatry are scattered across a wide range of journals, books, and other sources. They are not easy to find for those who are interested in the subject but unfamiliar with the research carried out in all these separate fields. This book, then, should help physicians, psychologists, teachers, and all those who are interested in the topic and have not lost their curiosity about the world and themselves.

This book should probably be read twice: once to get the main argument, and a second time to understand the details. Once the general ideas become clear, many things that may have seemed confusing will seem obvious. Readers eager to have fun immediately may want start with chapter 10 on semantic models or with the users manual for the brain described in chapter 12.

Ulm, Germany
March 1998

Acknowledgments

In preparing the manuscript, I had help from my family as well as from several friends and colleagues.

Within the past eight years, my research has been supported by the Alexander von Humboldt Foundation, the German Research Society (Deutsche Forschungsgemeinschaft, DFG), the German Society for Psychiatry and Neurology (Deutsche Gesellschaft fr Psychiatrie und Nervenheilkunde), and by the National Alliance for Research in Schizophrenia and Depression (NARSAD). The Psychiatry Hospital at the University of Heidelberg provided me with the environment that made my work possible.

The English translation of this book was first suggested by Michael Posner while he and his wife were on a visit to Germany. They dropped by at our home, and we had a good time showing them around some of the more picturesque parts of the country. I happened to show Mike my new book, which had just been published, and went through it with him briefly. He liked it and said he would love to see it come out in English. Two months later, therefore, I started translating it and, not long after that, received the support of The MIT Press—in particular Michael Rutter. Without his never-failing and always positive encouragement, the project probably never would have been completed (especially as I had changed jobs in the middle of the project). Many thanks to the two Michaels!

Brooks Casas, who had been one of my undergraduate students at Harvard and was spending a year in my Heidelberg lab, also worked with me on the translation. I greatly enjoyed his invaluable comments and missed his help when—after a successful year in Germany—he returned to Harvard as a graduate student. Special thanks to Brooks!

Finally, Katherine Arnoldi of The MIT Press and copyeditor Roberta Clark did their best to change all those passive-voice German sentences in my translation into something readable in English. Many thanks for the hard work you put into my book.

This book is dedicated to my children. They taught me a lot.

The Mind within the Net

1

Introduction

There are about twenty billion neurons in the brain, each of them connected to as many as ten thousand others. Given the magnitude of these numbers, understanding the functions of such a system mathematically might appear to be completely out of our reach. In fact, it seems unreasonable even to conceive of such an attempt. And even if it were possible to do so, how would thinking about the brain in these terms affect our understanding of human individuality and freedom? Does a mechanistic theory of the brain and its functions necessarily degrade us to the level of machines?

Don't despair!

Nor need we become confused by the labyrinth of questions about our brain and its twenty billion neurons. We can start simply, by looking at a few neurons, maybe three or five, and see how far we get. As we will see later, it would be a mistake to start with more. To make progress in understanding a complex phenomenon scientists have to make matters as simple as possible.

Let us take, for example, a physics problem. If you want to understand the principles of gravity (i.e., why and how things fall to the ground), you had better disregard the color of the particular objects and the composition of the air space through which they fall. In fact, you should probably think not in terms of any specific object falling at any particular location but of an abstract object, thereby simplifying matters considerably. Once you understand the principles of how objects fall in a vacuum, you can discover additional laws relevant to specific conditions. Knowledge of how air resistance affects objects, for example, can be combined with the principles of gravity to explain the falling of leaves or the flight of airplanes.

To put it a bit differently, imagine that you are strolling through a forest in the fall as the wind swirls hundreds of thousands of leaves around you. In the light of such complexity, you might be tempted to think it impossible to understand the motions of the many leaves. However, swirling leaves in the wind need not cause an epistemological nightmare. We know the principles that govern the actual fall of the many thousands of leaves by understanding a few laws of physics. We need not, therefore, assume the existence of some "vital force" in the wind or of a drive within leaves that motivates them to dance whenever wind is present. Of course, our understanding of the physical principles does not entail the belief that any physicist has ever predicted, or will ever be able to predict, the exact flight paths of all the leaves falling on a windy day in a particular forest.

By the same token, the principle of gravity tells us nothing about the color or form of a falling object, just as it completely disregards the qualities of the air. Thus, on the one hand, it accounts only to a certain degree for any particular real object falling on earth but, on the other hand, also applies to objects falling on the backside of the moon. Scientists must reduce the multitude of influences on the colorful, moving, swirling world around them to the few factors that are essential for studying a specific aspect of the world. That is, scientists simplify matters by reducing a complex reality to a simpler model of reality. It is therefore not unusual, and by no means unscientific, to study not twenty billion neurons, but only three. In fact, it would be against the very spirit and nature of science to start with many more.

To understand human beings better is a good thing. "Know thyself" the proverb inscribed on the Temple of Apollo at Delphi reminded the Greeks, and wise men ever since have striven for a better understanding of themselves. If we understand ourselves better, we will perhaps treat ourselves, and others, more wisely. It is strange that when we buy a fairly complex tool or machine—a personal computer for example—we take it for granted that we will get a thick manual of instruction. However, although our brain is many orders of magnitude more complex than any computer, we assume that there is no manual for it.

History

More than a hundred years ago, people began to think about how groups of neurons might give rise to higher mental functions. The Italian physician Camilo Golgi (figure 1.1a) originally set out to stain the meninges—the layers of tissue in which the brain is wrapped. Experimenting with silver salts, he discovered that some of the cells in the brain became black, while most of them remained unstained. Thus the famous Golgi method of staining was discovered (figure 1.2). Its most important virtue is that

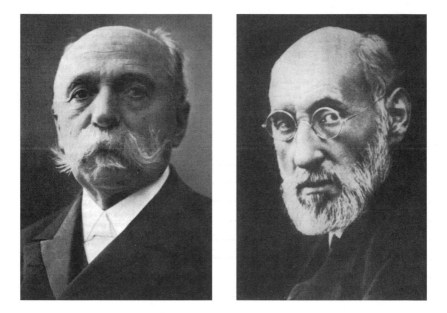

Figure 1.1
(a) The methodologist Camillo Golgi (1843–1926) and (b) the anatomist Santiago Ramón y Cajal (1852–1934). Golgi's method of staining is unique, because it not only shows the neurons in striking detail but also stains only about one in a hundred neurons, leaving enough surrounding translucent space to permit close examination of the stained neurons. Golgi's method is still used without much change, and we still do not know why it stains only in a fraction of the neurons. Ramón y Cajal used Golgi's method to discover small gaps between the ends of any one of the treelike cells and other cells. He interpreted these gaps as real gaps—rather than as artifacts of staining or other accidental phenomena—and recognized their importance for understanding how the brain is built.

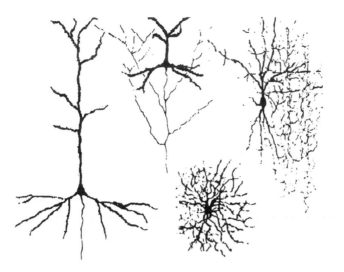

Figure 1.2
Neurons, as drawn by Santiago Ramón y Cajal from microscopic observation of
Golgi-stained brain tissue.

it works on only about 1 percent of the cells, coloring in unprecedented
detail all the small structures of the cell body, while adjacent cells remain
invisible. If all the cells in brain tissue became black in this way, we would
be unable to distinguish any one cell from all the others. But as only
about one in a hundred becomes black—the reason for this is still
unknown—we can see those few cells and their connections in beautiful
detail.

Working with Golgi's method, the Spanish neuroanatomist Santiago
Ramón y Cajal (figure 1.1b) developed the idea that the nervous system
consists of single cells, the *neurons* (as these cells were baptized by the
German anatomist Wilhelm Waldeyer in 1891). After carefully scrutiniz-
ing thousands of brain slices, Ramón y Cajal hypothesized that the brain
is not a unitary entity, like a sponge, but consists of many small elements,
the neurons.

Golgi and Ramón y Cajal both received the Nobel prize in 1906 while
they continued to dispute each other's ideas. Golgi still insisted that the
brain is not built out of neurons, but is, rather, a *syncytium*, a spongelike
structure. Ramón y Cajal's hypothesis nonetheless won out and by the
turn of the century was widely accepted by the scientific community.

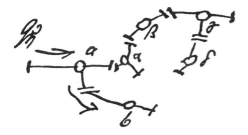

Figure 1.3
Neural network drawn by Sigmund Freud in 1895. The arrow on the left denotes incoming energy, which is redirected within the network. Several authors have argued that a large part of Freud's psychoanalytic theory can be traced back conceptually to his understanding of the neurophysiology of his day, that is, to ideas about the flow of energy in neural networks (Pribram & Gill 1976, Sulloway 1982, Spitzer 1984). For example, neurophysiologist Freud held that energy can be redirected (*displaced*), thereby changing the connection between an idea and its energy (*cathexis*). He also used the term *regression* to describe what happens when energy flows backwards through the network.

In the waning years of the nineteenth century, two Austrian physicians, Sigmund Freud and Siegmund Exner, thought that networks of neurons could explain normal as well as disordered mental phenomena and made drawings showing how such networks might function (figure 1.3). These early attempts to develop network models of mental functioning, however, remained speculative neurophysiology. Although researchers could see neurons, they had no idea how they worked or what they were processing.

In the ensuing fifty years the phenomena of membrane potential, action potential, and synaptic transmission—the transmission of signals through the release of chemical substances across the gaps between neurons—were discovered. More recently, neurophysiologists have learned that the release of chemical substances at the synapse is subject to change, depending upon the experience of the organism. By about 1980 the basic physiology of the neuron had been worked out.

At least as important as the discoveries of the mechanisms of neuronal excitation and inhibition was the idea that neurons do not process energy but, rather, *information*. This completely novel conception was developed by the neurophysiologist Warren McCulloch and the mathematician Walter Pitts. It threw new light on the question of how neurons work and what they do and provided a totally new framework for research into how information is processed by neurons and neural networks.

McCulloch and Pitts answered the question of how neurons process information by assuming that neurons are logical switches. The groundwork for this idea had been laid in the last century, by Gottlieb Frege (1879/1977; cf. Kneale & Kneale 1984), who identified logical elements and rules as the building blocks of any complex proposition. In their landmark paper, McCulloch and Pitts (1943/1989) demonstrated that neurons can be used to implement the basic operations of propositional logic: the operators *and, or,* and *not.* This finding provided the foundation for their claim that any complex proposition could be represented by neurons. This assertion was, of course, a major breakthrough.

McCulloch and Pitts's paper broke new ground theoretically and provided the basis for an entire new field of inquiry. It was also highly speculative; it even included discussion of how the new theory could be applied in psychiatry. Dysfunctional states ranging from tinnitus to delusions thereby came within the scope of a neurobiological and neurocomputational theory that banished ideas about "ghosts" in the head: "In such systems," they wrote, "'Mind' no longer 'goes more ghostly than a ghost.' Instead, diseased mentality can be understood without loss of scope or rigor, in the scientific terms of neurophysiology" (McCulloch & Pitts 1943/1989:25).

It later turned out that the ideas of the two scientists about how neurons actually operate were all wrong. Neurons are *not* logical switches like transistors and computer chips. Nonetheless, the insight that neurons process information was born and has remained fruitful ever since. It provided the entirely new vista from which we have studied neurons ever since and posed the fundamental research question: If neurons process information, how do they do it?

Groundbreaking research on the functions of neural networks was carried out during the birth of the field of neurophysiology in the late 1950s and early 1960s. However, in the ensuing decade, as the major limitations of the early models were pointed out—for example in the influential book by Minsky and Papert (1969)—work in the field tapered off (cf. Spitzer 1996a, Zell 1994).

Since the middle of the 1980s, neural network research has bounced back and is now very strong in such diverse fields as computer science, physics, psychology, neuroscience, psychiatry, linguistics, artificial intelligence, medicine, and engineering.[1]

Neural Networks in Intensive-Care Units

Currently, simulated neural networks are used in applied as well as research settings. They are quite often employed by engineers and technicians when there is a vaguely defined or complex problem to be solved with limited computing power (cf. Ritter et al. 1991, Sanchez-Sinecio & Lau 1992, Schöneburg 1993, Spies 1993). If a given problem does not have a worked-out algorithm—that is, it cannot be tackled in a step-by-step fashion in which all the possible steps are known—or if a problem requires application of judgment, gestalt pattern recognition, or rules of thumb, simulated neural networks are likely to provide a solution. Quite possibly, there is a neural network in your camera or in your microwave oven (Anon. 1994). Other applications of neural networks are the computer models used in research on machine vision and automatic pattern recognition.

These problems arise in the most diverse domains of science and in studies of the smallest to the largest objects. In high-energy physics, for example, when subatomic particles are made to collide, new particles come into existence and are detected by photographing their traces in so-called cloud chambers. In multiple experimental sessions, thousands of photographs are generated; they must be examined one by one by research assistants searching for an unusual trace indicative of an unusual particle. The task of examining these photographs has been, in part, taken over by simulated neural networks trained to recognize unusual patterns. In astronomy, too, neural networks help with the task of classifying newly discovered galaxies. The flood of images generated at

---

1. There are a number of introductory books and overviews of neural network research. The two volumes by Rumelhart and McClelland (1986) have become classics and are still highly recommended as introductions to the subject. Kosslyn & König (1992) provide a brilliant account of neural network research in psychology, and Anderson (1995) has probably written the best general introduction. The edited volumes by Anderson and Rosenfeld (1988), Anderson et al. (1990), and Arbib (1995) contain neurobiological and neurocomputational resources for in-depth reading.

astronomical observatories around the globe also need to be rapidly classed as clusters, spirals, clouds, or other types of galaxies. Interestingly, astronomers have still not agreed on an international classification system for galaxies, although they have learned that neural networks can do the job of classification as well as any human expert (Lahav et al. 1995).

In the field of medicine, too, where many of the tasks performed by doctors lack an algorithmic solution, problems of pattern recognition and judgment are ubiquitous. For example, neural networks are increasingly being used to interpret electroencephalographic (EEG) curves (Gabor & Seyal 1992), sleep EEGs (Mamelak et al. 1991), chest x-rays (Boone et al. 1992), microscopic tissue samples in gynecology (Boon & Kok 1993) and other specialties (O'Leary et al. 1992), and clinical and radiological data from cancer patients (Kiernan 1994, Maclin et al. 1991, Ravdin & Clark 1992, Wilding et al. 1994, Wu et al. 1993). Even in psychiatry, neural networks have provided guidance for decisions about admission, diagnosis, and length of stay (Florio et al. 1994, Lowell & Davis 1994, Modai et al. 1993, Somoza & Somoza 1993).

All these applications have one common feature: They require a complex pattern to be analyzed on the basis of previous experience. Neurologists, cardiologists, and radiologists have examined thousands of EEGs, electrocardiograms (ECGs), and x-rays; working from their experience, they are able to evaluate new patterns quickly, picking out essential features and disregarding artifacts. Exactly what allows these specialists to detect essential features is often unclear; that is, the meaning of *experience* and *essential* cannot be precisely quantified and expressed algorithmically. For this reason, it was long believed that these capabilities could be studied only in a human context; that is, by interpreting the activities of the human mind. This may not be so. Looking at some applications of simulated neural networks can demonstrate the incorrectness of that assumption.

In medicine use of neural networks does not stop at the door of the intensive-care unit (cf. Tu & Guerriere 1993). They are also employed to evaluate Doppler ultrasound signals and decide whether or not microembolisms are present (Siebler et al. 1994). If the results of numerous laboratory tests of, for example, blood-lipid levels, are entered into a neural network, it can predict the risk of heart attack in a given individual (Lapuerta et al. 1995). A neural network can also diagnose heart disease from ECGs more reliably than a conventional computer program can. If a heart attack occurs and the patient is successfully resuscitated, neural networks trained with a large enough data base can predict the patient's survival on the basis of clinical and laboratory variables (Ebell 1993).

One emergency room physician at a North Carolina hospital trained a neural network by inputting large quantities of experiential data on diagnoses and severity of injuries (Rutledge 1995). In due course, the network learned to predict from complex clinical data the clinical outcome of patients brought in by the ambulance. This capability can be important, particularly when available resources are limited and have to be distributed in a way that achieves the most benefit for the most patients. After a large road accident, for example, seven people with major injuries may require intensive care when only four beds in the unit are available. In such a situation, assigning patients who will derive the most benefit from the care will make the best use of a scarce resource. In the case of any one patient, moreover, the physician may find it extremely difficult to make such a rational judgment on the basis of the patient's injuries, laboratory results, age, and general clinical condition. Moreover, no human being is free from subjective feelings and private values that may influence a decision when, for example, a bleeding child is brought in. These subjective factors make reaching a decision that will result in the best possible outcome difficult, if not unachievable.

Because a neural network can, in principle, store more experience than any physician, it can usually come up with a rational decision in such a case within seconds after clinical and lab data are entered. The idea of leaving such decisions to a computer is, admittedly, hard for many people to swallow. Why?

Enlightenment!

Over the centuries, we have become accustomed to the fact that the earth is not the center of the universe. For little over a century, we've had time to get used to the idea that the human animal may not be the apex of creation. Compared to the uneasiness generated by the ideas of Galileo Galilei and Charles Darwin, our reactions to the mysteries of the mind are even more unsettling. The last bastion of human uniqueness, it seems, is about to be conquered by science.

Even if we are not the center of the world and the apex of evolution, we might argue, we at least have our minds—minds governed by laws quite different from those controlling matter. Because the natural sciences are about matter, and not about mind, the latter has often seemed secure from scientific scrutiny. In short, although we've had to sacrifice being the center of the universe and the crown of creation, at least our minds have been secure. This view of ourselves has been radically challenged by the research of the past decade.

We know very well what is good for our car, our garden, our stomach, and our heart. But what is good for our brain? Even the question sounds a bit strange if we are thinking not about vitamins, low cholesterol, and moderate alcohol consumption but about the right *food for thought*. Which thoughts, perceptions, sensations, feelings, and so forth are good for our brain? The question makes no sense to us. Why?

Until a few years ago, we regarded the brain as a rather static organ, unlike other parts of the body. If we train a muscle, it gets bigger; even adult bones are constantly growing new cells, shuffling bone matter around to provide the most stability at the least material cost. (It is not only astronauts who have to fight this feature of the bones.) Neurons, in contrast, cannot divide. Neuronal tissue in humans is a type of *postmitotic tissue;* that is, its cells have lost the ability to divide to form new cells. We are born with a set of neurons that begin, slowly, to die immediately thereafter at the rate of about ten thousand a day. Even though only 1.3 percent of our original neurons are dead by the time we are seventy—so that we still have almost all of the twenty billion we started with—the idea that we are losing brain matter remains a frightening thought. No new cortical gyrus grows when we do difficult math problems; it appears, then, that our brains are not adapting to the ever-changing challenges of life. All we have is a three-pound mass of unchanging, slowly dying, forever-inexplicable matter. Of course, from this perspective, the question of the best food for thought makes no sense at all.

But this view is plainly wrong! We know that our brain is our most flexible and adaptive organ. In contrast to a conventional computer, our brain "hardware" cares a great deal about what "software" is running on it, because "bio-hardware" constantly adjusts itself to the software. It is as though a personal computer (PC), in order to run more efficiently, continually reconfigured itself to respond to the demands of the software and the files it processes. PC users, plagued by system crashes and carelessly programmed software, can only dream of such a computer. In biology, these "computers" are a reality.

A blind person learning to read Braille must sense small protrusions on the paper—up to six per character—with the tip of the right index finger. Someone reading a Braille book touches more than a million little dots and processes them into characters, words, sentences, paragraphs, and the meaning of the story (figure 1.4). Wouldn't it be nice if the small piece of cortex that takes care of processing sensory information from the tip of the right index finger could grow in size?

According to research carried out in the past fifteen years, this is exactly what happens. In the brains of people who read Braille, the area devoted to processing sensory information from the tip of the right index finger is larger than the corresponding area for the left index finger. By contrast, the cortical areas used to carry out the processing of sensory information from a limb shrink in size after that limb is amputated. This capacity of the brain to respond to changes in the input by changes of the corresponding hardware is called *neuroplasticity* (see chapter 7). It is present not only in children, but also in adults.

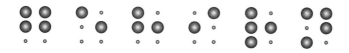

Figure 1.4
The word *brain* written in Braille, the writing system used by the blind since the middle of the last century.

Although brains and computers are often mentioned together—because both process information—they are different in many respects. Let us have a look at these differences.

Brains versus Computers

What is 4,257,891 divided by 306? Most people not only need paper and pencil to come up with an answer to this question but also quite some time. A computer does such a task within a tiny fraction of a second. On the other hand, most people know thousands of faces and can recognize one of them within a few hundred milliseconds—a task that is presently beyond the reach of even the most advanced supercomputers. This example highlights the fundamental differences between biological information-processing systems and conventional digital computers. These differences can be spelled out in terms of three dimensions: speed, reliability, and architecture.

Speed

Compared to the switches of the integrated circuits in a computer, neurons are terribly slow. The central processing unit (CPU) of a conventional PC may have a clock speed of 200 megahertz; that is, it can do two hundred million computations in one second. In contrast to such raw speed, neurons are slower by at least six orders of magnitude; at maximum speed even the fastest neurons in the human cortex can perform no more than about two hundred computations per second.

It should be noted that this difference in processing speed is highly problematic for researchers in artificial intelligence (AI), the field investigating how conventional digital computers can perform higher cognitive functions. Human beings can perform certain high-level cognitive tasks such as reading a word or recognizing a face in a remarkably short time (a few hundred milliseconds). Because neurons can carry out only about a hundred computations within this time frame, it would seem that the "programs" that run on our neural hardware are extremely simple. A human word-reading program or a face-recognition program, therefore, must not be longer than about a hundred lines (i.e., consist of no more than about a hundred steps). Since even simple computer programs often contain thousands of lines of code, it follows that the "algorithms" running on biological information-processing systems must be quite different from those employed on conventional computers. In the field of AI, this is known as the hundred-step problem (cf. Rumelhart 1989:135).

Reliability

For a PC to run properly, it must not make any mistakes. This was highlighted most clearly in 1995 when a faulty computer chip made headlines around the globe. The Intel Corporation had produced a new central processing unit for personal computers that, according to calculations performed by the company, on average made a single error in nine billion computations (Arthur 1994, Cipra 1995). The error was so minute that it remained undetected during the initial production and testing phase of the new chip. It occurred only when certain programs were running, and even then happened very rarely. Nonetheless, when the news of the error broke, there was an outcry among computer users, and Intel was forced to replace the faulty chips, with no charge to the customers and at high cost to the company.

If we were to cry out whenever a neuron in our brain made a mistake, we would be constantly screaming. With respect to reliability, neurons differ from computer chips by nine orders of magnitude (i.e., a factor of one billion!), as the mathematician John von Neumann estimated in his famous Yale lectures on *The Computer and the Brain* (1960). Thus reliability is the most pronounced difference between neurons and computers. The difference in speed, of a factor of about one million, pales in comparison with a difference in reliability of something like a billion. Even if von Neumann's estimate turns out to be too high (cf. Mainen & Sejnowski 1995), we can safely conclude from the marked difference in reliability and speed that neurons operate very differently from computers.

However, on the flip side of the high error rate of neurons lies a remarkable fact about neuronal information-processing systems (i.e., brains) in contrast to silicon-based digital computers: Brains are remarkably insensitive to hardware problems. Unlike PCs, brains can still function even when large numbers of their components, the neurons, have broken down, whereas a conventional computer simply stops working completely if only a single wire has broken. There may be no noticeable subjective or objective decrease of function in a human brain that has lost a large portion of its neurons and connections. The slow and gradual change of function in biological brains that is caused by an increasing number of hardware errors has been called *graceful degradation* (Rumelhart & McClelland 1986).

Architecture

Brains and computers differ not only in speed and reliability, but also with respect to their internal structure, which is often referred to as their *architecture*. In computers, *data* are stored at specified *addresses,* while in brains there is no difference between data and addresses: the stored data *are* the addresses. Furthermore, in computers data are processed by *programs,* and there is a *central processing unit.* In neuronal systems, there is neither a distinction between data and programs nor a central processing unit. Finally, whereas conventional computers process information bit by bit in a serial fashion, in the brain billions of neurons work in parallel.

Recap

Ideas about how neurons work together in networks are almost as old as the idea that the brain is composed of neurons. However, it took the concept of information to throw light on what neurons actually do—process information.

The common task of human perception—of the physician making a diagnostic decision, the astronomer classifying galaxies, and the particle physicist searching for new forms of matter—is *pattern recognition.* Such patterns may be the signals traveling from the eye to the brain along the optic nerve, or clusters of symptoms, or pixels on a computer screen. Neural networks can carry out the task of pattern recognition and are being used around the world to an increasing degree whenever a problem is ill defined, calls for the application of rules of thumb and judgment, and has no worked-out algorithmic solution. They are most frequently met with in medical contexts.

However, we have a hard time getting used to the idea that a simulated neural network running on a computer can carry out tasks we think of as requiring uniquely human capabilities—tasks, for example, that used to be carried out by doctors. For many of us, the hardest idea to swallow may be the notion that thought itself can be the subject of scientific inquiry.

As pointed out above, although brains and computers share the ability to process information, they differ greatly in speed, reliability, and architecture. Because neurons are slow and prone to error, they make lousy information-processing hardware, although they compensate for these limitations by their sheer number. Moreover, in contrast to conventional computers, the hardware of the biological brain is highly plastic and constantly adjusts itself to the demands of the "software" running on it—that is, the experience of the organism.

In light of the pronounced structural differences between computers and brains, it is factually wrong to equate them with each other, as people who know little about either or both of them sometimes do. It should be clear from the discussion that human beings are not "mere computers" just because both the brain and the computer are information-processing devices. Quite the reverse is true: the more we learn about brain-style computing, the better we recognize the differences between the brain and the computer. These differences will become obvious in various passages of this book as we investigate network models of information processing that can cast new light on our brains and, therefore, on ourselves.

This book is divided into three parts. In the first part I provide an introduction to some of the basic principles of neural networks. In the second part, I report on a number of the most important discoveries that have been made by using computer simulations of neural networks, in particular discoveries that have significant consequences for our understanding of how the biological brain operates. In the third part, I describe in some detail several applications of network models that throw new light on normal and abnormal states of mind. In my view, insights gained from these models may change radically the way we think about ourselves and others. Throughout the book, to make the discussion as accessible as possible to a variety of readers, I avoid the use of mathematics in favor of examples and intuition.

I

Basics

The following three chapters provide the basic information needed for discussion of higher mental functions in neurobiological and simulated neural network terms. In chapter 2 we describe in a detailed, step-by-step fashion how small networks made of a few neurons actually process information. In order to function properly, such networks have to be "programmed." In chapter 3 we see that whereas in conventional computers such programming is carried out by the storage of rules, neural networks are programmed by learning from examples. In this respect, neural networks are like children, who do not become educated by learning and applying rules through preaching or programming but by observing, experiencing, and practicing many examples. Finally, in chapter 4, we tackle the question of how information is coded and why vector coding is advantageous in terms of the required hardware. It turns out that neural networks do linear algebra; that is, they compute with vectors.

2

Neuronal Teamwork

Every living cell is capable of responding to its environment. Heat, cold, the presence of certain chemical substances, or merely touch can change the permeability of the cell's membrane to ions and thereby induce changes in the membrane potential. Moreover, these changes in membrane potential propagate along the cell membrane. In the course of evolution, however, one type of cell became specialized in its excitability and its ability to conduct changes of electrical potential along the membrane. These cells are the neurons (figure 2.1).

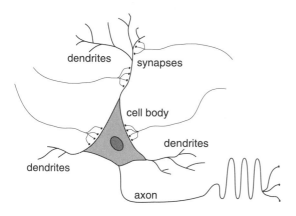

Figure 2.1
Schematic rendering of a neuron. The wide, treelike branches are called *dendrites* (from the Greek word *dendron*, tree). At the dendrites, as well as at the body of the cell (the *soma*, again, from the Greek word for body), the neuron receives signals from other neurons by way of the *synapses* (Greek for coupling), small protrusions at the ends of fibers. Each neuron has one *axon*, a long "wire" through which it sends out signals.

The neuronal functions of excitability and conductivity of signals are based on the movement of ions, that is, electrically charged atoms. All cells of the body use at least one-third of their energy to pump sodium ions out of, and potassium ions into, themselves. This causes an electrical potential of about seventy millivolts at the cell membrane (and a negative charge inside the cell); this is the so-called *resting potential*. In addition to sodium and potassium, other substances are constantly exchanged between the cell and its environment. The involved processes and structures—ion pumps, ion channels, and receptors—interact in complex ways, which has the net effect that the membrane resting potential can become unstable under certain circumstances. In other words, if the resting potential is disturbed, it may change rapidly and either increase or decrease. Although this process can occur in all cells, neurons have become specialized to use these changes in membrane potential for the processing of information.

If the resting potential of a neuron is decreased by about twenty millivolts, rapid changes take place inside the membrane and cause the negative potential to decrease further and even to become positive for a brief period of time. These processes are like an avalanche: once started, they are inevitable and continue automatically, guided by their own nature. This *depolarization* of the membrane is followed, within one to ten milliseconds, by the re-establishment of the resting potential, that is, by a *repolarization* process. This very brief burst of the membrane potential into the positive range followed by the immediate restoration of the resting potential is called an *action potential*. Action potentials follow a simple all-or-nothing rule: there are no graded—that is, small or large—action potentials (Kandel & Schwarz 1995, Nichols et al. 1995, Schmidt & Thews 1995).

The membrane potential at which the avalanchelike action potential is automatically triggered is called the *threshold* of the neuron. If a neuron gets excited, its resting potential is shifted more and more toward the threshold, until it reaches threshold and fires off an action potential. Action potentials start at certain positions on the cell's membrane and travel along the axon of the neuron, which then conducts the potential (and hence the information that something has happened at the cell where it originated) to other cells.

Neurons as Information-Processing Units

The neuron is the information-processing unit that transforms many input signals into a single output signal. These input signals are carried to the neuron by the axons of other neurons. A run-of-the-mill neuron of the human cortex receives between a thousand and ten thousand incoming axons from other neurons. The incoming signals are action potentials that all look alike and carry information by their mere presence or absence, like the dots and dashes of Morse code. For example, if light falls on a patch of neurons in the light-sensitive rear of the eye (the retina), cells in the retina send action potentials to the brain.

The signal-carrying axons from other neurons end with small button-like protrusions, the *synapses*. Unlike the connections between electrical wires, which ordinarily work equally well under any circumstances, the transduction of a signal at a synapse can be good or poor, a fact that is important for the proper functioning of the nervous system. In fact, it is crucial that the signals coming into a neuron from other neurons have different effects, which are caused by differences in the efficacy of the respective synapses. In other words, the ability of a signal to be conducted to other neurons depends critically on the synapse through which it must travel.

In computational terms, the incoming signal can be described by a number (figure 2.2). In the simplest case, we can look at a neuron at any given moment and state whether or not an action potential is being conducted through a synapse of the neuron. The incoming signal, called the *input* of the neuron, may be described, again in the simplest case, by either the number 1 or the number 0. Of course, it is also possible to take a dynamic perspective and to characterize the input in terms of action potentials per unit of time. When this is done, the input is a variable that denotes the frequency of the firing input neuron.

The quality of the synaptic transmission can also be represented by a number. If the signal travels freely through the synaptic cleft and has a high impact on the resting potential of the neuron, we can say that the action potential has a full impact on the neuron. If the signal is conducted poorly, its impact on the neuron will be small. If the synapse has an inhibitory effect on the neuron, the input must be multiplied by a negative

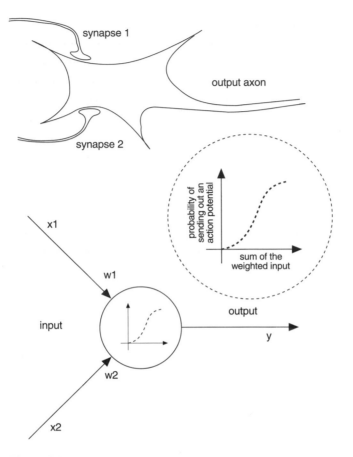

Figure 2.2
Action potentials traveling through the axons to the synapses. Each potential is
multiplied by a weight representing the strength of the synaptic transmission at
the synapse. Out of up to 10,000 incoming axons, only two are depicted; they
are described computationally as x1 and x2 (input 1 and input 2). These inputs
are weighted during the process of synaptic transmission; that is, input x1 is
multiplied by the weight w1, and input x2 is multiplied by w2. The synaptic
transmissions cause the cell membrane to depolarize. Mathematically speaking,
all the weighted inputs are summed up. If the membrane potential reaches a
threshold, the cell fires. This is equivalent to comparing the summed weighted
input with a fixed value (the *threshold*). If the summed weighted input is larger
than the fixed value, the neuron sends out a 1 (one). If it is smaller, nothing
happens. In real neurons, there is no threshold but rather a sigmoidal function
establishing the probability of neuronal firing for any given amount of weighted
input (activation function).

number representing the inhibitory input. Mathematically, this effect is captured by simply multiplying each action potential by a number that specifies the strength of each synapse. We can use any number between −1 and +1 to describe inhibitory as well as excitatory synapses of various strength. The strength of a synapse is often referred to as its *weight*.

Incoming action potentials, weighted by the strengths of the synapses through which they travel, lead to more or less depolarization of the neuron's membrane resting potential. Whenever the resting potential drops below a certain threshold, the neuron sends out an action potential. In mathematical terms, the neuron sums up the weighted input signals (i.e., the products of all incoming signals, zeros and ones, and their corresponding synaptic weights) and compares the sum with a threshold. Whenever the weighted input is larger than the threshold, the neuron fires an action potential—that is, sends out a 1. If the weighted input is smaller than the threshold, nothing happens . In biological neurons, the threshold will be probabilistic; that is, when graphed it will not look like a step, but rather have a sigmoidlike shape. This curve is called the activation function.

Computationally, the function of a neuron can be completely described by the input, the synaptic weights, and the activation functions of the neurons.

A Simple Network for Pattern Recognition

All living organisms face the problem of recognizing patterns and producing specific and appropriate responses to them. Sensory cells transmit uninterpreted signals from the environment in the form of action potentials. These "incoming nerve currents," as the psychologist William James termed them, have been replaced in modern neurophysiology by a stream of zeros and ones. However, the basic problem remains the same: How does the organism produce, from an uninterpreted stream of data, meaningful information about the environment? In particular, how does it respond in a way that takes into account these data and benefits from them? To take an example from vision, the retina is bombarded by dots of light, which are transmitted to the brain as spatiotemporal patterns of action potentials. However, the problem for the organism is how to

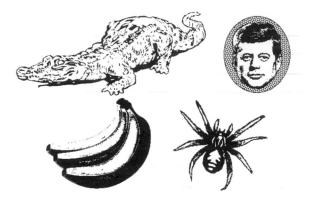

Figure 2.3
Patterns each consisting of from 10,000 to 20,000 black or white dots (picture elements, pixels).

use these patterns of electrical activity to come up with meanings, such "there is something to eat over there" and "to the left there is some edible stuff, but right behind there is a predatory animal" (figure 2.3). In order to survive, the organism has to come up with such "ideas"; it has to recognize patterns quickly and reliably. How does the nervous system accomplish this feat?

To answer this question, let us look a very simplified case (see figure 2.4). Consider a layer of light-sensitive sensory cells consisting of only three neurons, the input neurons of the network. Let us further assume that in the environment of the organism three different, important patterns (A, B, and C) occur, to which the organism has to respond differentially. These patterns are perceived by the organism when, falling on the sensory cells of the organism's eye, they become represented. Finally, let us assume that the organism has to produce three different kinds of behavior, that is, three different outputs. This is accomplished by the firing of three different output neurons. Output neuron 1 may represent flight (perhaps the motor neuron of a leg muscle); output neuron 2 may represent eating (such as a neuron controlling the tongue); while output neuron 3 may signal digestion by firing the vagus nerve. The task of the nervous system is therefore to produce, as quickly and as reliably as possible, a mapping of the three input patterns to the three output neurons. How does it produce such a mapping?

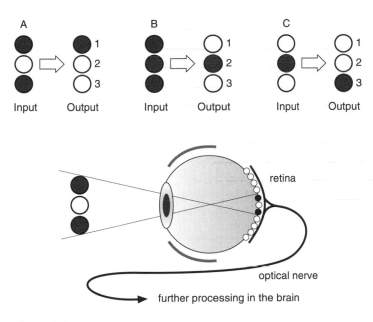

Figure 2.4
Desired input-output-mapping (top). A very simple but also rather typical problem of pattern recognition is depicted. The patterns A, B, and C have to be
recognized; that is, if pattern A is present on the retina, output neuron 1 should
be active; if input pattern B is present, output neuron 2 should be active; and if
output pattern C is present, output neuron 3 should be active. As we see in
chapter 4, such patterns consisting of black and white dots can be written down
as vectors. Thus, input pattern A can be written as the vector (1,0,1), B as (1,1,1),
and C as (0,1,0). Accordingly, the output the nervous system generates can also
be characterized as vectors: as (1,0,0), (0,1,0), and (0,0,1). At the bottom is a
schematic representation of an input pattern falling on the retina of the eye.

First, think about how a conventional personal computer (PC) would
perform the task. A program for the recognition of patterns A, B, and C
might look something like the following serial code. "Go to the middle
neuron of the retina and determine whether it is active or not. If it is not
active, generate output pattern 1. If it is active, go to the top neuron. If
it is not active, generate output pattern 3; if it is active, generate output
pattern 2." This algorithm is rather simple, but if the patterns get more
complicated (i.e., if the number of pixels is increased), the algorithm gets
very long and complex. For example, for such an algorithm to detect all
the characters in a 5 by 7 grid, it would need to consist of several pages
of code. To recognize faces, it would probably need to be as long as a

book. Because, as we have seen above, neuronal switching takes several milliseconds, such serial algorithms would be terribly slow if they were carried out by the brain. It would take the brain seconds or minutes to run a program of thousands of lines of code, whereas we can actually perform the recognition task within fractions of a second. Furthermore, serial algorithms are prone to error: when a computer works its way through a complicated decision tree, a single mistake can cause the process to take a completely different path and, hence, to produce a wrong result. The erroneous recognition of a pattern in the environment, however, may have disastrous consequences for the organism.

In contrast to serial algorithms, neural networks accomplish pattern recognition quickly and robustly. To understand how they work, we need only remember a little elementary school mathematics.

To produce the mapping of the above-described input and output, a neural network would utilize three input nodes and three output nodes (figure 2.5). Each input node is connected to every output node. Let us further assume that every output node has an activation threshold of 0.8;

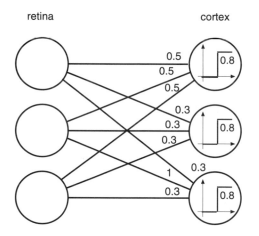

Figure 2.5
A very simple neural network that recognizes the patterns depicted in figure 2.4, that is, that implements the corresponding input-output mapping function. The network has two connected layers, an input layer and an output layer. It is characterized by the strengths of the connections (represented by the numbers) and by the activation function of the output neurons. In this network, the functions of real biological neurons are reduced to the bare minimum, making it possible to see clearly the principles of neuronal functioning.

that is, each of the output nodes becomes active whenever its weighted input is larger than the threshold. If the weighted input is smaller than the threshold, the neuron remains at its resting potential.

The differential strengths of the synaptic connections between the neurons of the input and the output layer are crucial to the effective functioning of the network. Let us look at what happens because of these differences in synaptic strength. If pattern A is perceived, the activity of the input layer corresponds to pattern A; the top and the bottom neurons are active, whereas the middle neuron is not. This pattern is transmitted to all output neurons through the connections. Each output neuron, however, processes this input differently, because each output neuron has connections to the input neurons of a different strength. The top neuron in the output layer, for example, receives the input 1 from the top neuron of the input layer through the corresponding synapse, which has a weight of 0.5. The weighted input, therefore, is $1 \times 0.5 = 0.5$. The weighted input coming through the other two synapses is $0 \times -0.5 = 0$, and $1 \times 0.5 = 0.5$, respectively. The sum of these weighted inputs, therefore, is 1. This is larger than the threshold of 0.8, which is why the neuron will become active.

Similarly, we can calculate the weighted input of the middle neuron (0.6) and that of the lower neuron (−0.6). Neither of these neurons will become active. (Readers can use figure 2.5 to do the calculations themselves.) The net result is just what we wanted the network to do—produce an active top output neuron when Input A is present. How about pattern B? The weighted inputs of the top and the bottom neurons are 0.5 and 0.4, respectively. Only the middle neuron receives a weighted input (0.9) that is larger than the activation threshold. Pattern B, therefore, will cause only the middle neuron in the output layer to fire. Pattern C will also be recognized properly by the network, because at presentation the sums of the weighted input of the upper, middle, and lower neurons are −0.5, 0.3, and 1, respectively. Therefore only the lower output neuron will fire when presented with input Pattern C.

Shared Labor by Parallel Processing

The simple example we have examined demonstrates how pattern recognition can be accomplished by a simple network of two layers. It is important to realize that all three output neurons receive all of the input at the same time; that is, they work in *parallel.* Pixels are not processed one by one, as in the serial PC model described above. Instead, the entire pattern is processed by each of the output neurons, which is why the brain's form of processing is sometimes called *parallel* as well as *distributed.* Neural network models are therefore also called *parallel distributed processing (PDP)* models (cf. McClelland & Rumelhart 1986).

When contrasted to serial processing, parallel processing has a number of important advantages. Notice that the patterns are recognized in a single computational step that is much faster than a serial algorithm working its way through the parts of the patterns one by one. If the patterns are more complex and consist, for example, of characters or faces, the recognition process remains, in principle, just as fast; it simply uses more neurons. (As we have already seen, we have plenty of them!) More complex patterns need no more time to process than simple patterns, because they are processed in parallel. In principle, a face made up of ten thousand pixels (cf. figure 2.3) could therefore be recognized in a single computational step, given the fact that the pyramidal neurons of the human cortex can each receive up to ten thousand input fibers. In short, pattern recognition can be very fast if done by parallel processing, even though the processing units are relatively slow.

We can hardly overemphasize the difference between information processing in neural networks and rule-based logical serial systems. The network, in contrast to the serial algorithm used by a conventional computer, contains neither rules nor calculation procedures. Its "knowledge" resides entirely in the weights of the connections. Although neural networks do not *contain* rules, what they do can be readily described by rules. This distinction may sound sophistical, but it has far-reaching consequences for our understanding of ourselves.

Until a few years ago it was generally assumed that the concepts of folk psychology somehow refer to things actually going on in our brains. When we spoke of thoughts, hopes, feelings, sensations, memories, and so on, we usually presupposed that there were brain states that in some way resemble these thoughts, hopes, feelings, sensations, and memories. For example, the structure of thoughts, which may be experienced as internal speech, was likened to the processing of memories by the use of symbolic formal operations. Internal images and symbols were thought to become activated and newly associated by thoughts and volitions, and the result of such processes were the mental acts experienced by an individual. Accordingly, mental operations have often been simulated by computer programs and flow charts. Thought was thus conceived of as the manipulation of symbols.

If we assume that the brain does not operate like a conventional computer, but rather like the neural network we have described, we gain an entirely new framework for understanding mental operations. Instead of rule-based algorithms working with symbols, they consist of subsymbolic processes, which can be described by rules and symbols only to a limited degree. Moreover, the internal representations involved in these processes constantly change during these subsymbolic operations. Such rules as exist *are not in the head* but are merely post hoc ways of describing mental functions (cf. Bechtel & Abrahamson 1991, Churchland & Sejnowski 1992, Churchland 1995, Clark 1993).

Language Acquisition by Children and Networks

Human language is arguably the most prominent example of a rule-based system, which human beings appear to use routinely in the production of such high-level mental functions as thinking and communicating. We all know implicitly a complicated set of rules. Each of the about eight thousand languages on earth comes with such a set of rules. Notwithstanding the obvious differences, there are some general principles to which all human beings adhere when speaking. Most noticeable is the astonishing fact that children are enormously creative during the process of acquiring language. Although they obviously use the many examples they hear to perfect their language skills, the linguist Noam Chomsky (1972, 1978, 1988) has convincingly argued that these examples are not sufficient for the child to generate the general rules necessary to speaking correctly. They simply do not hear enough examples; moreover, those they hear are sometimes contradictory. The child could never, from the examples alone, generate all the necessary rules. Chomsky has proposed, therefore, that children must acquire language through some inborn competence, some form of language instinct (cf. Pinker 1994).

Let us take a close look at an example. When children learn to speak, they must acquire, among other things, the rules that govern the generation of the past tense from the word stem. Although they do not know these rules explicitly—none of us can consult a grammar book in our head—they can use them creatively. One of these rules, for example, specifies how to convert the word stem (*sing, chant*) into the past tense (*sang, chanted*). In English, there are two ways to form the past tense. Many verb stems are converted to the past tense by adding the ending *-ed* (*chant* becomes *chanted*). However, there are exceptions to this rule, and a fair number of verbs have irregular forms of the past tense (e.g., *sing* becomes *sang*). While regular verbs can be changed from present to past by the application of a single rule, irregular forms have to be learned one by one.

Psycholinguistic studies on the development of language skills in children have demonstrated that children acquire the past tense in certain steps or phases. First, they learn to change irregular verbs; this probably happens by imitation, as irregular verbs are also frequently used verbs (e.g., *to have, to be*). In a second phase, children appear to acquire the rule that governs production of the past tense in regular verbs but tend to use it indiscriminately; they apply it to irregular as well as regular verbs. In this phase, errors like *singed,* or even *sanged,* are common and children are able to creatively generate the past tense of nonexistent verbs. When asked, for example, "What is the past tense of *quang?*," they reply "*quanged.*" This capacity to create past tenses for words they have never heard before has been regarded as crucial evidence that children have acquired a rule. Only in the third phase are children capable of forming correctly the past tenses of regular as well as irregular verbs; that is, they have learned both the rule and the exceptions to the rule. They know that it is *take, took* but *bake, baked*. Once you start to think about how to produce the past tense, you realize how complicated a task it really is. Moreover, you realize the enormous difficulties almost all children master in the first few years of their lives.

About a decade ago, neural networks were applied to the problem of past-tense acquisition for the first time by Rumelhart and McClelland (1986). They programmed a neural network with 460 input and 460 output nodes in which every input node was connected to every output node, resulting in 211,600 connections ($460^2 = 211,600$). The input patterns consisted of 420 word stems; the task of the network was to learn the corresponding 420 forms of the past tense. Learning (see chapter 3 for details) was performed by presenting the input layer of the network with a soundlike pattern of the stem that caused random activation of the neurons in the output layer. Because the desired output (i.e., the sound pattern of the past tense) was known, the actual and desired outputs could be compared. The difference between the output actually produced and the desired output was used to make small changes in the weights of the connections between input and output neurons. These small adjustments in weight in the desired direction gradually taught the network to respond with the correct past tense when presented with the stem.

In fact, after 79,900 trials, the network had learned the correct correspondence between input and output; that is, it had come up with the synaptic weights needed to produce the sound pattern of the past tense when presented with the sound pattern of the stem. Even when presented with new verbs somewhat similar to the nonexistent verbs given to children, the network operated almost flawlessly: it produced the correct past tense of regular verbs in 92 percent of the cases and, even, the correct past tense of irregular verbs with 84-percent accuracy.

What was most notable about the model was that its learning curve for regular and irregular verbs resembled that of children (figure 2.6). The network acquired the past tenses of regular verbs steadily; that is, it produced a constantly decreasing number of errors. In contrast, it first produced the past tenses of irregular verbs increasingly well, then reached a stage at which performance actually decreased, only to increase again later.

The fact that the network model, like children, not only gradually improved its performance over time but also went through similar phases and produced errors that resemble those of children can be regarded as strong support for the idea that children and neural networks learn in a similar way. The striking parallels suggest, at least, that similar mechanisms are at work. This similarity has far-reaching consequences.

Notice, for a start, that there was no explicit learning of any rule, just a gradual change in connections. Moreover, the rule does not exist except

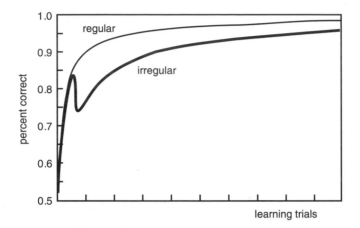

Figure 2.6
How children and neural networks acquire the past tense. The figure represents
the results of a computer simulation. The decrease in performance in producing
the past tense of irregular verbs, which has been shown to exist in children as
well, is clearly visible.

as a description of what has been learned. Whereas linguists like Chomsky and other members of his school of thought had assumed that rules
as rules must be explicitly represented in the brain for language acquisition to occur, the network model has proved that this is not necessary.
The network performed the task because the connections between hundreds of neurons changed their strengths, *not* because it followed a
learned rule. Nonetheless, the network produced the correct output (the
sound patterns of the past tense) for regular as well as irregular input
(the sound patterns of the stem). It treated regular and irregular verb
forms in the very same way. In the network—and by analogy in the heads
of speaking human beings—there is neither a rule nor an exception! (This
may be why so many of us find grammar difficult.) According to the new
view, the rules of grammar are not inside our heads. Rather, they are
spelled out after the fact, to describe what the networks actually do.
    Although a number of details of the model proposed by Rumelhart
and McClelland have been subjected to criticism (cf. Marcus 1995,
Pinker & Prince 1988, Plunkett 1995), the model is very plausible and
has been confirmed by further simulation experiments (cf. Hoeffner
1992). These simulations were able to prove, for the first time, that

rule-governed language behavior is possible without any explicit internal representation of the rules.

Is it true that we do not follow rules when we talk? Can we only state rules on a post hoc basis? If so, what does this imply about other rule-based human activities and behaviors?

Computer Simulations of Higher Cognitive Functions

There is an increasing number of studies showing how higher cognitive functions can be simulated by neural networks. These studies have sometimes come up with astonishing results. Such models offer advantages over explanatory hypotheses and theories. Unlike the latter, a simulation can be subjected to experimental manipulations and empirical tests of the effects of these manipulations.

In other words, the only way to test a theoretical explanation is to confront it with new real world data to see how more, or less, well the theory predicts the new data. A simulation model, however, allows us to introduce changes and observe the effects of these changes. In "playing" with the model, we can generate predictions about the real world and check them by comparing them with new observations and experiments. In short, the model allows us to *experiment with the mind*. For example, the parameters of the network—such as the patterns of connection, the activation function of the neurons, or its size—can, like the input signals, be manipulated, and the resulting behavior can be studied in detail. Such experiments are either impossible or very hard to carry out on real neuronal systems. A network can even be damaged to various degrees (neurons and connections can be set to zero) to test the effects of such damage on performance under different circumstances—for example, at different levels of informational load. We have already discussed an example in which the learning history—that is, the changes in performance over time—is highly informative, especially when there are specific differences that depend on input characteristics. The more detailed the predictions are and the more sophisticated the model is, the more informative are the results of such simulations. Of particular interest are the counterintuitive results that simulations may produce; these can direct researchers to phenomena and functional relations that would otherwise have escaped their attention. In short, the possibilities of network simulations are endless. They are limited only by the creativity of the experimenter.

Obviously, the fact that a certain task can be simulated on a computer running a neural network model does not mean that the task is implemented in the brain in the same way (cf. Crick 1988, 1989). In particular, the fact that a network simulation model *behaves* the way a real nervous system does cannot be taken as proof that biological nervous systems produce behavior in the same way. Notwithstanding these caveats, a network model can demonstrate operating principles that *might* be at work in real nature; in fact, such a model may be the only way to detect these principles. If a damaged model, for example, behaves in a way that is strikingly similar to a damaged real nervous system, and if the model generates unexpected predictions about the behavior of the biological system that, upon subsequent careful examination, are found to be correct, one can hardly escape the compelling plausibility of such a model.

DECtalk versus NETtalk

The final example we discuss in this chapter is another simulation regarding an aspect of language learning (cf. Churchland 1995). Like Rumelhart and McClelland's model, this simulation calls into question the view that language can only be mastered by the application of a complex set of rules.

A few years ago, the American computer company Digital Equipment Corporation (DEC) developed a program to convert written text into spoken language. Such a program is useful for blind people, who otherwise have to rely upon especially produced texts in Braille. The conversion of written text into sound, however, is more or less difficult in various languages. If the language has a good spelling-to-sound correlation, like Spanish or Italian, the task is relatively easy. English, however, appears hopeless in this respect. Not only foreigners learning English as a second language, but even British and American people, have difficulty learning to write correctly, which is why a large proportion of classroom time is devoted to the rote memorization of awkward spelling. The letter *i* may sound like the first *i* in *imagine* or like *ai*, as in *I* and *icon*; an *a* may be bright (æ) like the first *a* in *Adam,* dull (ə) like the second *a* in *Adam,* or like *ei* (*a*) in *aorta.* George Bernard Shaw once caricatured this puzzling feature of English by pointing out that the word *fish* could be written as *ghoti*—using the *f* from *enough,* the *i* from *women,* and the *sh* from *nation.*

Because of the complicated rules governing the transformation from spelling to sound in English, DEC's computer specialists had to take into account not just single characters, but also characters and their environment. They used the three characters to the left and to the right of a single character to figure out the correct sound pattern for that character. Of course, this turned out to be a complex enterprise, and the programming of the many rules involved took several man-years of programming. When run by a fast computer, the software did its tricks, however. The machine—called DECtalk—could actually read written English text.

A few years later, a neural network was used to accomplish the same task. The same hardware was used to scan the text and to synthesize the voice, but no algorithmic computer program with complex rules provided the software; instead, a neural network called NETtalk was used. The network was trained (see chapter 3) with text input and correct speech output for only ten hours; at the end of this period it produced output that was 95 percent correct. Additional training improved its performance to 97.5 percent correct. The network carried out the task just as well as the algorithmic machine that had taken years to develop.

Like Rumelhart and McClelland's model, NETtalk contains no rules; it functions properly because it makes a series of small corrections of weight during training. Like the tiny network of three neurons introduced at the beginning of this chapter, NETtalk's performance relies upon nothing but the correct mapping of input patterns onto output patterns achieved by correctly tuned synaptic connections.

It should be clear by now that these connections are crucial to the functioning of neural networks. Addressing the origin of connections, we have referred a number of times to "training," and stated that proper training causes these weights to come about miraculously. But how does this happen? And, more importantly, how are these weights produced in biological systems (if we assume that live systems work in a somewhat similar way)? In short, how does the brain learn? The answers to these questions are crucial for our understanding of education, in particular of how children learn and how they should be taught. We will address these issues in the next chapter. But, before doing so, let us look at an idea about how synaptic weights come about that appears plausible at first glance but that cannot be correct.

Beethoven, Karajan, Sony, and the Human Genome

One might suppose that the proper connections between neurons could be genetically preprogrammed. After all, why should an organism run the risks involved in learning? Why not just inherit the correct weights? But what are the correct weights? Well, that depends on the environment of the organism! Moreover, the environment may change or the organism may move from one environment into a different one. In some areas it may be beneficial to respond to the presence of red berries with appetite, while it may be deadly to do so in other areas. If the organism were preprogrammed with a fixed set of parameters determining an equally fixed repertoire of behaviors (like the knee-jerk reflex, which *is* prewired), the organism would have no flexibility to respond differently to different environments and circumstances. In short, genetically programmed connections in the central nervous system of complex organisms like human beings is not desirable.

Furthermore, a little mathematical calculation allows us to estimate that the human genome is not large enough to store all the information needed to code all the connections in the human brain. The human genome consists of about three billion base pairs. Each single base can be one out of four possible bases, which makes for an informational content of each base of two bits and an information content for the entire human genome of six billion bits. When you buy a computer, memory storage capabilities are often given not in bits, but rather in bytes (eight bits equal one byte). The information content of the human genome therefore is six-eighths of a billion bytes, that is, 750 megabytes (MB).

We can compare this capacity with the standard size of compact discs (CDs). When the standard was first set, the small round silver disk was to have a diameter of 11.5 centimeters (cm), which allowed it to hold 550 MB of information. Conductor Herbert von Karajan, as well as the wife of the chairman of Sony, objected to the standard, because the ninth symphony of Beethoven, which lasts for about 74 minutes, did not fit on such a CD. The standard was therefore changed; the disc's present size is 12 cm, which allows it to hold 74 minutes of music, equivalent to 680 MB (cf. Schlicht 1995).

The nucleus of each cell in the human body, therefore, has an information storage capacity that is only slightly larger than that of a CD. But how much information would be needed to genetically preprogram all the connections in the human brain?

Let us assume that there are ten billion (10^{10}) neurons in the forebrain and that each of these neurons is connected to one thousand (10^3) other neurons. The number of connections, therefore, is 10^{13}, that is, ten trillion. Even if we characterize these connections as only one bit of information each (i.e., we state only whether the connection is present or absent), this results in 10^{13} bits of information needed—that is, 1.25 X 10^{12} bytes or 1,250,000 MB. With its capacity of only 750 MB, the human genome could contain only a fraction of all the information needed to preprogram these connections in our brains. Moreover, this estimate is conservative, in that the number of cells, as well as of connections per cell, is likely to be larger and in that connections are not just present or absent but rather graded.

The upshot of these considerations is clear: even if the entire human genome were used to code all the connections between neurons in our brains, it would be several orders of magnitude too small. The brains of human beings, it follows, cannot be prewired. Instead, we learn from experience; that is, our experiences wire our brains. How this is done is the subject of the next chapter.

Recap

Simulated neural networks are information-processing systems that consist of a large number of processing units. Because these units are more or less similar to biological neurons, we sometimes refer to them as neurons and use them to construct neural networks to model human cognitive functions.

Information in these networks is processed by the activation and inhibition of neurons. Neural network research is biologically motivated;

that is, it has the aim of characterizing neuronal function computationally. By abstracting from a neuron's biological features—such as form, color, microscopic structure, cell physiology, and neurochemistry—we can conceive of it as an information-processing device. Within this neurocomputational framework, the function of a neuron is to calculate the products of the input signals and the weights, to sum all these weighted inputs, and to compare the result with a threshold weight.

Even simple networks can recognize patterns faster and more efficiently than serial computers can; and all it takes for the processing of more complex patterns is a larger number of neurons. Because information processing in neural networks is distributed across many neurons working simultaneously, the type of information processing performed by them is often called *parallel distributed processing* (PDP).

At one time, researchers assumed that mental operations are carried out by the operation of rules upon fixed mental representations. In the past few decades, however, our image of what the mind is and what it does has changed from one that is static and rule-based to one that is dynamic and process-based. It has become increasingly clear that biological mental operations are similar to the operations performed by computerized neural networks.

We have seen that rules merely describe what brains and networks do; they do not exist as explicit entities within these systems. By looking at two examples of apparently rule-based behavior—the production of the past tense from the word stem and reproduction by a computer of the sounds of English speech—we have seen that such tasks can be carried out by networks trained only by examples and not by the storage of explicit rules.

Finally, we have demonstrated that the connections between the neurons in a human brain cannot possibly be genetically determined, because the entire human genome is by far too small to contain all the necessary information. Instead, humans learn through interactions with the environment that change the connections in our biological brains. The precise mechanism of this learning is the subject of the next chapter.

3
Learning

Even simple organisms learn. The higher on the evolutionary ladder an animal is, the more flexible it is. Flexibility, however, is only one side of the coin. Its flip side is the energy and time it takes to learn. Some animals have such a simple structure and live in such undemanding environments that they need not learn. A well-known example of this is the tick, as described by Jakob von Uexküll. This animal cannot see or hear and perceives only two parameters of its environment: temperature and butyric acid—both keys to its ability to find prey.

The tick rests motionless on the tip of a branch of a tree, until a mammal passes by underneath. Then, the animal, awakened by the smell of butyric acid, lets itself fall from the tree. The tick falls into the fur of its prey, through which it makes its way to the warm skin, where it drives in its stinger and begins pumping blood into its own body. The tick does not possess an organ of taste. (Uexküll 1940/1970:145)

The environment of the tick, from the tick's point of view, consists solely of the two parameters useful for detecting sweating mammals (figure 3.1). (Sweat contains butyric acid.) Those parameters leave no room for either learning or adaptive behavior; if mammals ceased to sweat, ticks would die out. Compare this highly restricted environment with the rich surroundings of mammals, with their vivid colors, shapes, smells, sounds, movements, and changes. Such a world is characterized not by two parameters, but by a large number of them.

The tick does not need to learn, because its world is limited to two parameters, the values of which wholly determine its behavior. The tiny amount of information it needs has been hardwired into the tick's nervous system by the process of evolution. The data are genetically determined and cannot be changed during the organism's lifetime.

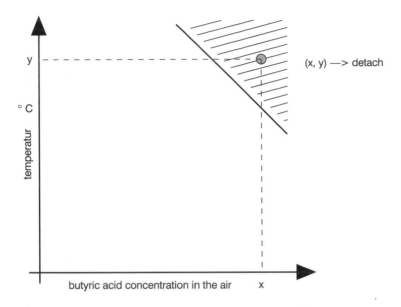

Figure 3.1
In computational terms, the environment of the tick. It consists of only two
dimensions: temperature and butyric acid concentration.

Associations and Hebbian Learning

More than a hundred years ago, William James, America's most prominent psychologist, clearly foresaw later discoveries about the function of
the brain's outer layer, the cortex, and the way in which neurons learn.
In 1890, before neurons had been discovered as the functional units of
the brain, his major work, *Principles of Psychology,* appeared. Two years
later, he published an abridged student edition, entitled *Psychology:
Briefer Course,* which became known among students as the *Jimmy,* in
contrast to the larger *James* of 1890. The following quotation is from
the *Jimmy's* chapter on associations.

The amount of activity at any given point in the brain-cortex is the sum of the
tendencies of all other points to discharge into it, such tendencies being propor-
tionate (1) to the number of times the excitement of each other point may have
accompanied that of the point in question; (2) to the intensity of such excite-
ments; and (3) to the absence of any rival point functionally disconnected with

the first point, into which the discharges might be diverted. (James 1892/
1984:226)

In this paragraph, James described the principles of cortical network organization even before the idea of the neuron as the unit of brain function had been succinctly formulated. If we replace his "point in the cortex" by "neuron," he is saying that the activity of a neuron equals the sum of its input, weighted by past simultaneous excitations of the connected neurons. Moreover, James emphasizes here the role of inhibitory neurons for the activation of a given neuron (cf. chapter 5). He even provides the first statement of a learning rule: "When two elementary brain processes have been active together or in immediate succession, one of them, on re-occurring, tends to propagate its excitement into the other" (James 1892/1984:226).

Half a century later, the Canadian physician and psychologist Donald Hebb (1949/1989), with the help of a growing body of physiological knowledge, built on these ideas. In 1949, he published his highly influential *Organization of Behavior,* in which he speculated upon the workings of cell assemblies and proposed a mechanism by which associations of neurons could be influenced through experience. He saw clearly that such a mechanism was necessary to any biological explanation of learning. Hebb outlined the operating principles of the association of single nerve cells, the *synapse,* and developed a scheme of how such associations could be influenced by meaningful associations; that is, something to be learned: "When an axon of cell A is near enough to excite a cell B and repeatedly or persistently takes part in firing it, some growth process or metabolic change takes place in one or both cells such that A's efficiency, as one of the cells firing B, is increased" (Hebb 1949/1988:50).

The Hebbian learning rule states that the connection between two neurons increases in strength whenever both neurons are simultaneously active. Obviously, this happens at the level of the synapse, which somehow gets "greased" whenever the two neurons are both active. Within a few decades after Hebb's suggestion, this simple rule provided the conceptual basis of thousands of research papers in neurobiology and computational neuroscience. However, it was another twenty-four years before the physiological basis of *Hebbian learning,* as it is now known, was finally discovered.

Learning Synapses

In the middle of the 1970s, the psychiatrist and neurobiologist Eric Kandel made some remarkable discoveries on the physiology and bio-chemistry of memory while working with the Californian sea snail *Aplysia*. The nervous system of *Aplysia* consists of about 20,000 neurons. On the one hand, this system is complex enough to manifest all the mechanisms of learning, while, on the other, it is simple enough to allow the researcher to study them in detail. Using this animal model, <u>Kandel was able to demonstrate for the first time that synaptic changes parallel behavioral changes, that is, learning</u> (cf. Kandel 1991: ch. 65). Once it became evident that synaptic changes and behavioral changes co-occur, research on similar mechanisms in higher organisms became a major focus of research.

In higher animals the hippocampus plays a major role in learning and memory (see figure 9.2). In the 1970s the first demonstrations of the synaptic changes that occur in the hippocampus were published. When input nerve fibers to the hippocampus are stimulated by brief pulses of electricity, a long-lasting increase of the connection strength between the input fibers and their target neurons results (Bliss & Lømo 1973). This finding provoked numerous studies of hippocampal neurons. The hippo-campus was used as a model, not only because it was known to be involved in learning and memory but also because its input and output connections, as well as its internal pathways, were relatively well known at the time. This knowledge allowed the researcher to stimulate groups of cells through two different input pathways. When a strong stimulus was applied through one, the cells were greatly excited, while a small stimulus applied through the second pathway produced only minor ex-citations. Applying either stimulus alone produced no interesting results, let alone any change in the hippocampus. When the strong and the weak stimuli were applied simultaneously, however, the weak stimulus had a larger effect on the cells' activity.

A series of experiments by Bliss and Lømo showed, that such changes occur only if both stimuli hit the target neuron at the same time. If the timing is different, nothing happens. This suggested that simultaneous activation of the cells is crucial to the effect, and that connections are strengthened only between cells that share information or are somehow involved in a process occurring simultaneously. *Long-term potentiation* (LTP), as the effect became known, occurs only at neurons that are active at the same time.

In order to demonstrate this directly, researchers had to record from single cells as well as from their respective input fibers. To do this, they prepared thin slices of hippocampal tissue whose single cells could be tapped by electrodes that could both stimulate them and listen to their responses. If *either* the cells or their input fibers were stimulated—that is, if stimulation occurred only at the presynaptic or postsynaptic site alone—nothing happened. Only if both the cells and their input channels were stimulated did the expected effect occur; that is, the effect of the input signals on the cells was increased (see figure 3.2). These studies convincingly demonstrated that Hebb's proposed mechanism was not mere speculation but was actually present in real neurons (Kelso et al. 1986).

Long-term potentiation of synaptic transmission is nothing more than a mechanism that signals a temporal coincidence of two inputs. In other words, this mechanism implements a neuronal coincidence detector. LTP has the following three fundamental characteristic features (cf. Bliss & Collingridge 1993).

1. *Cooperativity:* Several input fibers must be active at the same time for LTP to occur. A weak signal alone does not produce LTP.

2. *Associativity:* LTP does not occur at any single synapse but, instead, at synapses that are active together. Thus a weak signal may be amplified when a strong signal is simultaneously present. This feature not only implies that LTP is the equivalent of classic conditioning at the cellular level, but also that it can be regarded as the mechanism of associative memory systems.

3. *Specificity:* LTP occurs only at the synapses of the simultaneously active input fibers. Hence, it is specific to these inputs.

Several scientists have doubted that LTP really exists or have argued that it might be caused artificially by the electrical-stimulation procedures; that is, they think it's a methodological artifact (cf. Rose 1992:238–40). It is therefore of interest to know that activation patterns similar to those used in the experimental studies of LTP have in fact been

Input   Output

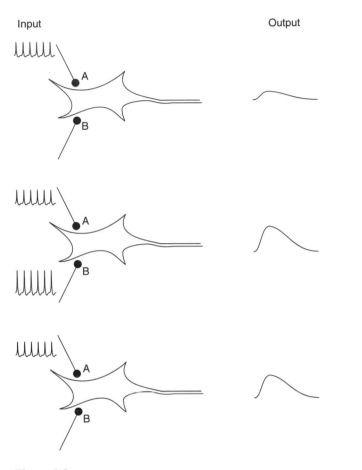

Figure 3.2
Schematic rendering of long-term potentiation (LTP) at two synapses, A and B.
(Top) A weak stimulus (via synapse A) alone produces only little output (i.e., a
small activation of the cell, depicted as the change in the target cell's membrane
potential over time). (Middle) If the weak input (A) arrives at a cell that is already
being stimulated by another input (via synapse B), the strength of synapse A
increases. (Bottom) Consequently, the same input transmitted through synapse A
has a larger effect on the cell after LTP has taken place. In sum, LTP provides a
mechanism through which synaptic weights can change.

recorded from the hippocampus of living animals during learning (Eichenbaum & Otto 1993).

Because LTP had been demonstrated only in the hippocampus, some have argued that the phenomenon has little validity for other brain structures (e.g., the cortex). However, this is not so. Although, as hinted above, for a time LTP could be demonstrated only in the hippocampus, this was not because it only occurs there but because it could only be studied there. At the time, the knowledge of the exact wiring of the structures under investigation necessary for stimulating one cell through two separate input pathways was lacking. It took almost two more decades for LTP to be demonstrated in the cortex, which is a much more complicated structure, in terms of connectivity, than the hippocampus (Bear & Kirkwood 1993; Iriki et al. 1991). Most important, LTP has recently been demonstrated in cortical areas that are known to reorganize themselves spontaneously when input signals change (Aroniadou-Anderjaska & Keller 1995). We will discuss these processes in detail in subsequent chapters.

Excursus: Glutamate and the 1992 Molecule of the Year

More than half of all the neurons of the cortex use the neurotransmitter glutamate. Such neurons are therefore called *glutamatergic*. Within one to three milliseconds of its liberation at the synapse, glutamate causes excitation in the membrane on the other side of the synaptic cleft (the postsynaptic site). Whenever we perceive something, think, feel, dream, or perform some other mental operation, glutamate—the major currency in the brain's information stock exchange—is liberated at the synapses.

At any given synapse, the presynaptic site at which the transmitter is liberated can be distinguished from the postsynaptic site, where the transmitter causes changes and where the information is carried further forward to the next neuron. Two types of receptors can be found at the postsynaptic site of a glutamatergic synapse: the so-called *NMDA-receptors* (which received their name because they can also be stimulated by the synthetic agent N-methyl-D-aspartate) and the *Q/K-receptors* (which are sometimes called *non-NMDA-receptors*).

If glutamatergic synaptic transmission occurs at a neuron that is not active at the time of transmission, only the Q/K-receptors are activated. They become permeable to sodium ions (Na^+), which results in activation of the cell. In this state the NMDA-receptors are blocked by a magnesium ion (Mg^{++}). In contrast, if the cell is already activated (by another excitatory input), the magnesium ion is forced out of the NMDA-receptor and no longer blocks it. Thus glutamate is able to affect the NMDA-receptors of an activated neuron by allowing an influx of calcium ions (Ca^{++}) through the open NMDA-receptor, which causes changes that result in an increase of the synapse's efficacy. NMDA-receptors, therefore, are specially adapted to become active only when two things happen simultaneously: (a) the postsynaptic neuron is activated; and, (b) there is an input coming in. Thus, these receptors have the features needed to produce long-term potentiation; they are molecular detectors of coincidental events (cf. Bliss & Collingridge 1993).

Excitatory synapses are located at small spinelike protrusions on the dendritic branches of the neuron and, to a lesser degree, on the body of the neuron. This spatial arrangement may have the advantage of restricting LTP to very localized effects on a single synapse and preventing it from spreading to others. If the calcium ions were to spread within the neuron—as well as to come in through open NMDA-receptors—their effects would not be localized and, therefore, could not carry synapse-specific information.

Which changes cause increases in the strength of the synapse, the "greasing" of the synaptic transmission by LTP? According to Bliss and Collingridge (1993), at least four different mechanisms are conceivable: (1) At the presynaptic site, extra neurotransmitter is liberated when an action potential arrives; (2) at the postsynaptic site, either the number of receptors for the transmitter or their efficiency increases; (3) outside the synapse, the biochemical degradation of the transmitter is slowed, thereby allowing it to affect the synaptic cleft and its receptors for a longer period of time; and finally, (4) morphological changes in the synapse cause an increase in synaptic function. It is likely that LTP is accomplished by way of *all* these mechanisms.

In any event, we know that LTP is caused by the influx of calcium ions at the postsynaptic site. While the effects of this influx have not been completely worked out, experiments have shown that it is crucial to the occurrence of LTP (figure 3.3). Within the postsynaptic dendritic spine, the incoming calcium causes the synthesis of the gas nitrogen monoxide (NO), which is a small molecule that can pass through membranes easily. Nitrogen monoxide is known to be poisonous; until a few years ago it was unthinkable that such a substance is not only present in the brain but also plays a major role in learning. Because of these highly surprising findings, nitrogen monoxide was named the 1992 Molecule of the Year.

The newly discovered function of nitrogen monoxide at the synapse solved a mystery that had puzzled neuroscientists for some time: how postsynaptic processes in a dendritic spine can have effects at the presynaptic site—that is, the site at which the transmitter is liberated. There is no way for larger molecules to travel out of the postsynaptic site and into the presynaptic site to cause the effect needed, for example, to increase the amount of liberated transmitter. However, a small gaseous molecule like nitrogen monoxide—and most likely also carbon monoxide, another poisonous gas—can easily travel through membranes by diffusion and is thus ideal for the job. Research has shown that both gases cause an increase in transmitter liberation at the presynaptic site. These gases may actually travel some tens, or possibly hundreds, of microns and can thus also reach adjacent synapses, where they may have a small effect.

Researchers have worked out the detailed mechanisms of LTP by adding to the cell substances known to block biochemical processes. If LTP is disrupted by a given agent, it is likely that the process blocked by it plays a role in LTP. For example, inhibitors of protein synthesis can decrease or even completely abolish LTP, which indicates that protein synthesis plays a role in the process. In sum, research on LTP at the biochemical level has demonstrated that this mechanism can make synaptic change—that is, learning—possible, although some details must still be worked out (cf. Baudry & Davis 1991, 1994).

NMDA receptors have also been linked to neuronal growth processes during embryonic brain development (Komuro & Rakic 1993). Because alcohol in the concentrations reached during heavy drinking inhibits NMDA receptors, it has been suggested that alcohol interferes with

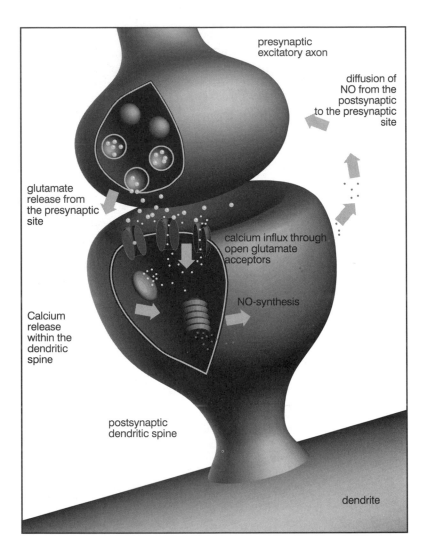

presynaptic
excitatory axon

diffusion of
NO from the
postsynaptic
to the presynaptic
site

glutamate
release from
the presynaptic
site

calcium influx through
open glutamate
acceptors

NO-synthesis

Calcium
release
within the
dendritic
spine

postsynaptic
dendritic spine

dendrite

Figure 3.3
Schematic rendering of the biochemical processes involved in synaptic learning.
The axon of a neuron coming in from the upper left ends in a synapse button at
a dendritic spine. In the usual case, the liberation of glutamate causes only the
activation of Q/K-receptors at the postsynaptic site. This causes a depolarization
of the cell membrane and, hence, transmission of the incoming signal. If, however,
the postsynaptic cell is already activated at the time of the incoming action
potential (i.e., if the presynaptic and the postsynaptic neuron are active at the
same time), the magnesium ion is forced out of the NMDA-receptor, so that it
no longer blocks the receptor. The NMDA-receptor can then be stimulated by
glutamate, which causes a cascade of effects: (1) calcium ions flow into the cell,

normal neuronal development (Lovinger et al. 1989). This finding explains why pregnant women should not drink alcohol.

Supervised Learning

Just as synaptic weights are not inherited and fixed in brains, they are not fixed in artificial neural networks. Instead, neural networks are *trained*, during which process the weights change. In other words, neural networks, like brains, learn by experience.

Such networks can learn in two ways that can be described, broadly speaking, as learning through *self-organization* and learning through *supervision;* they differ in that the first requires no external trainer, whereas the second does. In self-organization, which will be described in detail in chapter 5, specific structural features of the network and regularities in the input lead to the spontaneous organization of internal representations in the network. In the second case, the untrained network is presented with input. Since the synaptic weights of an untrained network are, by definition, small random numbers, the output produced by such a network will not be the correct or desired output. However, a training algorithm can compare that output to the desired output, calculate the difference, then change the synaptic weights slightly to reduce the difference so that the output produced comes a little closer to the desired output. This method, which leads to the step-by-step reduction of the difference between the actual and the desired output is called the *delta rule* (because the Greek letter delta is the symbol for difference).

In practice, this happens as follows. At the start of a simulation, the weights are set to small random numbers (e.g., between −0.2 and 0.2). Before training, the network therefore has no strong connections but only weak excitatory and inhibitory connections. In the process of training, the synaptic weights are gradually changed in small increments until they produce the desired output. In this process, some synapses will increase,

and there is additional liberation of calcium from stores inside the cell; within the cell, calcium causes (2) the phosphorylation of enzymes and (3) the synthesis of nitrogen monoxide (NO) and (4) of proteins. The net effect of all this is that the synaptic strength increases. The next action potential will have a slightly stronger effect upon the neuron than the previous one.

others will decrease in strength. Although it is possible to change the weights in a single step, such a procedure has, as we shall see below, major disadvantages.

Once the first input pattern has been presented and the weights have been changed accordingly, another input pattern is usually presented. This leads to yet another change of the weights to produce an output closer to the desired output for this new input. In a large-scale network simulation, several hundred or even several thousand input patterns may be presented to the network in this way; then the entire set of inputs is fed through the network again.

If the synaptic weights were changed completely upon presentation of a single input, one particular input pattern would be learned instantaneously. Presentation of the next input pattern, however, would lead to changes that would destroy what had just been learned. Only when the weights are changed slowly is such interference prevented, so that all the synapse strengths are changed in a way that finally maps the correct outputs onto the entire set of inputs (figure 3.4).

Moreover, if the synaptic weight were changed in large increments, it might miss the target, figuratively speaking, by overshooting or by undershooting it. Large changes might therefore lead to wide oscillations of the network around the desired output, rather than progress toward a stable input-output mapping. Finally, large-scale network simulations with many patterns—like those for generating the past tense—have exhibited a feature that depends on the slow change of weights: that is, the ability to *generalize* from input patterns. In past-tense production, the network produced the correct output not only for patterns with which it was trained, but also for patterns it had never encountered before. Such generalization only occurs if the weights change slowly; in effect, the network gets the gist of the desired input-output mappings instead of a fixed number of single mappings. If the weights were fitted exactly to a limited set of input-output mappings, only those mappings would be reproduced. When, in contrast, the weights are changed gradually, they are not fitted to any specific patterns but to what these input patterns have in common. Needless to say, the ability to generalize in this way is crucial for living organisms that must adapt to new situations—that is, have to generalize from the finite set of experiences to the many new situations they may encounter. The better the organism's generalization, the better it can make predictions and the more adaptive its behavior will be. In the example of learning to produce the past tense upon input of the stem, many of the verbs presented added the ending -ed to the stem. The gradual change in the weights enabled the network to learn to recognize this common feature and, hence, to produce the rule. *In sum, small changes of the weights cause the network to extract general features from the input and generate rules from examples.*

For quite a long time after its invention, learning by means of the feedback of errors was restricted to two-layer networks. In the early 1980s, however, researchers developed mathematical learning procedures that allowed them to train networks with, for example, three layers. The important *backpropagation of errors,* the most widely known and used procedure for training neural networks, now permits production of so-called *hidden layers* between input and output layers. Networks with hidden layers will be discussed in chapter 6.

Age and the Learning Constant

The proverb that "you can't teach an old dog new tricks" means that elderly people have a hard time adjusting to a new environment, in marked contrast to children, who seem to experience no such difficulty. As everyone knows, children learn rapidly. Why is this so? Why does the ability to learn decrease with age?

Thinking back to the learning network just discussed, we recall that the difference between desired and actual output was calculated during each learning trial and that the connection weight was then changed by a small amount in the right direction. But how small exactly is this small amount? This question can be answered by a single number, the *learning constant.* It represents the fraction of the amount of change in the right direction needed to produce the correct output. If the learning constant is 1, the change is made in a single full sweep; that is, the weights are changed so that the correct output is immediately accomplished. As we have just seen, however, this is disadvantageous for learning. In actual computer simulations of learning by neural networks, the learning constant is set to a fraction (e.g., to values between 0.1 and 0.2). A learning constant of 0.2, therefore, implies that the synaptic changes during one trial will bring the actual output 20 percent closer to the desired output.

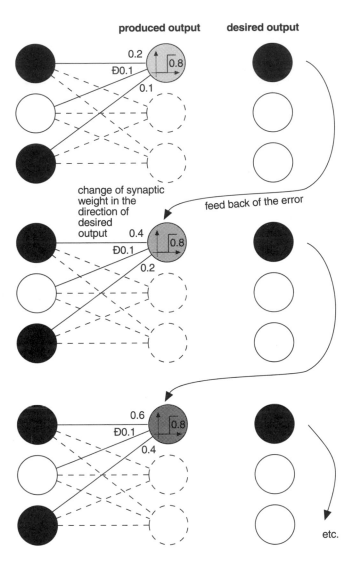

produced output   **desired output**

Figure 3.4
Supervised learning in a small neural network. (Top) A pattern is presented to an untrained network with random small synaptic weights. The output that is thereby produced at the top neuron $(1 \times 0.2 + 1 \times 0.1 = 0.3)$ is different from the desired output (at least 0.8). The actual activation of the top neuron is coded in gray, with larger activation represented by a darker level of gray. The desired output pattern (with the top neuron becoming activated) is shown on the right. The error is then fed back to the network, and the information is used to change the weights by a small amount. In this case, the connection strength from the active input neurons to the top output neuron is increased. Thereafter, other

The learning constant therefore determines how fast learning occurs. However, how fast *should* learning occur? Whereas we have provided several arguments for why slow learning is advantageous, it takes little effort to endorse just the opposite position: of course, rapid learning is advantageous for living organisms; the organism that quickly comes to grips with its environment will have an edge over one that does so slowly. In short, there exists a tension, a problem, for every learning organism. It must learn quickly for obvious reasons, but it must learn slowly in order to generalize in a way that will produce the optimal solution without oscillating around it or forgetting it because of some other stimulus.

Do biological systems have a learning constant? We all know that we sometimes learn faster than at other times. If we were to describe our learning ability by a number, we would have to state that this number varies according to our mental condition, motivation, physical needs, and so on. We will come back to the effect of these factors in a later chapter. In the following section, we discuss a general principle that explains why learning decreases with increasing age—which is by no means always disadvantageous!

Reality as the Basic Set and Experience as a Part Subset
Let us again summarize the general problem regarding the speed of learning faced by every organism. The central nervous system of the organism has to generalize across single events and, thereby, filter out general structures of the environment from the "throng and turmoil of the senses." This happens if, and only if, every single impression causes only a small change of the synaptic weights in the organism's brain. If the organism learns too quickly, it will learn single events quickly but fail to detect the general structure in the many input patterns. In contrast, if synaptic changes happen slowly and in small steps, it will detect and learn about the general structures in the input, not merely single cases. This is immensely important for the organism, because the storage of

patterns are fed into the network (not shown). When a new training cycle begins, the pattern is presented to the network again, and the weights of the connections are again changed in the desired direction. Through numerous repetitions of this process, the network learns the desired input-output relations.

general principles is more economical than the storage of numerous single events, and because principles can be used for predicting future events.

We can conceive of the environment of a given organism as the set of all possible situations it might experience and regard the organism's actual experiences as a subset of this set of all possible experiences. Within this general framework, we can view a nervous system as an apparatus that formulates estimates of the environment's general features; that is, that predicts general features from the empirical data base of its experience (again, a subset of all possible experiences). From this limited experience, the organism has to come up with the best possible representation of the real world—the true values of many parameters it can only predict on the basis of limited data. We all, for example have seen thousands of clouds, but we do not memorize them all. Instead, we have a general notion of a cloud and how it looks, and this general idea allows us to recognize as clouds things that we have never seen before. Similarly, we have seen millions of small blades of green grass, sensed millions of sand grains under our feet, and heard millions of words. None of these experiences has been stored as an individual fact. What remains in the grid of our experience are the general ideas of how grass looks and sand feels; and we have stored words and the rules for using them, again, in relation to the general ideas that words represent.

What we have learned, therefore, are general structural aspects of the world, parameters that describe input patterns. Clouds have a certain shape, color, and brightness; grass and sand have color and temperature, as well as certain surface features. Linguists conceive of the setting of parameters during language development in a similar way. These parameters, for example, determine whether the sequence of the words in a sentence matters (as it does in some languages) or not (cf. Bloom 1994).

In this general view of experience, the interactions of an organism with its environment can be generally conceived of as the sampling of data in order to predict the true (i.e., adaptively valid) values of parameters (McClelland et al. 1995; White 1989). As stated above, this task can only be accomplished if every single experience (every single input pattern) has only a very small impact on the changes in the network. If the changes are too large, estimates may oscillate around the true values rather than approximating them. Again: the system only works when learning happens slowly.

The Accuracy of a Prediction Increases with the Square Root of the Number of Observations

This adaptive advantage of slow learning is in conflict with the adaptive advantage of learning quickly. Time is costly for any organism, as during learning the organism is prone to error. Hence, there is evolutionary pressure to learn fast.

We know from statistics that there is a relationship between the size of a sample (n) and the accuracy of the prediction we can make using data from the sample. The rule states that the accuracy of an estimate (a prediction) increases with the square root of n. For example, if you want to know how tall men are, you can measure the heights of twenty-five men and compute the mean. Your estimate of the height of male human beings will not be bad, but it will also not be completely accurate. If you measure the height of a hundred men instead of twenty-five, your estimate will be closer to the truth; that is, the error of measurement will be smaller. If you take ten such measurements of the mean of twenty-five men and another ten measurements of the mean of a hundred men, the estimation error will be about twice as large for the sample size of twenty-five as for the sample size of a hundred. In short, to double accuracy, you have to quadruple the sample size.

This implies that out of a hundred measurements the first twenty-five contribute to the estimate of the true value, with respect to the size of the error, as much as the remaining seventy-five do. If I want to know the value of a parameter that I do not know, and if I have to form a judgment that is in line with every measurement, I would do well to rely heavily on the first few measurements, as they go a long way toward reaching an accurate estimate. The first twenty-five measurements will get me close to the true value, while the next seventy-five measurements will only halve the remaining distance to it.

Because accuracy increases more slowly than sample size, it often takes only a small sample size to estimate a certain parameter within an acceptable level of exactitude. For every organism (and for every neural network, too) this implies—to use the same numbers—that the first twenty-five experiences of an input pattern bring about the same growth of knowledge as the next seventy-five experiences (input patterns).

For these reasons, when setting up network simulations, it makes sense to adjust the learning constant to the phase (or stage) of learning. At first, it is useful to have a high learning constant, so that synaptic weights will change quickly in the desired direction. Once the network has formed weights that are close to the optimum, however, learning should slow down.

By the same token, it should be advantageous for every organism to be capable of adjusting its learning constant. It should learn quickly at the start and slow down later. In other words, the learning rate of any organism should be age dependent; that is, it should decrease with increasing age. Organisms must obtain a rough estimate quickly, then fine-tune their representations of environmental parameters in order to make increasingly accurate predictions and judgments.

These concepts drawn from statistics and computational neuroscience can easily be related to psychological observations. As noted above, it is common knowledge that children learn quickly, whereas elderly people learn more slowly. The reason is quite simple: if an organism's survival depends on knowledge of its environment, it is good to learn about it quickly and then to slow learning down to render the knowledge increasingly accurate. In this way, the true values of environmental parameters can be estimated quickly and with ever-increasing reliability.

Applied to human beings, this means that in a stable environment older people are better adapted than younger ones. The old master of violin building makes better violins than the young student of the trade. If, however, all of a sudden the customers want music synthesizers, the student will adapt to the change more readily. The problems of elderly people can therefore be clearly related to the fast pace of change in our society. The presupposition of a stable environment, which was a given during the evolution of human beings, is no longer granted. In many areas of human activity, stability is no longer achieved, desired, or even perceived. People can therefore easily get into a situation in which their acquired knowledge and skills are no longer needed, or in which they continue to filter from the environment rules and values of parameters that no longer hold true.

The decrease in the learning constant with increasing age can be related to neurophysiology as well as to social and psychological data. For example, we know that acetylcholine plays a major role in learning and memory (cf. chapter 10). If acetylcholine modulates human learning capabilities—that is, the learning constant of neurons in the cortex—we would expect to find a decrease in its concentration over a lifetime. Such a decrease would make sense from an evolutionary point of view. In fact, just such a decrease in the acetylcholine content of the human cortex of has been reported (Feuerstein et al. 1992). Moreover, this decrease has been demonstrated to be specific to acetylcholine and not a nonspecific effect of aging on the availability or presence of certain substances in the brain. Allgaier and colleagues (1995) measured another neuromodulator, norepinephrine, and found no age-related changes in it (cf. chapter 11). In sum, it is conceivable that reduction in acetylcholine content is the mechanism through which the learning constant in the human cortex decreases over the life span. This mechanism probably evolved because of the statistical nature of learning and predicting, and because of the evolutionary pressure to learn quickly and reliably.

Why Children Play

Not only human children play. In other higher animals too, youngsters spend a lot of their daily time and energy at play. Why is this so?

Let us have a look again at the argument from evolution, which can be found in many versions in the literature on neural networks. It states that once the organism has learned a particular behavior it is better adapted to the environment; that is, its chances of survival increase. And, as mentioned above, learning is constructed gradually through repetitive experience (play) with input-output relations until small synaptic changes produce the correct output with increasing probability.

The problem with this view is that a wrong output may have disastrous consequences for the organism. How can learning by the feedback of errors occur if the animal's errors result in its death? It can only learn this way if errors produce no adverse consequences for the organism; that is, if the organism can experiment with different behaviors without being harmed. This is why there is play. Within play, input-output mappings can be repetitively changed, tried out, and learned without danger of suffering major injury from the wrong behavior. Play is thus the

<u>consequence of the capability to learn</u>. And, because we generally assume that humans are the species best able to learn, we should expect humans to be the most playful species. We simply, most dearly, *need* to play!

Practice, Don't Preach

If simulated neural networks are similar to biological brains—that is, if organisms learn from examples (unlike computers, which are programmed by inputting rules)—and if the human child differs from youngsters of other species by needing to learn many more behaviors, then education has a great deal to do with practice and observation and very little to do with preaching. Children learn from examples. They do not learn rules, they distill them (i.e., produce the rules by themselves) from the examples with which they are presented. For example, if you repeatedly tell your daughter, with elevated voice and pointing index finger, to do her homework, clean the bathroom, or be nice to others, she may extract from your example the rule that her parent is someone who always has an elevated voice and index finger (the general feature of your preaching).

We must not, therefore, cling to any idea of a utopian future in which human beings are programmed by teaching and insight to produce desired behaviors. Human beings cannot be programmed like computers! As we shall see below, the fact that children not only learn but also undergo brain development at the same time causes them to automatically extract (or filter out) input that is best suited to them at a given age. However, the particular content of this input is determined by the episodes of the child's experience. If daddy always shouts in his attempts to teach his small son what to do and what not to do, the boy will learn that daddy shouts or even that all daddies shout. Compared to the striking regularity of such an input, the impact of the individual things his father tells him to do or not to do is almost negligible.

<u>It follows that children need no preachers but only good examples</u>— many of them and as many different ones as possible. Children who observe a large variety of good examples will over time acquire a set of general experiences that helps them get around in and do well in this world.

It also follows that children need structure in order to learn. The worst thing that can happen to a neural network, as well as to a child, is random input. If the input is random, no structure can be extracted from it and nothing can be learned.

Computer Models and Biological Neurons

One might argue that nodes in networks simulated on a computer and real live biological neurons are completely different. With special respect to learning, the argument runs as follows: the kind of supervised learning used in network models does not occur in living neurons. In brains, there is no trainer; nor do errors travel backwards. Moreover, errors are not computed by biological neurons in the way described above, for the very good reason that the desired output in most cases is neither known nor represented anywhere in the brain. A comparison between desired and actual output cannot, therefore, be performed. In sum, none of the building blocks of the backpropagation learning rule appears to be implemented in biological nervous systems. Network models—it might be argued from this point of view—may be useful for technical applications of pattern recognition, and for classifying anything from the smallest particles to patients in intensive care to the largest galaxies; but they will never tell us anything about the brain, let alone anything about its higher cognitive functions. This critique has been, and still is, frequently heard (cf. Crick 1988, 1989). It aims at the biological plausibility of neural network models, rather than at their technical feasibility. Network models, say these critics, are acceptable in engineering but of no use in the neurosciences.

As we shall see, there are several reasons why this argument is not valid. First, the phenomenon of feedback is ubiquitous in the central nervous system. Second, researchers have developed training algorithms that do the same thing as the backpropagation of errors but are more biologically plausible (Zipser 1990, Zipser & Rumelhart 1990). Finally, whenever network simulations display striking and unexpected similarities to biological observations, the models gain plausibility, sometimes becoming quite compelling. Let us look at such a model.

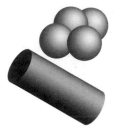

Figure 3.5
Examples of shaded surfaces from which our visual system can construct three-dimensional shapes with ease.

Shape from Shading

One of the problems the human brain has to solve is how to extract three-dimensional form from the shaded two-dimensional representation on the retina. To simplify matters, we will leave out color perception and all clues to depth except shading. Assume that we see two-dimensional images in shades of gray on the retina but perceive them as three-dimensional objects. How do our brains do the trick of producing the three dimensions from these elusive shades?

This task is a difficult one for conventional computers, because there are many shapes and the effects of different ways of illuminating them are almost unlimited. However, Lehky and Sejnowski (1988, 1990) were able to train a three-layer network with a large number of examples of shaded forms (a few of them are shown in figure 3.5) to produce the desired output, which consisted of the three-dimensional shapes. After training, the network was able to come up with the correct shape of an object when presented with a shaded image. Moreover, the network's nodes (artificial neurons) displayed unexpected features that turned out to be similar to features found in the real neurons of the visual cortex. For example, most neurons of the network's hidden layer developed a preference for a certain direction and, thus, became increasingly like the orientation-specific cells of the primary visual cortex. In the 1960s these cells were described in cats and monkeys by David Hubel and Torsten Wiesel (cf. Hubel 1989); they received the Nobel prize in physiology for numerous clever experiments demonstrating that certain cells in the visual cortex fire only when a light or dark strip of a certain orientation is present on the retina. These cells have been called *simple cells* to distinguish them from cells that are activated only in the presence of more complex patterns.

The activation profile of complex cells has also been clearly described by Hubel and Wiesel. These cells become activated upon presentation of moving bars, the light of which strikes different parts of the retina. Hubel has speculated that cells of this type may process the output of the simple cells, an assumption that was confirmed by the model of Lehky and Sejnowski. The output neurons in the latter's simulated network displayed features similar to those of the complex cells of the visual cortex. The model thus shed new light on the findings of physiological experiments. If we take into account only the results from physiology, it would appear that the cells in the primary visual cortex do nothing but analyze motionless or moving bars. While such light or dark bars are in fact found in our visual environment (just think of doorsteps, trucks, or telephone poles), they may be only a small part of the story. In fact, the simulated network shows that measuring the cells' features and determining the stimulus that activates them the most does not tell us much about their function. After all, the network was trained to distill shape from shading, not to distinguish the direction of motionless or moving light or dark bars. As Churchland and Sejnowski comment:

In other words, the receptive field properties of the model's hidden units might seem to license the inference that the cells are specialized for edge detection or bar detection. Yet their demonstrable and acquired function is to extract curvature from shaded images. Their inputs were exclusively smoothly varying gray levels. Therefore, bar and edge receptive field properties do not necessarily mean that the cell's function is to detect bars and edges in objects; it might be an intermediate step to detect curvature and shape, as in the network model, or perhaps some other surface property such as texture. (Churchland & Sejnowski 1989:186)

The significance of this model can hardly be overestimated. First, it demonstrates that one need not simulate all the complex connections found in the cortex to produce features that are quite similar to those of the cortex. It thus demonstrates that models can be simple and still highly informative. Second, the model shows that biologically relevant results can be accomplished even when we use biologically implausible learning procedures. In other words, even though the brain has learned something in a different way than the network has (which is highly likely), the results of the learning procedures employed by nature and the computational neuroscientist may be strikingly similar. As Zipser correctly states, this is probably because the specific task to be learned forces any learning system to utilize certain crucial features.

Lehky and Sejnowski's model is not the only one demonstrating that computer simulations of neural networks performing a clearly defined task can produce functional features in the artificial neurons of the hidden or the output layer that are very similar to those observed in biological neurons. (For another instructive example, see Zipser & Andersen 1988.)

Recap

Simple organisms like the tick need not learn. Their environment consists of only a tiny aspect of the rich world we humans inhabit. All the relevant parameters controlling behavior in that simple world can be hardwired into the tick's nervous system. In organisms that have to extract complex features from their environment in order to respond to them with equally complex patterns of behavior, learning becomes important.

According to the Hebbian learning rule, the connection between two active neurons is strengthened through experience. Simulated neural networks are trained by the presenting them withation of examples of the input-output mappings to be learned. At first, they produce the wrong output, which is compared with the desired output; the difference is then used to adjust the weights of the connections to bring the actual output a bit closer to the desired output. This procedure is repeated several hundred or several thousand times and results in a network with well-adjusted weights; that is one that produces the desired output pattern for each input pattern.

The basis of such learning in physiological systems is synaptic change through long-term potentiation (LTP), a process that has been the focus of research in the biochemistry of memory and learning for more than two decades. LTP is the mechanism that enables neurons to comply with the Hebbian learning rule.

Supervised learning has to proceed slowly, so that not single events but rather the general structure of the input is learned. This necessity for slow learning, which contradicts evolutionary pressures on every organism to learn as quickly as possible, can be reconciled by changes in the rate of learning—starting out fast and slowing down later. In this way, the true values of the many parameters that characterize a specific environment are approached quickly and (a bit later) more exactly. In simulated networks, the speed of learning is determined by a number, the learning constant. The learning constant of the brains of humans and other species also decreases with age.

Children, like neural networks, learn by extracting rules from many examples, but they do so spontaneously and by themselves. Thus they need no preaching of rules but only good examples. Children also learn by playing, trying out a variety of complex patterns of behavior and social interactions in a playful way in a context where errors do not produce disastrous consequences.

4

Vectors in the Head

Every organism of sufficient complexity is faced with the problem of storing in memory the important aspects of its environment. The bee has to memorize where the honey is, the salmon must remember where it was spawned. Human beings can identify thousands of different faces, and dogs can distinguish and memorize a huge number of smells.

Any organism living in an environment that is structured to some degree needs to have an internal representation of that environment and its important structures to improve its responses to events as they unfold. But, although memory and the ability to learn are useful tools for survival, they come with certain costs in time and energy. For this reason, there is evolutionary pressure to construct these internal representations as efficiently as possible; this pressure has given rise to various *codes* that organisms use to represent the important aspects of their environment efficiently.

For example, it is highly inefficient to form an image of the environment on—to use a computer analogy—a pixel-by-pixel basis. Such an exact copy of, for example, the landscape of the environment, would take up a lot of memory space, which is why organisms are unlikely to store detailed copies of images they have perceived through their senses. Instead, they extract the essence of many scenes and store that; in computational terms, their nervous systems compress the information that is the basis of the codes used in the higher cognitive functions. Not only the storage, but also the processing of information is faster and more efficient when the system focuses on the essence—that is, on the most important aspects of what is to be processed. This is achieved by efficient coding of the spatiotemporal patterns perceived by the sensory organs and by using these codes in further information processing.

One highly efficient way to represent information is *vector coding*. A number of experimental studies, as well as certain theoretical considerations, suggest that the brain makes use of this type of coding.

Vectors

Nearly 150 years ago mathematicians William Hamilton and Hermann Grassmann first showed, independently of each other, how the mathematical principles of size and direction could be represented by arrows or vectors.

A *vector* is characterized by both size and direction, in contrast to a number, which is characterized by size alone. We learned in algebra class that you can add vectors by stringing them together and that they can be multiplied by a number to change their length (see figure 4.1). Who would have guessed back at school that these arrows could be used for anything other than calculating forces or solving geometry problems without a ruler and a pair of dividers?

In the current state of knowledge about the brain, we can characterize what the brain does, in computational terms, as vector algebra—a highly efficient method of coding.

Codes

Suppose, for example, that you want to transmit over the telephone an image of the Olympic symbol depicted in figure 4.2. There are several ways you might do that. (1) You could divide the image into tiny black and white dots and represent each dot by either the number 0 (for white) or 1 (for black). By sending a string of zeros and ones, you could transmit the image. (2) You could just extract the essential graphic features of the image and describe these in mathematical terms over the telephone. (3) You could extract from the graphic features the semantic content of the image and report that.

Clearly, the three codes differ strikingly in the amount of time and effort they take to transmit the information: In the first case, transmission time would depend on the quality of the image; that is, on a computer screen, by the size of the grid that makes up the dots. If we use a fax machine, which uses a similar code, the image would come out in a

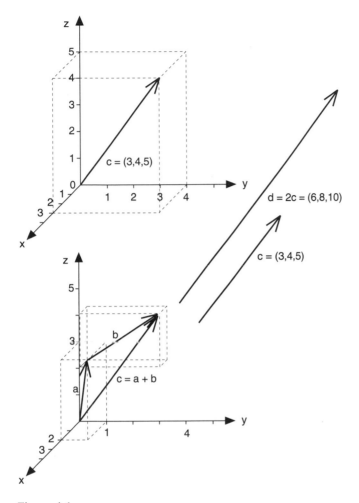

Figure 4.1
A three-dimensional coordinate system defining a vector by its three coordinates. (Top) The vector c = (3,4,5) is multiplied by a number (2) by multiplying each of its components with this number, which lengthens or shortens the vector by the amount specified by the number (shown at the right). (Bottom) Two vectors (a and b) are added by adding their components. The vector sum of vectors a = (2,1,3) and b = (1,3,2), therefore, equals c = (3,4,5).

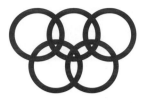

Figure 4.2.
This image can be coded and transmitted in different ways.
(1) As a bit map (pixel by pixel):
00000100000010000001000000
00001010000101000010100000
etc.
(2) As a mathematical description: Five circles each with a radius of 1 cm; coordinates of the centers: C1 = (1, 2.5); C2 = (2.5, 2.5); C3 = 4, 2.5); C4 = (1.8, 1); C5 = (3.2, 1).
(3) As a semantic description: "Olympic symbol."

somewhat degraded form at the other end and would also require us to transmit several thousand zeros and ones. In the second case, we could simply define the coordinates of five points and the radius and thickness of the equal-sized circles that surround these points. This method, which can be transmitted in only a few sentences, is quite parsimonious. But in the third case just two words would do the trick. In general, all three forms of transmissions can be termed a *code,* that is, the form in which information is represented.

Symbols versus Vectors

Let us consider how we might convey information about color. We could give each shade of color a name and use such names. Artists, of course, do this; they employ not just the word *red* but many words denoting different shades of red (e.g., Grumbacher red, scarlet, cadmium red, alizarin crimson, and Windsor red). Even the most elaborate semantic system for naming colors, however, pales beside the millions of colors the human visual system can discriminate.

Colors as Vectors

The system for representing color information in the video memory of computers is quite different from the artists' system. Computers make use of the fact that every color can be produced by mixtures of just three different components: the primary colors red, green, and blue (figure 4.3). By adding together bright dots of these components, for example, white light is produced. If only the red and the green dots are lighted and the blue dots are switched off, yellow appears on the screen. Different shades of any color are produced by varying the brightness of each of the three components. The total number of colors a screen can display depends upon the number of different shades of each component available to it, which, in turn, depends upon the amount of memory available to each dot on the screen. The display of the computer I used to write this book, for example uses twenty-four-bit color: Each component—red, green, and

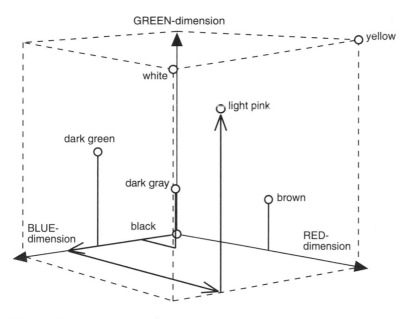

Figure 4.3
Every color can be regarded as a vector in a color space made up of the three components: red, green, and blue (RGB space). Each color is a point in this room, which can be conceived of as the vector sum of the component colors. To obtain the color rose, for example, you have to mix quite a bit of blue light, a lot of red light and quite a bit of green light. This is equivalent to adding three component vectors. If we assume 8-bit quantization for each dimension (i.e., 256 different possible values for each component), then rose may be coded as the vector "r 255, g 200, b 200." In RGB space, black is coded as (0, 0, 0), white as (255, 255, 255), yellow as (255, 255, 0) and dark gray as (45, 45, 45).

blue—can take a value between 0 and 255 (i.e., 2^8 = 256 possible subtly different shades). Because the components can be mixed freely together, the resulting number of colors that can be represented is 256 × 256 × 256 (or 2^{24} = 16,777,216). This is actually more colors than the human visual system can discriminate and far more than we can designate with our color vocabulary.

Any given color, it follows, can be represented in two different ways: by a name, and by an ordered set of three numbers representing the brightness of the three color components. The word *purple* and the color code *r 250, g 5, b 83,* therefore, represent the same color but do so in completely different ways. We term the first a *local* representation and the second a *distributed* and *dense* representation. The words in any human language denoting some aspect of the world are prime examples of local representation systems, whereas vector color coding is a good example of distributed dense coding. Vector coding is distributed because each color is represented by a value for each of the three dimensions (red, green, and blue); it is dense because there is no more economical way to code colors. The words of a language are local because every item represented occupies a specific point (or entry) in the lexicon.

The advantages of vector coding are evident. Every color can be represented with ease; the accuracy of the system depends only on the gradation of the component colors. In fact, the system is so efficient that it was invented by nature long ago.

The human eye uses similar principles for color perception, although the basic dimensions are somewhat different. In the human eye, there are four different types of receptors: three cones (one each for red, green, and blue) and a receptor for brightness, the rods. The latter are most sensitive for green-blue light and are responsible for night vision. Because the human visual system can discriminate among approximately seven million colors, we can easily calculate how fine the gradations of these receptors have to be to achieve this and level of sensitivity. For the sake of simplicity, let us assume that all four receptors contribute equally to perception of the four-dimensional human color space. If we assume further that the activity of all the receptors combines freely, then the number of gradations multiplied by itself four times must equal seven million. As the fourth root of seven million is approximately fifty-four, each of the four types of receptors needs to signal only about fifty different shades of red, green, blue, and gray.

Vector spaces, as we just have seen, need not be limited to three dimensions. Features of the environment may be represented by more than three dimensions, although we have a harder time imagining multi-dimensional space. In principle, feature spaces can have any number of dimensions, depending upon how many basic features are needed to represent an object of interest Churchland (1995) provides a nice example of how efficient such n-dimensional spaces are for coding information. Suppose that smells, like colors, are coded as vectors. Furthermore, assume that a bloodhound can discriminate seven basic smells, each of which contains thirty different gradations. Such a relatively simple system, then, could encode 30^7 (almost thirty billion) different smells.

Codes as Optimization Strategies

If the number of components in a vector coding system increases, the number of the possible combinations explodes exponentially. A few hundred neurons, each with only a few gradations, could produce a code able to represent every single atom—there are only about 10^{80}—in the universe. Such dense coding, however, would have an important disadvantage: whenever a single dimension was lost, the information in an entire segment of the n-dimensional room would disappear. Color-blind human beings (who mostly suffer from the inability to discriminate red and green), therefore, suffer not just from the loss of two colors but from the loss of an entire dimension of their visual space. At equal luminance, light green and light red cannot be discriminated by these people; nor can dark red and dark green. That is why traffic lights always display the different colors in the same order and display a green that is brighter than the red—to provide additional information for those who cannot distinguish between these colors.

Thus, if information in the human brain were coded as parsimoniously as possible, the loss of a single neuron would inevitably lead to loss of a great deal of information. However, as there are billions of neurons in the brain (why so many if a few hundred are enough to code everything?) and, as we have already learned, brain function degrades gracefully when neurons are destroyed, we may infer that parsimony is not the only principle governing evolution of neuronal code. The other, just as important, principle is *robustness*.

There is a trade-off between parsimony and robustness. To ask for the right code for a given purpose, therefore, is to ask for the optimum at which evolution arrived. On the one hand, it is necessary to code a certain feature of the environment as efficiently as possible—that is, with the least costs to the organism in energy, matter, and time. On the other hand, the code should be robust (i.e., safe against failure), so that faulty neuronal hardware does not cause information loss (cf. Hinton 1992). Because the human brain is remarkably resilient under conditions of neuron loss, it is highly unlikely that important aspects of the environment are coded by single cells.

Several lines of independent research suggest that the problem of efficient and robust coding is solved in the brain cortex by the principle of the *population code*. Information is not represented by a single neuron, but rather by a group of neurons. This design ensures that the loss of a single neuron does not cause information loss. Population codes are redundant. However, this redundancy does not imply that the neurons in such a group all represent the same content. In contrast, each neuron of the group codes the information, as it were, from its own perspective, and these perspectives change gradually within the group. It is the sum of the activity of all the neurons in the group that fully represents the information. Let us look at an example.

Vector Populations and the Population Vector

In order to understand how these codes work, we will look closely at how the direction of arm movement is coded in the motor cortex of the monkey. Monkeys, like humans, can carry out precise grasping movements. The question therefore arises: How does the brain represent the direction of such movements through the activity of neurons? In other words, how is the direction of a movement coded in the motor cortex?

Physiologists once thought that the motor cortex does nothing but generate action potentials that travel down the spinal cord in order to excite other neurons, which then drive the muscles. This view of the motor cortex as a mere electrical engine is wrong. We now know that neurons in the motor cortex can represent certain aspects of a movement task, including the direction of a stimulus; that is, they can represent perceptual information. This has been shown, for example, in experiments on cats in which the direction of the stimulus and the direction of the movement were separated (cf. Martin & Ghez 1985, Smyrnis et al. 1992). Just as the primary visual cortex contains not simply an image of the retina but rather a representation of the complex features of the stimulus, the motor cortex is more than just a generator of action potentials for muscle movement. Studies by Schieber and Hibbard (1993) have further shown that even the movements of a single finger are represented by distributed populations of neurons in the motor cortex.

Groundbreaking work on the problem of how direction is coded in the motor cortex has been carried out within the past decade by Anastopoulos Georgopoulos and his coworkers (1986, 1988). Because these studies have such far-reaching implications, we will discuss them in some detail.

Georgopoulos began by training rhesus monkeys to position a lever over one of several lights on a table when it lights up. The lights were positioned in a circle, so that they were equally far, in various directions from the center of the circle. Whenever the animal performed the correct movement, it was rewarded by a sip of juice. The monkey then had to reposition the lever over the middle of the circle, which activated a new light signaling it to move the lever in another direction. There were eight lights, each one 12.5 centimeters from the center of the circle.

By placing electrodes into the motor cortex of the monkey, researchers recorded neuronal activity directly while the monkey carried out the task (figure 4.4). They recorded simultaneously from almost three hundred neurons during the movement experiment. It turned out that about three-quarters of the neurons recorded showed direction-dependent activity; that is, most neurons had a preferred direction. Single neurons, however, were not active for only one discrete direction but, instead, fired whenever the arm moved within certain ranges of direction.

To better understand how these neurons code direction, the vector concept came in handy, because a vector, by definition, has direction as well as size. The activity of any single neuron can therefore be represented

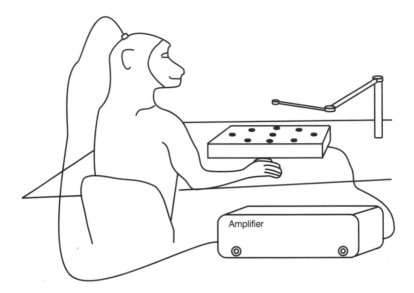

Figure 4.4
Experimental procedure of Georgopoulos et al. (1989). At first, the lever is in its resting position over the center of the circle. Then one of the eight lamps on the circle lights up, either brightly or dimly, which is the sign for the monkey to move. The monkey was trained to move the lever either to where the lamp lights up or to a lamp that is positioned 90 degrees counterclockwise from it.

by a vector—that is, by a quantity pointing in a certain direction. The idea is rather simple: A neuron represents a direction by firing whenever the arm is moved in that direction. If the neuron were active only when movement occurred toward a specific point in that direction, the usefulness of the vector idea would be trivial. However, this is not so. Before we look at how direction is coded in the monkey's brain, we need to examine why the one direction–one neuron strategy would be highly disadvantageous as the basis of a code. Such a code would be highly prone to hardware error, as whenever a neuron died movements could no longer be made in the direction it had represented.

As Georgopoulos and coworkers learned, the actual activation of neurons was different from such an error-prone coding scheme. Any given neuron was most active when the arm moved in its preferred direction; if the arm moved in a direction slightly off the preferred direction, however, the neuron's firing rate decreased slightly. Whenever the arm moved in a direction totally different from the neuron's preferred direction, the neuron showed little or no activity. By using vectors, the researchers were able to quantify these observations precisely as follows: Every direction-sensitive neuron becomes maximally active in a certain direction, which we may call its *preferred direction;* if the direction of the movement differs from the preferred direction by the angle α, the activity of the neuron equals the product of its maximal firing rate (size) and the cosine of α (direction) (figure 4.5).

Note that Georgopoulos and his colleagues first gathered their data and then developed the model to account for them. Once the model was developed, however, it turned out to be highly useful for describing neuronal activity. The different levels of activity of many neurons for a given movement could be simply summed up by taking the sum of the

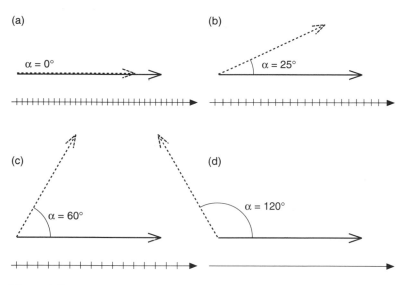

Figure 4.5
Schematic rendering of the activity of a neuron (a) when the movement occurs in its preferred direction; (b) when the movement occurs in a slightly different direction; (c) when the movement occurs in a rather different direction; and (d) when the movement occurs in a completely different direction. The horizontal arrow represents the preferred direction of the neuron, whereas the dotted arrow represents the direction of the movement. Angle (between both vectors determines the activity of the neuron (shown as short perpendicular lines on a time arrow below each angle.

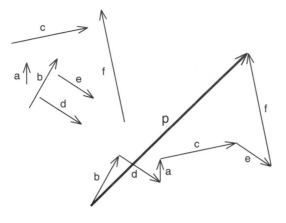

Figure 4.6
Sum of the activity of several direction-sensitive neurons (schematic representations). The length of the vector represents the activity of the neuron. The
direction of the vectors represents their preferred angle, which had been detected
before by noting the direction of movement that most strongly activates each
single neuron. All of the direction-sensitive neurons together code a single direction, which is the vector sum of the individual neurons. This is itself a vector (p),
which is figuratively created by stringing all the vectors together. The summation
vector points in the direction represented by the population of direction-coding
neurons; it is called the *population vector.*

activation vectors (figure 4.6). This sum is itself a vector and points
exactly in the direction of the movement.

Georgopoulos and coworkers (1988, 1993) used the concept of the
population vector to describe the relationship between the activity of
several hundred neurons in the motor cortex, on the one hand, and the
direction of an arm movement, on the other hand (see figure 4.7). In their
model, the population vector is defined as the sum of the activation
direction vectors of single neurons.

It is also possible to use the population vector to predict the direction
of an actual movement. To do this, the monkey was trained to wait for
a second and then to carry out the movement. Within this second, the
population of neurons that represents the direction of the movement to
be carried out became active. In other words, the population vector can
be used to monitor and describe processes that occur during the planning
of a movement, that is, before the movement is actually carried out. It

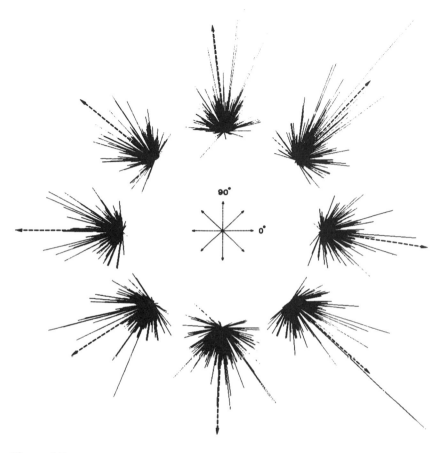

Figure 4.7
Direction-sensitive activity of more than 200 neurons in the area of the motor cortex of the monkey while the animal carries out, one at a time, the movements shown by the small arrows in the center of the figure (from Georgopoulos et al. 1989). The activity of each neuron is represented by a line pointing in the direction that is coded by the neuron (i.e., the direction of movement in which the neuron is maximally active). The longer the line, the more active is the neuron. The sum of the activities of all neurons, the population vector, is shown as a dotted arrow. It represents the direction coded by the entire population of neurons and points in a direction very close to the direction of the actual movement.

has also been demonstrated that the accuracy of prediction increases as researchers record from larger numbers of neurons (Lurito et al. 1991).

In further experiments that have become classics in the field of neuroscience, Georgopoulos and coworkers (1988) demonstrated that the population vector can be changed systematically during the planning phase of a movement. The monkey was trained to move its arm and the lever when the light came on to either the location of the light or to a location 90 degrees counterclockwise from the light. When the light came up dimmed, the animal moved its arm directly to the light; whereas when the light was bright it moved the lever in the direction that was 90 degrees away from the stimulus. It was hypothesized that if the monkey's cortex uses a population vector to code direction, and if this vector is also used to plan arm movements, the population vector would turn away from the stimulus in the bright-light condition (cf. figure 4.8).

To investigate this hypothesis directly, the research team recorded the activity of neurons in the motor cortex of the monkey every 10 milliseconds while the monkey was planning the movement and then moving its arm. The recordings demonstrated that whenever the monkey moved the lever directly to the light, there was a build-up of a population vector pointing in the direction of the movement during the planning phase. When this vector reached a certain length (i.e., when the combined activity of the neurons reached a certain level), the arm movement began. If the monkey was signaled to move its arm in the direction 90 degrees counterclockwise from the stimulus, something else occurred. After the bright stimulus light appeared, there was a build-up of a vector that at first pointed in the direction of the stimulus and then rotated by 90 degrees away from it. In other words, the activity of the neurons representing the movement shifted gradually, at first representing a movement in the direction of the stimulus and then rotating away from it. This counterclockwise rotation of the internal representation happened within 225 milliseconds of the time the light came on, *before* there was any actual movement, which started 260 milliseconds *after* the light. The planning phase could not be detected in the behavior of the animal, as it happened internally, but could only be observed with electrophysiological methods. The researchers further observed that the representation of the direction did not abruptly flip to the new direction but rather rotated

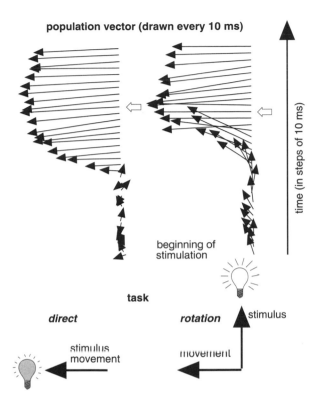

Figure 4.8
Length and direction of the population vector during a mental rotation (after Georgopoulos et al. 1989). *Task:* When a dimmed light came on (left) the monkey had to move the lever directly to the light. When a bright light appeared, its task was to move the lever to a direction 90 degrees counterclockwise from the light. The length and direction of the population vector, as calculated from the activities of several hundred neurons, is shown every 10 milliseconds, from the onset of the stimulus (the lighting of the lamp) until after the onset of the movement (indicated by the little arrow). The rotation of the population vector (on the right) can be clearly seen. "When the population vector lengthens, for the direct case (left) it points in the direction of the movement, whereas for the rotation case it points initially in the direction of the stimulus and then rotates counterclockwise (from 12 o'clock to 9 o'clock) and points in the direction of the movement." (Georgopoulos et al. 1989:234).

toward it. A rotation, but not a flip, implies that the population vector acquires direction gradually between the stimulus and the response. About halfway through the planning time, for example, the population vector points in a direction about 45 degrees counterclockwise from the stimulus (Lurito et al. 1991).

Let's think a minute about what these experiments demonstrate. Using sophisticated methods, neuroscientists can watch the planning of a movement before any behavior is visible. By observing neurons that represent a parameter (the direction of movement) and watching changes in that parameter, they can infer the nature of the code and measure the time it takes to initiate action based on the coded information—while the unaided observer can see no change in the animal's behavior.

The beauty and simplicity of the coding scheme may be deceptive, in that the results may seem trivial. They are not! Prior to these experiments, no neuroscientist predicted that changes in the direction of an organism's movement were internally coded by actual turns in the internal representations of those directions.

Measuring regional cerebral blood flow with modern functional imaging techniques have shown that in humans the primary motor cortex, as well as other frontal areas responsible for the planning of movements, is activated during a mental rotation task (Deutsch et al. 1988). Moreover, psychological experiments in which subjects rotate both actual and imagined images have shown that we rotate objects in our minds with an average speed of four hundred degrees per second (Shepard & Cooper 1982). This rotation speed, which varies considerably between individuals, is of the same order of magnitude as the rotation speed of the population vector measured directly in the monkey brain. Finally, experiments have demonstrated that humans rotate images of mental movements and of actual intended movements at very similar speeds, which can be interpreted as an indication that similar processes are involved in both tasks (Georgopoulos et al. 1993).

The experiments performed by Georgopoulos and his group are important because, for the first time, they allow us to observe changes in the activity of neurons over time and relate those changes to a complex cognitive task. In the experiment to which we turn next, a similar method was used to watch neurons learn something new about their environment.

Observing Neurons During Learning

Populations of neurons in the hippocampus, a structure crucial for learning and memory, have been observed during learning. Every time you get lost while driving your car, going around in circles until you gradually acquire some understanding of your surroundings, the neurons in your hippocampus are actively learning. We know that neurons in the hippocampus represent, among other things, the spatial features of an environment; they do so by firing whenever you are in a certain location. Such cells have been termed *place cells*.

Wilson and McNaughton (1993) implanted more than a hundred electrodes into the hippocampus of rats to record the activity of a large number of cells. For ten days the rats were allowed to move freely around half of a box measuring 62 by 124 centimeters. To encourage the rats to become acquainted with all areas of their half of the box, the researchers distributed chocolate pellets all around the floor. The walls of the box also contained various visual and tactile stimuli to help the animals orient themselves. The second half of the box was blocked by an opaque wall (figure 4.9).

Close inspection of the activation patterns of the neurons revealed that about 20 to 30 percent of the neurons were place cells; that is, cells had developed a preference for a certain place in the box and fired whenever the animal happened to be at that spot. The activity of the place cells, however, codes the spatial location of the animal, just as the direction cells code direction of a movement—not in a single highly specialized hippocampal neuron but by the weighted sum of the activity of all the place cells. For example, the neuron that fires most rapidly whenever the animal is in the rear left-hand corner of the box fires even when the animal only approaches that corner. The closer the animal moves to the corner, the more rapidly the neuron fires.

When the population vector of all recorded place cells is calculated, the actual location of the animal in the box can be determined quite accurately. At first glance, this may appear a trivial result; someone might say "I only need to look to see where the animal is." Nonetheless, the fact that neuroscientists can now record the activity of individual brain cells, recognize their code, and tell, by merely looking into an animal's brain, exactly where the animal is shows that enormous advances have

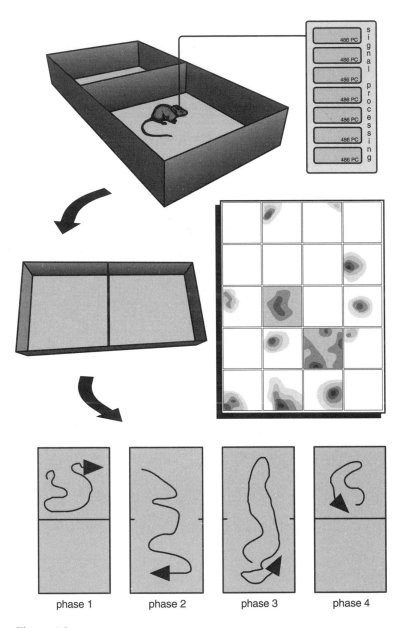

Figure 4.9
Schematic representation of the experiment carried out by Wilson and McNaughton (1993). (Top) The box, measuring 124 by 62 centimeters has a wall dividing it into two halves so that the rat can move about only in the front half. A recording device weighing about 10 grams, which does not interfere with

been made in the field of neuroscience. Like the observation of an animal mentally rotating the direction of a movement, such an accomplishment was unthinkable only two decades ago.

This research further demonstrates that as the number of recordings used to determine location increases the predictions become more accurate. When twenty to thirty neurons were recorded, the prediction error of the animal's location was about five centimeters; the error dropped to two centimeters when recordings from about forty neurons were used to calculate location.

In a subsequent experiment, Wilson and McNaughton (1994) addressed the question of what happens when animals explore a new environment (figure 4.10). This experiment was designed in four phases. In phase one, the animals just ran around in the known half of the box for ten minutes. In the second and third phases of the experiment—each lasting ten minutes—the wall was removed so that the animals could forage within the entire box. Finally, the wall was replaced, and the animals spent the final ten minutes of the experiment doing the same thing as during phase one. For the entire forty minutes of the experiment, the animals' movements were recorded by a video camera mounted above

the animal's ability to move around the box, is fixed to its head. The neuronal signals are amplified and processed by seven personal computers working in parallel, which gives an idea of the computing power needed to cope with the information recorded from the animal's brain. (Bottom) The box and the movement of the rat, as seen from right above, is depicted for the different phases of the experiment (the front part, above, is now the upper part). Each phase lasted for ten minutes. In phases one and four, the animal was allowed to forage only in the upper part of the box, whereas in phases two and three the wall was removed and the animal moved around the entire box. The panel of 20 squares shown on the right side in the middle of the figure schematically represents the original data from the paper of Wilson and McNaughton (1993:1057). These 20 squares represent the activity of 20 neurons on a gray scale keyed to the location of the rat in phase one of the experiment. For example, the neuron whose activity is represented by the left upper square is not active during this phase. The adjacent square to the right represents a neuron that becomes active whenever the rat is in the left upper corner (as viewed from above) of the box. The next square to the right shows the activity of a neuron that becomes active when the rat is in the right upper corner of the box, and so on. About half of the 20 neurons whose activity is plotted display a spatial preference; that is, they code for the location of the rat in the box.

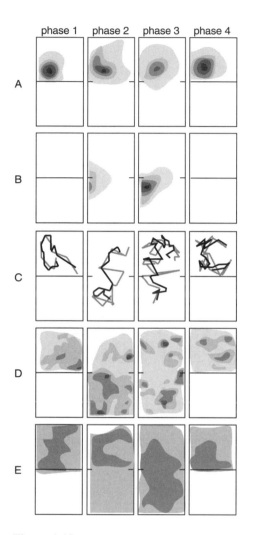

Figure 4.10

Data from the four phases of the experiment are shown by plotting them on schematic renderings of the entire box, as viewed from above. The top row (A) shows the activity of a single neuron that codes a location in the known part of the box. Row B shows the activity of a neuron that was not active during phase one of the experiment. However, during phase two, this neuron acquired a spatial representation of a location in the new environment. The middle row (C) depicts a part of the actual path of the foraging rat (gray), as well as the corresponding calculated path as derived from neuronal activity. With the exception of movements in the new part of the box during phase two of the experiment, the two paths correspond quite well. That is, the activation of neurons can be used to the box; the electrical activity of their hippocampal neurons were also recorded. It turned out that during phase one the neuronal recordings identified the location of the animals quite well, whereas in phase two, good results were obtained only when animals were in the part of the box they already knew well. When the rats moved into the new part of the box, their location could no longer be determined from the neuronal recordings.

After ten minutes, however, the situation changed. In phase three, some of the neurons in the hippocampus—mostly those that had so far apparently not represented anything—had acquired a spatial preference. It again became possible to calculate the spatial location of the animals from the activity of hippocampal neurons, which now provided the relevant information. The rats had apparently learned within ten minutes to orient themselves within the new area by forming neuronal representations of locations in it. Phase four demonstrated that the new learning did not make the rats forget what they already knew. The place cells coding the known part of the box were practically unchanged by the new experience and allowed researchers to calculate the animals' location as accurately as they had in phase one. In sum, when the animals entered the new environment, it was not yet represented by the neurons in the hippocampus; but new experience drove rapid changes in some neurons and within a few minutes produced new representations.

As only active neurons can learn—because learning requires LTP and because LTP requires some activity at the synapse—it follows that the activity of the inhibitory interneurons (see chapter 5) must be reduced for learning to take place. This is, in fact, what actually happens. During phase two, when the animals began to explore the new environment, the

predict the location of the animal. In row D, the error of these predictions is plotted. The darker the area, the larger the error. It is evident that the error increased during phase two of the experiment, that is, during the phase in which spatial representations had not yet been formed. The bottom row (E) shows the activity of an inhibitory interneuron. The neuron obviously does not represent any location. It appears to modulate the activity of other hippocampal neurons. During the second phase of the experiment, its activity decreased whenever the animal entered the new half of the box, thereby enabling the neurons to become activated more easily (after figure 2 in Wilson & McNaughton 1993:1057).

activity of the interneurons decreased by about 70 percent; this reduction occurred whenever a rat wandered into the new part of the box. When the rat returned to the known areas the activity of the inhibitory inter-neurons returned to normal.

Recap

Information can be present in different forms. Thus, different aspects of the environment, or of the organism's behavior, can be coded in different ways. A *code* or a *representation* (the two words are used as synonyms) is the form in which information is stored and processed. Features of the environment can be represented parsimoniously by vectors in a *vector space,* which is generated by *basic dimensions.* A few dimensions with a few graded values for each dimension is all it takes to represent millions of characteristic features. Any particular feature can be represented as a point in vector space.

A code must not only be parsimonious, but also robust—that is, it must work even when errors occur (for example, when parts of the hardware fail or are damaged). Population codes provide such robust-ness. In such a code, a feature of the environment, or of the behavioral response to it, is represented by a large number of neurons. In neural networks, the feature or behavior is represented by the sum of the directionally weighted activities of single neurons. This sum of vectors is called the *population vector.* If the feature represented is, for example, the direction of a movement, then the population vector points in that direction. If the feature is a point in space, the population vector com-posed of *place cells* points to the actual location of the animal.

Research in which population vectors have been observed and calcu-lated has allowed us to peek into the brain of an animal—as it were—and to draw inferences from neuronal activity about the direction of a move-ment and the location of the animal. The concept of a vector thus has proven to be highly useful for interpreting the activity of a large number of neurons.

II

Principles

Having examined several basic features of neural networks—how they work, and how they learn—we can build on these basics by looking at some of the principles of information processing in biological systems. We do so in chapters 5 through 8 by considering certain neurophysiological data and theories and using them to flesh out the network models. In other words we will build some biology into the very simple network models we began with, making them more realistic and able to perform more functions.

This process will let us see which tasks are executed by which anatomical or physiological features. Neurobiological knowledge comes to life in such simulations, allowing us to see features of systems that can emerge only when the elements of the system interact with one another and with the environment. Because such dynamic features cannot be discovered by any static method, simulations are crucial.

5

Maps in the Cortex

How can simulated networks learn without being told the correct output in every trial by a teacher? In particular, how do the real neurons in real brains learn by real experience?

In the early 1980s, the Finnish engineer Teuvo Kohonen experimented with a new type of neural network set up to simulate some of the basic features of the neocortex. Remarkably, these networks display the capacity for *self-organization*—the ability to learn without a teacher. To understand how Kohonen's network works, we first need to consider some essential facts about the human cortex. Next we introduce Kohonen's network, along with model simulations that exemplify the features of this kind of networks and its biological importance.

Anatomy of the Cortex

The human cortex contains both excitatory and inhibitory neurons. The bulk of cortical information processing is performed by so-called *pyramidal cells,* which make up about 70 percent of the neurons in the cortex; they sometimes have the triangular shape from which they take their name (see figure 5.1). Pyramidal neurons are glutamatergic in that they use the excitatory amino acid glutamate as their transmitter. About 20 to 30 percent of the cortical neurons are inhibitory neurons, which use the transmitter gamma-amino-butyric acid (GABA). Because their circuitry causes them to form connections between excitatory neurons, these *GABAergic* neurons are called *inhibitory interneurons.*

Isocortex—The General Purpose Machine
The human cortex can be described as a folded surface 1.5 to 5 mm thick and about 0.25 m^2 wide (Cherniak 1990, Guyton 1992). It is composed

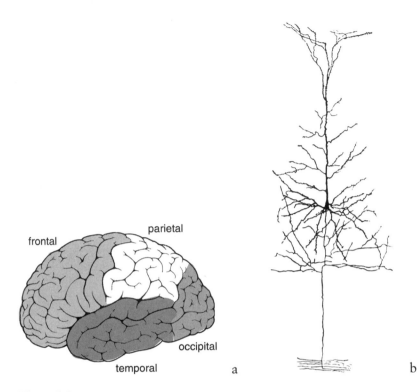

Figure 5.1
(a) View of the human brain from the left, showing the gyri (convoluted surface) of the cortex. Each half of the cortex can be divided into the frontal lobe, the temporal lobe, the parietal lobe, and the occipital lobe. (b) The neuron, drawn by Ramón y Cajal, is the workhorse of the human cortex, the pyramidal cell (from Cajal 1988:389).

of neurons that are highly interconnected, in part through inhibitory interneurons. One cubic millimeter of cortex contains about a hundred thousand neurons—except for the primary visual cortex, which contains about twice as many neurons per volume (cf. Rockel et al. 1980). A cubic millimeter cut from the cortex contains the ends of about sixty thousand neuronal fibers (Creutzfeld 1995).

Pyramidal cells have specific topographic connections to other cells called *projections*, which serve as the brain's rapid information conductors. Their glutamatergic transmission is performed by ion channels; that is, the transmitter glutamate permits the influx of ions and consecutive changes in the membrane potential within one to three milliseconds. GABAergic neurons are somewhat slower, and their projections may be a little more "diffuse," but both types of neurons work rapidly and do the bulk of cortical information processing (cf. Morrison & Hof 1992, Nauta & Feirtag 1990).

More than 90 percent of the cortex of the human brain has a remarkably uniform structure and is called *isocortex* (from the Greek *iso,* uniform); because it is the most recent in evolutionary terms, this part of the cortex is also called the *neocortex*. The uniform structure of the neocortex extends in both the horizontal and the vertical directions. The neocortex has six horizontal layers (see figure 5.2), and its functioning depends on its vertically oriented columns of cells (see below).

In evolutionary terms, the neocortex is a highly successful structure that serves all kinds of purposes. Isn't it remarkable that regardless of whether the rat sees, the monkey moves, or the human thinks, the cortical matter carrying out these functions has the very same structure? The functional principle of the cortex, once it evolved, became versatile enough to solve a large variety of computational problems. Clearly, the functional principle underlying cortical activity must be very general; otherwise it would not be as adaptable as it is.

What is the nature of this general structure?

Columns of Information Processing
A closer look at figure 5.2 reveals both a horizontal and a vertical structure. Most of the synaptic connections of a large cortical pyramidal cell (from layer 5) are located between 0.3 and 0.5 mm from the vertical axis of this cell, which suggests a cylindrical architecture of cortical information processing. Several decades ago, electrophysiological investigations of the visual cortex, as well as biochemical studies, demonstrated that the functional unit of the cortex is the cortical column (cf. Mountcastle 1957; Hubel & Wiesel 1962).

These columns can be regarded as the smallest processing units in the cortex. However, it is still unclear whether they are structurally fixed or are, perhaps, just functional assemblies around a momentarily active neuron—that is, the structure of a neuron's functional environment only while it is performing its task.

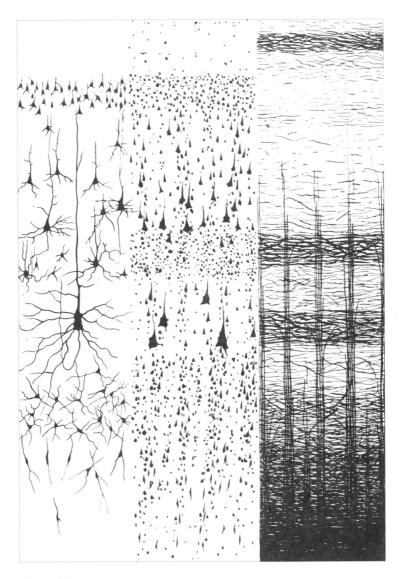

Figure 5.2
Neurons under the microscope. Different stains can be used to stain different structures. The figure shows, left to right, the cortex as stained with the Golgi stain, the Nissl stain, and the Weigert stain. This widely reproduced semischematic figure from a chapter by Rose in the *Handbook of Neurology* (Bumke 1935) dates back to the early–twentieth-century neuroanatomists Otto Vogt and Korbinian Brodman. The six layers sometimes cannot be readily distinguished under the microscope. We have already discussed the Golgi stain. The Nissl stain

But how can we study the functional environment of a neuron? The trick here is to combine several methods of investigation in a creative way. For example, researchers can use tiny electrodes to stimulate a single neuron and measure the output of nearby neurons to learn whether (and how) the stimulated neuron has affected them. With enough time and some luck, they can identify and study cells that are functionally connected. For example, they may find that when one cell fires, it causes an adjacent cell to fire as well; or it may stimulate the adjacent cell so that it fires more easily upon subsequent stimulation. In yet another case, stimulating one cell may inhibit the firing of another cell.

Once such functional relationships between and among cells have been characterized, scientists must ask where exactly these cells are located relative to one another. Remember, all that has been done so far is to characterize some cells according to their function. Experimenters still do not know what the cells look like, where exactly they are in the cortex, or, in particular, how and where their fibers connect. To discover these facts, they first inject dyes of different colors into the neurons they had just studied electrically, then prepare thin slices to examine under the microscope. The connections that have been functionally characterized can then be anatomically described.

Using this procedure permits the functional environment of a cortical pyramidal cell (i.e., its connections to other cells), to be described as follows (cf. Thomson & Deuchars 1994).

1. A pyramidal cell may directly activate its neighboring cells. This activation occurs via NMDA-receptors and hence is modified by its use.

(center), was invented in the 1880s by Franz Nissl, who then was a student in Munich; he was chairman of the Psychiatric Hospital at the University of Heidelberg from 1904 until 1918 (cf. Mundt 1992). His technique uses the fact that the axons have to be nurtured by the cell body. Because the axons of nerve cells can be quite long—think of a three-mile-long piece of spaghetti—the neuron sitting at one end has to synthesize the proteins and send them throughout the length of the axons. This implies that neurons have a higher rate of protein synthesis than other cells (such as the glia cells surrounding the neurons). The machinery of protein synthesis, the messenger RNA, is the substrate to which the Nissl stain binds. Thus the staining delineates all the neurons but not their fibers. On the right, Weigert staining of the cortex has just the opposite effect; that is, it reveals the fibers but not the cells.

This type of strong activation happens mainly between neurons in the vertical direction (see figure 5.3).

2. This type of connection is limited horizontally to a small cylinder—a column—of less than 100 %m in diameter.

3. The activity of such a column, once excited, is a self-limiting physiological process. After a brief feedforward burst, the activity breaks down. The column is then refractory for about 10 milliseconds, after which it can again be excited. This self-limiting mechanism ensures that pyramidal cells are not engaged in continuous mutual excitation, which would be of no computational use.

4. In addition to the strong connections within a column, there are weaker connections between more distant pyramidal cells. These connections are not strong enough to lead to the firing of the cell, but they cause the cell to be activated more easily by later stimulation. These connections cause something like a excitatory halo around an excited column; that is, such an activated column causes adjacent columns to be activated more readily by, for example, a similar signal.

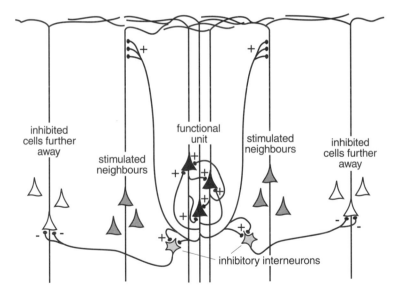

Figure 5.3
Local circuitry of cortical neurons. A neuron and its immediate neighbors form a functional unit; that is, they fire together (black). Somewhat more distant neurons (gray) become somewhat excited, whereas inhibitory interneurons (star-shaped, light gray) cause inhibition in the more distant neurons (white).

5. GABAergic interneurons are activated by pyramidal cells and cause inhibition of other pyramidal cells located at a distance. Taken together, these excitatory and inhibitory connections of a pyramidal cell implement the *center-surround structure* described decades ago (cf. Spillman & Werner 1990).

The cortical column shown in figure 5.4 can be regarded as the functional unit of information processing. This does not imply that a single neuron is not itself such a unit but, rather, that information processing occurs at several levels (and at several scales) of neuronal organization. Some data suggest that computations may be carried out even at the level of single dendrites (Borst & Egelhaaf 1994, Shepherd & Brayton 1987), although we may assume that many computational features of the neocortex are best captured by taking the column as the unit of function. The following simulation takes this position and assumes that the column, with its center-surround structure, is the basic unit of cortical processing.

Self-Organizing Feature Maps

The self-organizing feature maps developed by Kohonen (also called *Kohonen networks*) consist, in their simplest form, of an input layer and an output layer (see figure 5.5). These layers can be two-dimensional; that is, in contrast to the simple pattern-recognition network discussed in chapter 2, which is just a string of neurons, they are sheets of neurons. The output layer, sometimes referred to as the Kohonen layer, also has a special internal structure.

In a Kohonen network, each neuron of the input layer is connected to every neuron of the output layer. In addition, there are interconnections among all the neurons within the Kohonen layer, as suggested by the structures depicted in figures 5.3 and 5.4. Every neuron in this layer excites the neurons in its surround to some degree and inhibits the neurons that are farther away (*lateral inhibition*). Each neuron in the Kohonen-layer, hence, has a center-surround environment (see figure 5.6). Because of this architecture, the neurons of the Kohonen layer can fine-tune their synaptic weights by self-organization so that the representation of certain features of the input are located at specific points on

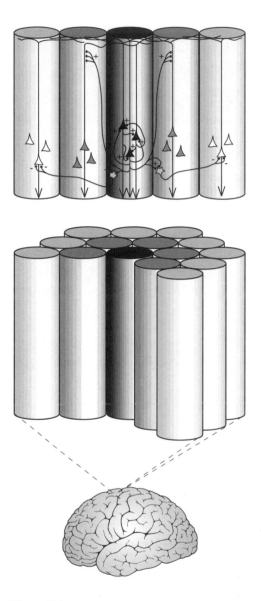

Figure 5.4
Principles of connectivity of cortical neurons into functional modules conceived
as columns. The entire neocortex consists of this structure.

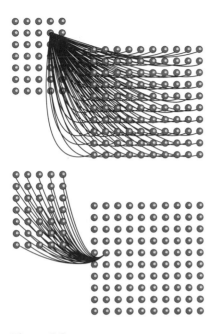

Figure 5.5
Simple Kohonen network. The input layer consists of a grid of 5 × 7 neurons, the output layer of a 10 × 10-neuron grid. Each neuron of the input layer is connected to every neuron of the output layer. If all of them were drawn, the figure would be entirely black and nothing could be seen. This is why, in an analogy to the Golgi stain, only the connections of a single input neuron with all output neurons (top) and all the input connections of a single output neuron (bottom) were drawn. The connections among the neurons of the output layer are not drawn (cf. figure 5.6).

the output layer. In short, the Kohonen layer forms a topographical map of the important features of the input.

The center-surround environment in the Kohonen layer implements competition among the neurons of this layer whenever a pattern comes in from the input layer. A complete copy of this input pattern arrives at every neuron of the Kohonen layer, as in the miniature pattern-recognition network described in chapter 2.

If the Kohonen network has not yet been trained, the connecting weights will be small and random. At each neuron, the entire input pattern will therefore go through synapses of slightly different and random strengths. In computational terms, each neuron of the Kohonen

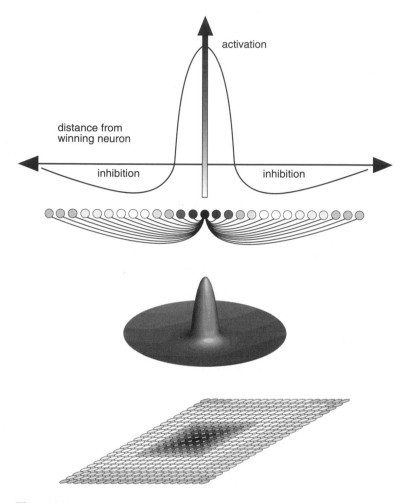

Figure 5.6
Center-surround architecture of the Kohonen layer. Each neuron is connected to
every other neuron in this layer: excitatory connections to close neurons and
inhibitory connections to distant neurons. The top of the figure depicts a cross
section of this function. In order to characterize the function across the entire
two-dimensional layer, we have to rotate it around the y axis (center). The
function now looks like a Mexican hat; in fact, it is actually called the Mexican
hat function. The drawing at the bottom depicts an active neuron coded on a
gray scale. Again, the active neuron excites nearby neurons and inhibits more
distant neurons.

layer will perform thirty-five multiplications (35 inputs X 35 weights) and sum them up. Thus far, the network functions just like the simple network in chapter 2, except that it is bigger.

Additional interesting properties, however, result from the internal connections of the Kohonen layer. In any of the hundred output neurons, the weighted input may be larger than its threshold, causing the neuron to fire. When it does so, it excites its adjacent neurons to some degree and inhibits neurons that are farther away. The active neuron is therefore called the *winning neuron,* because its firing inhibits most of the other neurons of the Kohonen layer; it alone becomes active and, thus, "wins" when a given input is presented.

In order for a Kohonen network to learn, the connections between the input layer and the Kohonen layer have to be adjustable by *Hebbian learning.* When such learning is implemented, the following occurs: the active input neurons that represent a pattern strengthen their connections with the winning (that is, active) output neuron, thereby increasing slightly the weights of the connections between them. This process of tuning the weights produces, over time, a highly specific representation of the input pattern.

Example: A Simulated Network for Letter Recognition

To understand the process of map formation in a Kohonen network, let us look at a simple network that learns to recognize the characters of the alphabet. The input patterns consist of graphic renditions of each capital letter on a 5 × 7 grid (see figure 5.7). To recognize these patterns the

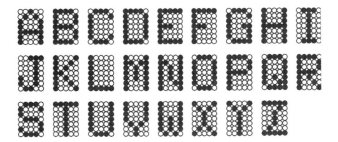

Figure 5.7
The 5 × 7 grid used in the computer simulation of letter recognition.

network must transform the graphic representation of the characters into a symbolic form; that is, it must code each character pattern as, for example, the activity of a neuron or a group of neurons. In the case of a self-organizing feature map, the task of character recognition is complete when every input pattern reliably produces a different winning neuron in the output layer. Once the network has been trained, the pattern of a given character should always excite a specific neuron in the Kohonen layer. In anthropomorphic terms, the neurons in the output layer each become responsible for a specific input pattern.

When a new letter pattern is represented at the input layer, each neuron in the output layer gets a copy (i.e., receives a signal from every neuron of the input layer) that varies according to the weight of its connection. To put it another way, before training a given pattern will activate all the neurons of the Kohonen layer to a different degree because of the different and random weights. One neuron of the Kohonen layer will—by sheer coincidence—receive the strongest input, fire, and thus be the winning neuron, thereby inhibiting most of the other neurons in the layer and exciting to some degree closer neurons. Finally, by firing it will increase its connections with the active input neurons.

What determines which neuron will win? Obviously, this depends upon the fit of the input pattern to the synaptic weights. If the synapses through which activity passes happen to be strong, while those through which no activity passes happen to be weak, the input will get through the strongest synapses with the least amount of decrease. In terms of linear algebra, this can be stated clearly and simply. Thinking of the input patterns as well as the connection weights as vectors, the winning neuron will be the one whose weight vector most closely resembles the input vector.

What does learning do to the entire Kohonen layer? First of all, learning in Kohonen layers occurs only in the winning neuron. Let us look at the winning neuron more closely. Its synaptic weights obviously fit the input better than the weights of the other ninety-nine neurons. However, when the network is only beginning to receive input, we cannot assume that the winning neuron's weights are optimal—they are just a little better than the weights of any other neuron. However, its weights change during activity, assuming a slightly better fit. And, because the winning neuron also has activated its surrounding neurons, there is an increased likelihood that input patterns similar to the one that activated the winning neuron will activate those surrounding neurons. As similar patterns become represented nearby, the resulting inhibition of all the other neurons will ensure that they will not be activated by these patterns. As a result of all these processes, the Kohonen layer changes after several hundred presentations of the input patterns. It forms stable representations of input patterns that are reliably activated when presented with the patterns. In short, the network has learned the input by forming neuronal representations. Furthermore, these representations are not distributed randomly across the Kohonen layer. Instead, a map of the graphic similarities of the input has been formed as similar input patterns are coded by neighboring neurons (figure 5.8).

Similarity and Frequency
Learning in a Kohonen network can be summarized as follows.

1. The input signal is present at the input layer, which transmits the signal to all the neurons of the output layer.

2. Because of their internal connections, the neurons of the output layer determine among themselves the "winning neuron"—that is, the neuron that is most excited by the input. The surrounding neurons also become slightly activated.

3. Now Hebbian learning occurs: the weight vector of the winning neuron (i.e., the neuron of the Kohonen layer with the weight vector closest to the input vector) is changed by Hebbian learning and becomes even closer to the input vector. All other neurons in the network remain unchanged.

4. The process starts over again (at step 1) when the next input pattern is presented to the input layer.

After several thousand such trials, the weight vectors of single neurons become increasingly closely attuned to certain input patterns. This, of course, only happens if there are regularities in the input. If every new input pattern is novel, nothing can be learned!

The maplike order of the representations of input patterns in Kohonen networks is a feature that deserves closer inspection. It does not just mean that every input gets represented by an identifiable neuron, a spot on the map; localized representation is only one of the map's characteristics. The second important feature is that similarity of input patterns is coded

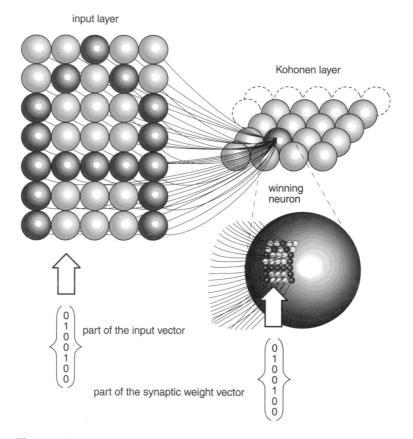

input layer

Kohonen layer

winning
neuron

$\left.\begin{matrix} 0 \\ 1 \\ 0 \\ 0 \\ 1 \\ 0 \\ 0 \end{matrix}\right\}$ part of the input vector

part of the synaptic weight vector $\left\{\begin{matrix} 0 \\ 1 \\ 0 \\ 0 \\ 1 \\ 0 \\ 0 \end{matrix}\right.$

Figure 5.8
(Top left) The letter *A* is represented by the neurons of the input layer of the Kohonen network (dark: active neurons; light: inactive neurons). (Top right) The part of the Kohonen layer that contains the winning neuron (dark) is shown. Also shown are the connections between every neuron of the input layer and the winning neuron. The close-up of the winning neuron (center) shows the synapses of the thirty-five connections. Their strength is coded on a gray scale (the darker the synapse, the better the connection). This rendering of the input and the synaptic weights allows us to make a simple visual comparison. It is obvious that the sum of the weighted inputs is largest when the input pattern and the pattern of the synaptic weights are similar, if not identical. If the weight pattern is dissimilar to the input pattern, the input is not transmitted well at the connections and the neuron is unlikely to fire. The input pattern, as well as the weight pattern, can be characterized by a vector, using 1 for every active input neuron and 0 for every inactive neuron, in a fixed order. Similarly, we can represent the weights as a vector by simply writing them down in a fixed order. The figure displays only a few of these vectors, which are each made up of 35 numbers. Only vectors for the second column are shown, in the interests of spatial economy.

by the distances between representations on the map. Similar inputs are represented by adjacent neurons on the map; dissimilar inputs, by distant neurons. Finally, frequent input patterns are represented by larger areas of the map (consisting of more neurons) than infrequent patterns. In a Kohonen network, therefore, the similarities and frequencies of input patterns are mapped as topographical features of the representations in the output layer (figure 5.9). This is no small accomplishment!

Similarity and frequency are thus the principles governing formation of representations of input patterns in self-organizing feature maps. What drives self-organization, therefore, is the internal order of the input patterns. It has been shown that Kohonen networks can extract regularities from input signals—that is, detect these similarities—and thereby represent the input in a highly ordered manner.

It is important to note that the principles of frequency and similarity refer to the spatiotemporal structure of the input patterns. In the alphabet-simulation example, *O* and *Q* are similar, as are *E* and *F. I* and *J,* however, are less similar (figure 5.10).

Receptive Fields

When input patterns are represented on a two-dimensional, self-organizing feature map, the Kohonen layer automatically selects those features of the input that vary the most. The network uses this dimension of greatest variability to order representations and spontaneously generate so-called receptive fields. The order of these receptive fields is a function of the features of the input patterns. As has been demonstrated, frequent input patterns cause the generation of larger receptive fields than infrequent input patterns do. Kohonen was further able to show that a two-dimensional output layer can represent not only simple feature spaces but also complex features made up of any number of dimensions. In other words, Kohonen networks are capable of abstraction; they can extract the general features of a succession of single events and can use the regularities behind (or within) the events to generate a meaningfully structured internal representation of them. We also have just seen that frequent inputs occupy more space on the map. Kohonen networks therefore classify inputs according to their probability in the environment, which is a first approximation of relevance.

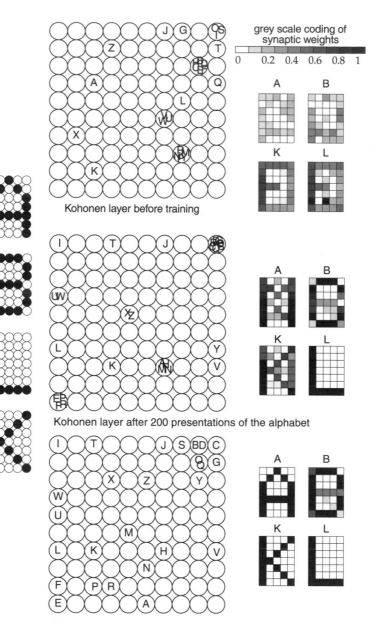

grey scale coding of
synaptic weights

Kohonen layer before training

Kohonen layer after 200 presentations of the alphabet

Kohonen layer after 700 presentations of the alphabet

Figure 5.9
A Kohonen network undergoing training. In the left margin, four of the 26 input
patterns shown in figure 5.7 are repeated. The center section of the figure shows

Cortical Topography

Topographic maps of ordered representations of features were first demonstrated in the human brain by the neurosurgeons Wilder Penfield and E. Boldrey (1937). Because the neocortex has no sense of pain, brain surgeons can operate on conscious patients, using only local anesthesia to numb the skull. This is important when, for example, removing a tumor. On the one hand, the mass must be completely excised (in order

the Kohonen layer before training (top), after 200 presentations of the alphabet (middle) and after 700 presentations of the alphabet (bottom). The four rectangles to the right of the network are graphic representations of the weights of the winning neurons when the letter patterns on the left were presented. The upper left rectangle, for instance, shows the weights of the connections between the neurons of the input layer and the winning neuron when an *A* was input. Each small square represents the strength of the connection between this neuron and one neuron of the input layer. In this manner, the upper middle gray square shows a medium strong connection of the *A* neuron of the Kohonen layer (labeled *A* because it was the winner when an *A* was present in the input layer) to the upper middle neuron of the input layer. The adjacent white square tells us that the connection of the *A* neuron to the upper second right neuron of the input layer is very weak (and so on). Looking at the graphic representation of the weights of this neuron makes it clear that before training its weights are far from optimal; that is, input patterns other than *A* will also lead to some activation of the neuron. The other three rectangles display the weights of three other winning neurons: the *B*, *K*, and the *L* neurons. Like the *A* neuron, these neurons (i.e., their weights) do not represent the input well. In the yet-untrained Kohonen layer, the characters of the alphabet are represented by a few neurons that do not discriminate well. For example, the neuron in the top right corner fires when several different characters are presented to the network. After 200 presentations of the alphabet, however, the network has changed (see middle network): The representations of the input have become distributed and more specific. Moreover, similar input patterns are closer together (e.g., the *I* and the *T*) than dissimilar ones (the *O* and the *E*, for example). However, there are still neurons with weights that can be activated by a number of input patterns (e.g., the upper right *CBDGOQS* neuron). After another 550 presentations of the alphabet (bottom), the situation has changed again; now almost all characters are nicely represented by corresponding winning neurons whose weights are specifically tuned to the input. Notice that the order of the winning neurons on the map corresponds to similarities in the input signals. Simulations were performed using an Apple Macintosh Quadra microcomputer running inexpensive and easy-to-use software designed to teach the neural-network approach to students (cf. Caudill & Butler 1992).

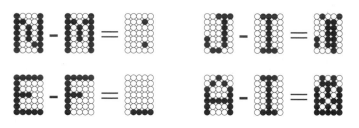

Figure 5.10
Graphic similarity of letters, as defined by the number of points that are different. The dissimilar points of two patterns are shown in black to highlight the difference between two patterns (i.e., the number of different points). The difference between *M* and *N* is 2 and between *E* and *F* is 4, whereas the difference between *I* and *J* is 15 and between *A* and *I* is 23.

to leave no cells to regrow the tumor), while, on the other, preserving the areas of the brain essential to speech, vision, and movement. Because it is impossible to determine the function of the various areas of the cortex by just looking at them, about sixty years ago doctors began stimulating points on the cortex, observing the effects on awake patients and questioning them about their experiences. In this way, they were able to map the areas of the cortex during the operation and gather information to use in carrying out the surgery.

During these operations, surgeons discovered that the part of the cortex that represents the body surface and is responsible for processing touch sensations has a maplike structure. This part of the brain forms a map of the body surface; for example, the shoulder is represented next to the upper arm, which in turn is represented next to the lower arm, and so on. Most important, they discovered that the parts of the body were not represented in relation to their size but in accordance with their importance. The hands and the lips, for example, process many more touch sensations than the back. Accordingly, the lips and the hands are allotted more computational surface on the surface map and signals from these parts of the body are processed more precisely than signals from the back. This is obviously highly adaptive for the organism's survival.

This discovery became widely known, not least because of an ingenious drawing of a man whose distorted proportions correspond in size to the cortical areas coding the touch sensations of various parts of the body (Penfield & Rasmussen 1950). The drawing of the homunculus representing the sensory and motor cortex quickly traveled around the scientific community; there is now hardly anyone who has not seen these little disfigured dwarfs with their big hands and lips (figure 5.11). Penfield's homunculi are so widely known—they appear in virtually every textbook on neurology and neuroscience—that the basic message sometimes gets lost. The important message is that there are maps in the cortex on which input signals (the sensations of touch) are represented according to the principles of similarity, frequency, and importance.

Not only the tactile sense but all the physiological senses are based on cortical maps. The human visual system contains more than a dozen retinotopic maps—that is, topographically ordered maps on which the points correspond to points of the retina. Like the body-surface homunculi, these retinotopic maps form a distorted image of the retina, with the part of the retina that gives us the sharpest images (the fovea) represented by the largest area of the cortical map. In addition, there are tonotopic maps in which the frequencies of tones heard are represented as an ordered frequency map.

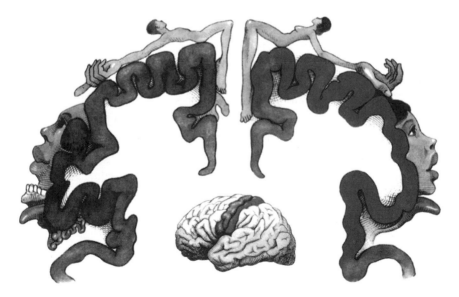

Figure 5.11
Motor (left) and sensory (right) cortical homunculus (from Posner & Raichle 1994).

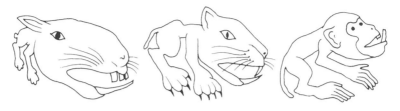

Figure 5.12
Sensory representation of the tactile body surface of rabbits (left), cats (center), and monkeys (right). As they are in figure 5.11, parts of the body are drawn in proportion to the size of the cortical area representing them (from Kandel et al. 1991:373).

Several experiments have shown that the sensory cortex of various animals is structured in a similar way (figure 5.12). Thus there is not only a homunculus but also, for example, a "ratunculus" and a "rabbitunculus." Animal studies demonstrate that the special capabilities of specific animals go together with large cortical areas. The whiskers of cats, for example, which are highly sensitive to touch, take up a large part of the cat's sensory cortex. Likewise, pigs have a large cortical area for smell, and sheep and goats have a large cortex for the lips.

Without understanding how Kohonen networks work, however, we remain unclear about how these cortical maps come about. It was thought for a long time that these maps are hardwired into the brain— that is, genetically programmed and "distorted" in a way that provides the most computational space for processing important information. However, as we have already seen in chapter 2, the human genome is not sufficiently large to carry all the information needed to wire the brain in this way.

Biological Example: The Auditory Cortex of the Bat
Biologists know that bats use ultrasound to orient themselves in the dark. They send out loud screams that are inaudible to human ears because of their high frequency but can be clearly heard by bats. The animals are able to perceive the temporal distance and difference in pitch (based on the Doppler effect) between the signal they send out and the signal they receive back. From the amplitude of the reflected signal they calculate the size of the reflecting object, and from the pitch of the signal they

derive its relative velocity. Detailed bat studies have shown that they can determine relative velocities (i.e., the velocities of objects in relation to their own speed) of as little as three centimeters per second. Given the speed of sound (three hundred meters per second), this implies that bats are able to detect changes in the pitch of an auditory signal of as little as 0.01 percent.

Human beings are also able to detect such small differences in auditory signals, but only in the frequency range of around 3000 Hz, the range of frequencies in the overtones of the human voice. At frequencies of 6000 Hz and above, differences in frequency can no longer be well detected. This is the reason, by the way, why the musical scale ends with notes having a frequency of about 4000 to 5000 Hz (Handel 1989).

The bat species *Pteronotus parnelli rubiginosus,* which has the discriminatory capabilities just described, sends out a tone of 61 kHz lasting for 30 milliseconds. It therefore has to process differences in pitch very accurately in the frequency range surrounding 61 kHz. According to experimental studies, these are the frequencies represented by more than half of all the animal's auditory neurons. The fine-grained analysis of sounds at the frequency band used for orientation is achieved by the highly distorted distribution of computational surface (i.e., cortex), which allocates by far the most hardware to sounds that have to be processed most accurately (cf. Ritter et al. 1991, Suga & Jen 1976).

The area of the bat's cortex devoted to special-frequency tone analysis corresponds to the cortical area for special visual analysis in humans. We know that one small area of the human retina processes information most precisely. We also know that a large part of the primary visual cortex is devoted to this small part of the retina, the *fovea.* When we look at an object, the visual signals from it fall onto the fovea. Because many cells carry out the analysis of signals from the fovea, we can see fixated objects quite sharply. In contrast, we perceive objects on the periphery of our visual field only vaguely, because relatively few neurons are recruited to analyze visual signals coming from that area of the retina.

In many other animal species, vision exhibits a similar area of sharpest sight (the fovea). The auditory sense, by contrast, has no such area (i.e., frequency band) of sharpest hearing, as we know from studies in dogs, cats, and monkeys. These species do not have a "preferred frequency," as it were, and, hence, do not need a larger number of neurons to code a special frequency band. In the auditory cortex, all audible frequencies are rather equally distributed. Like the cortical surface for touch sensation, the auditory cortex is a feature map, in that the pitch of the tone is coded topographically, with low tones coded more anteriorly and high tones more posteriorly (Merzenich et al. 1975). It just happens that no particular frequencies are especially represented by a larger number of neurons, as they are in the bat. We may conclude that in most mammals no particular frequency of sound is especially important for survival.

In bats, the situation is different. About half of all their auditory neurons are responsible for the analysis of tones in the narrow frequency band around 61 kHz (see figure 5.13). This makes sense, because the auditory input of the bat consists not of a more or less equally distributed mixture of all frequencies, but rather of a heterogeneous mixture of tones in which tones of about 61 kHz predominate.

By running computer simulations using Kohonen networks, Ritter and coworkers (1991) were able to show that a fovealike specialization of a cortical area can be produced by a skewed distribution of the input signals. In short, if input signals are distributed in a way similar to what the bat supposedly hears, a feature map remarkably like the cortical map experimentally found in real bats self-organizes. The simulation suggests, therefore, that because the bat hears particular tones very often, it forms special representations of those tones.

In the human brain, several neuroscience studies have demonstrated the existence of quite a large number of somatosensory, motor, retinotopic, and tonotopic maps (Killackey et al. 1995, Purves 1994, Sereno et al. 1995, Woolsley 1982). The structure and function of these maps is the subject of intensive neurobiological and neurocomputational research (cf. Schreiner 1995). There is no doubt that in human beings these maps are dynamic; that is, that they change when the input changes. (This phenomenon, called neuroplasticity, is discussed in detail in chapter 7.) The maplike form of representation has been clearly demonstrated for many areas of the cortex and is likely to be found in areas not yet studied. The principles that govern map formation have been investigated by using Kohonen networks; and, although the biological cortex is more complicated than a Kohonen network, the simulations show that only a

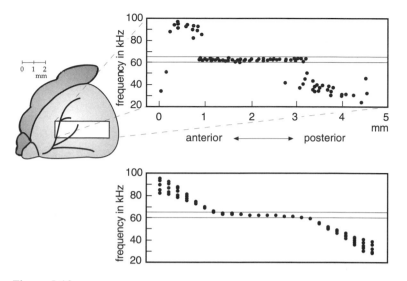

Figure 5.13
Schematic drawing of a bat's brain (left), looking at it from the side (after Suga & Jen 1976, Ritter et al. 1991). The area of the auditory cortex is drawn in white against the light-gray brain. The graph at the top shows the topographic distribution of frequency-coding neurons, with the x-axis giving the location in the anterior-posterior direction, and the y-axis giving the frequency of the neuron. One can see that about half the neurons code the small band around the "echo-navigation frequency" of the bat. The graph below is the result of a computer simulation using a Kohonen network with an output layer of 5 _× 25 neurons after 5,000 learning trials. The input consisted of soundlike patterns with an assumed frequency distribution similar to that of the bat. This input caused automatic formation of a map on which the most frequent input patterns are disproportionately well represented. In other words, the simulation suggests that the input heard by the bat causes its cortex to devote many more cells to frequencies around 61 kHz than to any other frequency.

few principles can capture basic neurocomputational capabilities of the cortex that would be hard to understand without such simulations. (See chapter 12 for further discussion of these general points.)

Networks of Maps: Modularity

In addition to discovering the maplike organization of representations, researchers using simulated neural networks have ascertained that networks employ the principle of *modularity.* Rueckl and colleagues

(1989) demonstrated that a network performs a given task more readily when the task is broken down into components, which are then processed by different parts of the network. Such a modular network architecture, as it turned out, needs fewer connections (and hence is computationally less intensive) and learns faster. In biological systems too, the principle of modularity is widely recognized. A large number of studies in cognitive neuroscience suggests that complex tasks involving language comprehension, attention, complex motor behavior, and visual perception are performed by modular systems (cf. Posner & Raichle 1994).

In real brains, it appears, information is processed by networks of networks. Within such a framework, modularity does not denote unconnected subsystems (as was proposed by Fodor in 1983) but, quite the contrary, the integrated actions of specialized subsystems. Many of these subsystems are either known to have or, at least, are likely to have a maplike structure. For example, in visual perception, information is preprocessed in the retina and the lateral geniculate corpus and is then fed to the primary visual cortex (V1), a retinotopic map. From there, information proceeds to other visual areas, which are designated V2, V3, V4, and V5. The color map, V4, is responsible for color vision. If you pay special attention to the colors of a scene, the neurons in this map work harder than usual (cf. experiments on selective attention described in chapter 7). If V4 is damaged by a stroke or a tumor, the visual world will lose color and turn black and white (cf. Zeki 1993).

The motion map (V5, also called MT) is responsible for perception of motion. When you concentrate on movement in a scene, the neurons in MT work harder than they ordinarily do. If MT is damaged, you no longer see seamless motion but, instead, perceive sequences of still images.

Information about the location of perceived objects in space is processed in yet other cortical areas (figure 5.14). Studies in the monkey have shown that visual input proceeds along two separate pathways, one of which calculates *where* it is, while the other analyzes *what* the input is. The "what-pathway" proceeds from the above-mentioned primary and secondary visual areas to the temporal lobe, whereas the "where-pathway" proceeds to the parietal lobe.

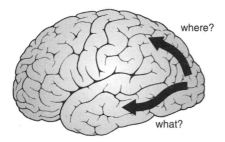

Figure 5.14.
Example of interconnected cortical modules: The "What-pathway" and the "Where-pathway" (cf. Ungerleider & Mishkin 1982).

In sum, the research indicates that information is processed within the cortex by closely cooperating modules. It is therefore *not* the case, as is sometimes assumed, that the entire cortex, or even the entire brain, is a single homogeneous neural network. Instead, it is made up of maplike networks that are highly interconnected and work together.

The current discussion about modularity started by Fodor in 1983 is not, therefore, about whether or not the brain has a modular organization (it certainly does) but rather about the degree to which it is modular and how certain modules work together (cf. Kosslyn & König 1992).

Recap

More than 90 percent of the human cortex displays a remarkably homogeneous structure consisting of six horizontal layers. In addition, neurons are functionally coupled in the vertical direction and thereby form columns. The neurons within a column are mutually excitatory and stimulate the neurons in adjacent columns to some extent, whereas they inhibit more distant neurons.

In Kohonen networks, these principles of cortical wiring and functioning are built into the model. Because of these principles, such networks display the ability to form maplike representations of structured input patterns. The maps of the most important input features form spontaneously, which is why Kohonen networks are also called *self-organizing feature maps*. In such maps, input patterns are ordered according to their similarity and frequency.

For decades, it has been known that the human cortex contains a number of maplike representations of, for example, the body surface, which is represented in accordance with the principles of similarity and frequency; for example, the representation of the hand is adjacent to the representation of the arm, which in turn borders on the representation of the shoulder (principle of similarity). The lips and the hands are represented by a comparatively larger cortical area than, for example, the back, because lips and hands receive many more highly relevant sensory inputs (principle of frequency).

A cortical map does not do its job of information processing by itself but works together with other maps. A map is a module in a larger ensemble of modules that, computer simulations have demonstrated, process information more efficiently than unitary networks.

The framework of self-organizing feature-map models sheds new light on the existence of cortical maps. Whereas earlier we might have thought that the maps exist (and are prewired) to process information effectively, the simulations turn this view upside down. Because some parts of the body provide a great deal of information to the cortex, as time goes by they are represented, through self-organization, by larger and larger feature maps. In chapter 7 we provide a more detailed discussion of the dynamic processes that lead to these changes.

6

Hidden Layers

When we touch a hot surface, we pull back our hand without giving it much thought. The action occurs by reflex, which presupposes neurons that report heat and are linked to neurons that activate muscles. The most widely known reflex is probably the knee jerk reaction. If you hit the tendon just below the patella, the lower leg performs an involuntary kick. This reflex requires just two types of neurons: The input is provided by tension-sensor neurons within the muscles that extend the leg, which send their output directly to neurons that activate the thigh muscles.

In simple organisms such as the sea anemone the input, processing, and output of information is all done by a single layer of neurons. These neurons fire whenever there is any significant stimulation at the surface of the organism, which causes muscle fibers to contract. In slightly more complex organisms, such as some jellyfish, the tasks are distributed to two types of neurons, sensory and motor neurons (figure 6.1). Such reflex arcs are made up of pairs of neurons transmit and process information rapidly and reliably, which is why they can be found in almost all nervous systems—including the human nervous system, as the knee jerk reflex shows.

The evolution of additional layers *between* the input and output layers was of great importance for the development of nervous systems, especially for those that later formed the ability to represent internally features of the external world. For reasons clarified by research on neuralnetworks, nervous systems with such additional layers (sometimes called *hidden layers*) can accomplish tasks that are beyond the reach of

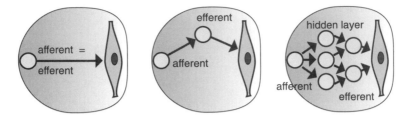

Figure 6.1
Nervous systems with a single neuron (left), an input and an output neuron (center), and a sensory and a motor neuron, as well as a layer of neurons between input and output (right). In the simplest of nervous systems, there is no distinction between fibers coming from the outside world (input, afference) and fibers that control responses (output, efference). Layers of neurons between the input and the output neurons appear to make the nervous system unnecessarily complicated. However, they are essential in many ways, as discussed in this chapter.

two-layer networks.[1] What is computationally important about hidden layers is best illustrated with a few examples.

The Exclusive-Or

The most widely known example of a problem that cannot be solved by a two-layer network is the problem of the *exclusive-or,* often called the *XOR problem.* Suppose you are hungry, go to a somewhat special restaurant, and find two items on the menu: sauerkraut and vanilla ice cream. Because you are really hungry, you definitely want something to eat; you may want either sauerkraut or vanilla ice cream but not both in one dish. The situation can be represented in a so-called truth table invented by the philosopher Ludwig Wittgenstein (table 6.1): 1 denotes the presence of an item or behavior; 0 denotes its absence.

The table defines the truth function of the exclusive-or, which can be represented by inactive and active neurons just as well as by the numbers 0 and 1 (figure 6.2). (As we saw in preceding chapters, the numbers 1

---

1. *A note on terminology.* Because in network simulations, the layers between input and output are not in contact with the "external world," and hence are "hidden" from it, they have come to be called *hidden layers.* As a matter of fact, there is nothing hidden about them, which may be why in German, for example, they are simply called *Zwischenschichten* (between layers).

Table 6.1
What do you want to eat? Truth table of the exclusive-or (XOR)

Sauerkraut	Ice cream	To eat
0	0	0
1	0	1
0	1	1
1	1	0

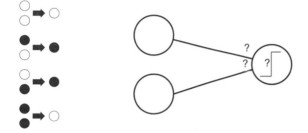

Figure 6.2
Function of the exclusive-or, as represented by the relation of ordered pairs of numbers (the arguments of the function) and the results (left), and as represented by an input-output mapping of the activity of two input neurons on one output neuron (center). The drawing at the right represents a two-layer network. How must the synaptic weights be set in order for the network to accomplish the task?

and 0 can symbolize an active and an inactive neuron, respectively.) How then would a small network represent this function?

By the end of the 1960s Marvin Minsky and Seymour Papert (1969) had demonstrated that it was impossible for a two-layer network to solve this problem. No combination of input vectors and synaptic weights (in mathematical terms, no linear combination), together with a suitable activation threshold of the output neuron, can represent the desired function. However, if a third ("hidden") layer of neurons is added between input and output—a layer that in this case can consist of a single neuron—the network can perform the XOR function. Why is this so?

The neuron of the hidden layer directly represents neither the input nor the output. Rather, it represents a generalization of the input: namely, sauerkraut *and* vanilla ice cream. Whenever this layer is activated the output neuron is inhibited and can no longer be activated by both inputs. It is important to note that neurons in hidden layers are capable of such generalizations and therefore can come up with more appropriate and more relevant representations of the external world than neurons that are directly connected to that world. In biological brains, this makes sense. The environment is full of complex, nonlinear combinations of features; the XOR problem is just the simplest case. Such cases certainly exists in nature, as we can easily see by thinking about the following examples: (1) An organism may eat all small or all red berries in an area except those that are red and small; (2) The alpha male of a group may respond with aggression when meeting the beta or the gamma male but not when meeting both.

Neural networks with hidden layers play a major role in current network simulation research, because they can represent many complex input-output relations (as the simple three-layer network in figure 6.3 demonstrates). The example discussed in the following section further illustrates the computational abilities of networks with hidden layers. It

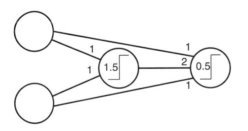

Figure 6.3
Three-layer network with synaptic weights and activation thresholds that can perform the function of the exclusive-or. The input layer consists of two neurons, the hidden layer and the output layer each have only one neuron. Let us calculate how the network works. If both neurons on the left are quiet, nothing happens. If either the upper or the lower neuron on the left are active, it sends out a 1 (one), which is enough to activate (via the synaptic weight of 1) the output neuron, which has a threshold of 0.5. The neuron of the hidden layer is not active in this case, since its threshold is 1.5. If both input neurons are active, the hidden layer neuron becomes active, which (because its connection weight is −2) strongly inhibits the output neuron, practically turning it off. The net effect is that if both input neurons are active, the output neuron is not.

turns out that such networks are capable of performing abstractions and forming prototypes.

Abstraction and Type Formation

Let's look first at a network designed to model the behavior of Little Red Riding Hood (cf. Jones & Hoskins 1987). As Little Red Riding Hood (LRRH) strolls through the forest, she may encounter one of three distinct beings.

LRRH must learn to run away, scream, and look for the woodcutter when she detects a being with big ears, big eyes, and big teeth (the wolf). She must learn to approach, kiss on the cheek, and offer food to beings that are kindly, wrinkled, and that have big eyes (grandma). And she must learn to approach, offer food to, and flirt with beings that are handsome, kindly, and have big ears (the woodcutter). (Jones & Hoskins 1987:156)

A two-layer network can learn to perform these functions. During training, input patterns (LRRH's perceptions of the features of the characters) are presented to the input layer, and the desired output patterns (the desired behaviors of LRRH) are compared with the actual output of the network. Then the learning rule as described in chapter 3 (cf. figure 3.4) is applied. The difference between the actual and the desired output is calculated, and each synaptic weight is either decreased or increased in order to achieve an output closer to the desired output. The size of the modification in each trial is controlled by the learning constant. After many trials, the learning rule results in a trained network able to produce the correct mapping of the input patterns to the output patterns. The network has learned the behavior of Little Red Riding Hood.

The behavior of LRRH may also be simulated by a three-layer network (figure 6.4). If the number of the neurons in the hidden layer is small, something important happens: These neurons tune their synaptic weights in a way that generalizes over the input patterns to form representations of clusters of these patterns that are relevant to a certain output. This clustering of input patterns to output-relevant features occurs more often when there are few neurons in the hidden layer. If that layer contains only three neurons, then these three neurons come to represent "wolf," "grandma," and "woodcutter" during the process of training. This happens spontaneously. Of course, the types *wolf, grandma,* and *woodcutter*

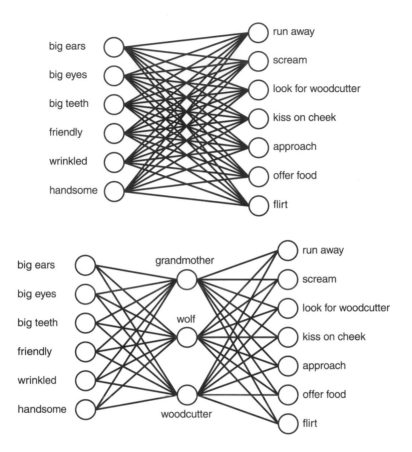

Figure 6.4
At the top, a two-layer network that implements the "functions" of Little Red Riding Hood. The three-layer network implements the same functions but, in addition, forms generalizations and needs fewer connections (after Jones & Hoskins 1987).

have been present (implicitly) in the input patterns from the beginning, as a concatenation of input features. After training, however, the hidden layer contains single neurons that map these specific clusters of features and thereby represent the outside world quite economically.

Economy is important to biological systems, as the maintenance of neurons and their connecting fibers consume valuable resources. As shown above, the functions of LRRH can be learned by a two-layer network, but such a network does not spontaneously generate neurons that represent anything general. In a two-layer network, there are input patterns (i.e., single events) but no notion that there is something "behind" these events, such as the wolf or the grandma. Moreover, whereas the number of neurons in the three-layer model is larger than in the two-layer model, the number of connections is actually smaller. Networks with more than two layers can therefore be more economical and hence, more effective, than two-layer networks.

The example demonstrates that neural networks with more than two layers, like Kohonen networks (with their special internal connections), can produce generalizations and form ideal types (or categories). The number of neurons in the hidden layer is obviously crucial for this process. If there are too many neurons in the layer, generalization may not develop; nor can they occur if there are too few neurons there.

Training an LRRH network with only two neurons in the hidden layer could produce an approach neuron and an avoidance neuron, thereby further clustering input and output. Such a highly general clustering, however, would no longer lead to a distinction between approaching grandma and approaching the woodcutter. In sum, a network with fewer than three neurons in the hidden layer could not capture the necessary distinctions and would produce a somewhat degraded output.

If there are more than three neurons in the hidden layer, the network can do its job of recognizing individual features, but it does not generalize. Instead it forms something like a look-up table for each input pattern. Such a network can accomplish its purpose, but it is less economical and more prone to error. If, for example, the ability to generalize is challenged by a slightly different input pattern, the look-up network may no longer produce useful output, whereas the network that has formed general concepts relevant to behavior may still work. To put it briefly, a three-layer network with the right-sized hidden layer will do its job most effectively (by generalization) and economically (by conserving connections) (cf. Crick 1989).

In sum, when certain boundary conditions are met, general representations and prototypes with the general features of input patterns may be spontaneously produced by neural networks. This process is essential for understanding how gestalt processes can come about in networks and how general concepts can be formed. It is important to recognize that abstract representations are not learned by neural networks as such (for example, by programming rules into the network) but are spontaneously produced whenever ordered input-output mappings are used for training.

Learning by the Feedback of Errors

In fact, a three-layer network cannot be trained by the delta rule discussed in chapter 3. Why not? The neural networks described are trained by the comparison of the actual output with the desired output, then multiplying the difference by a small number (the learning constant) and changing the weights by a tiny bit in the right direction. This can be done easily and unambiguously in two-layer networks, because it is clear which synapses have to be changed to what degree. In three-layer networks, however, there are two layers of synapses. Changes would need to be introduced in both synaptic layers, but it would be by no means obvious how these synapses should change. For this reason, the delta rule cannot be used to train three-layer networks.

The problem of training networks with more than two layers was solved in the 1980s by the invention of the so-called *backpropagation algorithm*. This algorithm works by changing the synaptic weights of the connections between the hidden layer and the output layer first, and then by propagating the error further back through the network, in order to determine the correct changes of the weights between the hidden layer and the input layer. The algorithm can even be used for networks of more than three layers, where it also works its way backwards from the synapses of the output layer to the synapses between the input layer and the first hidden layer. A thorough elucidation of this algorithm can be found in Rumelhart et al. (1986); Jones and Hoskins (1987) also provide a nice introduction to it.

The backpropagation algorithm has been criticized because it requires complicated mathematical calculations that are unlikely to be performed in real brains and so is not considered biologically plausible. However, as we saw in chapter 3, we can imagine examples demonstrating the value of the backprop-algorithm (as it is often abbreviated)—for example, the shape-from-shading problem. Furthermore, in network simulations biological plausibility is never the only relevant consideration. In fact, biological details may impair the simplicity and clarity of a model whose main purpose is to demonstrate principles of function and lead to new and often counterintuitive insights about such principles. The proof is not in the biological details but in the "pudding" of the computational insights. We should also note that researchers have devised learning algorithms other than the backpropagation of errors; some of these are biologically more plausible and, at the same time, achieve similar results.

Hidden Layers in the Brain

Within the past ten years, computer simulations of networks have demonstrated that neurons in hidden layers can generalize and form prototypes. In biological networks, we might expect hidden layers to perform the same, highly adaptive functions. And, in fact, during the course of the brain's evolution hidden layers have, to a great extent, arisen between the input and output layers. Such neurons are found in the *ganglia* (small convolutions of neurons and connecting tissue) of lower animals and in the brains of higher animals. In fact, in the terms of our discussion, a brain is, for the most part, nothing but a complex structure of nested hidden layers—the human brain being the most extreme example of this structure.

The optic nerve, our most important input channel, carries about two million fibers. All together, the sensory input fibers number in the order of magnitude of 10^7. On the output side, there are between two and three million fibers of the primary motor neurons traveling down the spinal cord to carry out the motor behavior that results from complex processing in the brain. In addition, there are the motor fibers of the cranial and sympathetic nerves as well as parasympathetic fibers to the internal organs controlling internal secretion, digestion, heart rate, and so on. Taken together, the number of these output fibers is in the same order of magnitude as the inputs.

Compared to the total of neurons in the cortex and all their connections, however, these numbers are small. If we assume that there are 10^{10} neurons in each hemisphere, then only 0.1 percent of these neurons receive direct input or send direct output (cf. Nauta & Feirtag). In other words, 99.9 percent of all cortical neurons receive their input and send their output to other cortical neurons. In short, our brains' neurons are engaged mainly with each other and to only a small degree with other parts of the body or the external world. Thus, in order to respond competently to well-known as well as novel inputs, our brains must be concerned to a very great extent with developing general structures and prototypes from the many input patterns it receives.

What do we know about these connections within the brain? Are there general principles of connection?

Cortico-Cortical Connections

We have already noticed the almost ubiquitously uniform structure of the neocortex and discussed the principles governing the fine-grained internal structure of single cortical areas. Next, we examine the connections between and among these cortical areas.

In chapter 5 we discussed the modular organization of the brain. Neuroscientists used to assume that information is processed by individual modules, which then feed the results to other modules. In this view, information is processed within a module, then passed on to be further processed in another (presumably higher-level) module. If this view were correct, we would expect to find more neuronal fibers within cortical areas than fibers connecting different areas. However, quite the opposite is the case. The majority of the axons of cortical pyramidal cells do not travel to adjacent cells but to cells in different areas. This is a striking observation!

The way in which different cortical areas are connected to each other is also remarkably uniform. Consider two cortical areas, A and B, that are processing information coming in from a sensory organ; let B be closer to the sensory input than A. B may therefore be called the *lower* area and A called the *higher* area, as regards the level of abstraction at which they supposedly operate and form representations (see figure 6.5). The connections between these two areas can then be described as follows:

• If area B sends axons to area A, then it also receives axons from this area (principle of reciprocal connections).
• Axons of pyramidal cells in layers II and III of the lower area (B) end in layer IV of the higher area A. This layer is generally considered the

Lower cortical area B   Higher cortical area A

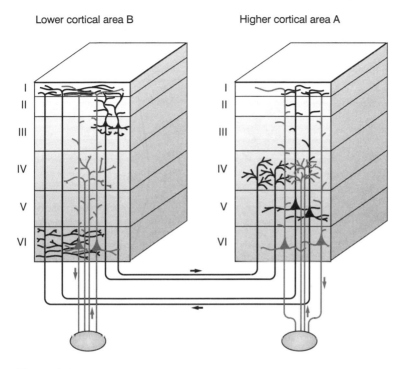

Figure 6.5
Origin and projection sites of cortico-cortical fibers within the different layers of
the cortex (after Mumford 1992:244).

input layer of the cortex because input from the sense organs (via the
thalamus), as well as input from other cortical areas, ends up in layer IV
of the higher area.
• The higher area sends fibers, which are the axons of pyramidal cells of
layer V, to the lower area; these fibers end in layers I and VI of area B.
Note too that the output fibers from the cortex to the thalamus originate
in pyramidal cells in layer V, which is therefore generally considered the
output layer of the cortex to lower—cortical as well as subcortical—areas
(cf. Mumford 1992).

There is no doubt that there must be fibers from lower to higher areas
of the cortex to ensure that information is transmitted from sensory input
areas farther up the processing stream. There is mounting evidence,
however, that downstream fibers (carrying information top-down) are
just as necessary as these upstream fibers delivering bottom-up informa-

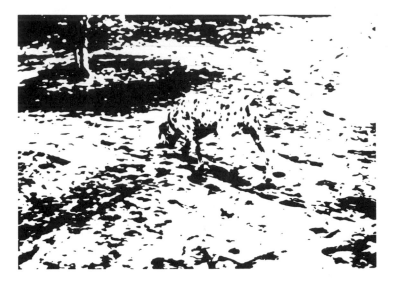

Figure 6.6
Example of top-down processes in perception. We perceive a dog, not so much because there is an image of a dog on our retina, but because the spots on our retina have undergone a process of interpretation by higher-level cortical areas. The most likely proposal to disambiguate the spots was thereby chosen and actually synthesized. This is why we actually *see* a dog, not merely spots that we interpret as dog (Mumford 1992:244, Rock 1984).

tion. We can best explain this supposition by looking at an example from perception.

If we use high-level concepts to analyze the picture, we perceive the many spots in figure 6.6 as a Dalmatian dog sniffing out a little wall on the ground around a tree. Our analysis of the visual input therefore consists to a large extent of a synthesis that uses stored information. The Dalmatian dog comes into existence by a process of disambiguation of a vague input pattern, because we already have a high-level concept of a certain type of dog.

The example shows that (1) by mere analysis of the input, even if highly sophisticated, the semantic content "dog" could hardly ever be generated. It takes synthetic processes using stored information to do this. (2) What we perceive is a *dog,* though it may take us a while. From a subjective point of view, it is wrong to describe the process by saying that we first perceive a few spots and then interpret them as a dog. <u>When we say that</u> <u>*we* interpret the spots, we are speaking incorrectly; it is not us, but rather</u> <u>a neural system that does the interpretation for us.</u> <u>We cannot help but</u> <u>perceive a dog, so the dog is not the result of a willful act but of a passive</u> <u>synthesis performed by neural systems within our brains</u> (cf. v. Campenhausen 1993, Gregory 1986, Gregory & Gombrich 1973).

Analysis and Synthesis

Gestalt psychology is full of examples (e.g., figure 6.7) demonstrating clearly that perceptual processes consist of neither pure analysis nor pure synthesis (cf. Metzger 1975) but, rather, of an interactive process involving bottom-up as well as top-down mechanisms.

Ping-Pong Style Information Processing

In contrast to the standard hypothesis that information is processed in one area and then fed to another one, Mumford (1992) suggests that the bulk of cortical information processing is carried out through the interaction of two reciprocally connected areas working at different levels. <u>In</u> <u>this view, the higher area uses stored templates to synthesize the most</u> <u>likely pattern to match the one coming up from the lower level and sends</u> <u>the pattern down to the lower level. In the lower area, the input pattern</u> <u>and the synthesized input from the higher area (this area's proposal for</u> <u>disambiguation of the input) are compared. This process either shows a</u>

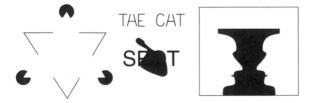

Figure 6.7
Examples of gestalt-generating processes in visual perception. To the left, we see a large white triangle, although there are only lines and circles with small cut-out sections. In the center, we can read *the cat* as well as *spot;* to the right, we can only see one interpretation—a vase or two faces—at any one time. Such processes of gestalt formation can also be observed in other sense modalities (cf. Kilgard & Merzenich 1995).

good match between input from "below" and synthesized interpretation from "above"—in which case the process comes to an end and the system reaches a stable state—or, if there is not a good match (i.e., the matching process leaves a large amount of information unexplained), the residual differences are fed back to the higher area. Using this new input, the higher area comes up with a new interpretation, and the process starts over again. Another template is used to synthesize another pattern, which is sent "down" for matching. The process lasts until a suitable interpretation is found.

This process of analysis by synthesis through close cooperation between higher and lower cortical areas serves to identify objects, or concepts (on a higher level), with data on a lower level.

After a few turns, either a good fit is found and the residual is acceptably small or the hypothesis is rejected and area A [the higher area] turns to other previously suppressed hypotheses. In the ultimate stable state, the deep pyramidals [of the higher area] would send a signal that perfectly predicts what each lower area is sensing, up to expected levels of noise, and the superficial pyramidals wouldn't fire at all. (Mumford 1992:247)

In this view, it is necessary for lower and higher cortical areas to work together to accomplish their job (figure 6.8). It is important to note that this principle appears to be applicable to a large number of different higher mental functions. (As we noted earlier, the principal circuitry of the cortex is strikingly uniform, regardless of the location and function of the area.) We will discuss additional examples of such higher-level functions in chapters 9 through 12.

Autism

To close this chapter, I discuss a network model of a childhood psychiatric disorder, autism. The concept of hidden layers and their functional characteristics, as highlighted by network simulations, provides a framework for understanding certain features of this syndrome.

Autism is a severe mental disorder (cf. Frith 1992). Children with the syndrome are impaired with respect to social contact, gesture, and facial expression. They also suffer from perseverations (constant repetitions of an action or utterance) and from inability to shift the attention away from single facts or events. These social and cognitive deficits were

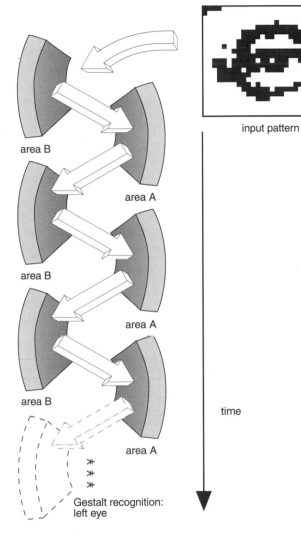

input pattern

area B

area A

area B

area A

area B

time

area A

※ ※ ※
Gestalt recognition:
left eye

Figure 6.8
Interaction between a "higher" and a "lower" cortical area during information processing. Input patterns are analyzed in ping-pong style, that is, by syntheses in the higher area that are fed back down to a lower area, where they are matched with the input. After a few turns, the two areas have worked out between them an interpretation that makes sense, that is, that fits the input.

illustrated in the movie *Rainman,* in which Dustin Hoffman plays an autistic grown-up who memorizes parts of the telephone book. Such *idiot savant* capabilities are displayed by quite a few autistic people. They may involve language (e.g., ceaseless repetitions of difficult words) or the memorization of simple spatiotemporal or symbolic patterns (telephone numbers, pictures drawn from memory, meaningless strings of words, etc.).

Because of its severity, it has long been thought that autism must have an organic cause; that is, that it results from some sort of brain pathology. Psychiatric researchers have therefore investigated the brains of deceased autistic patients with great care. They found decreased numbers of neurons in some brain areas, though not, to their surprise, in areas of the brain usually involved in learning and memory—the hippocampus, the amygdala, and the entorhinal cortex. Instead, they found an *increased* number of neurons in these areas. Because this finding could not be explained or related to the features of the disorder in any meaningful way, it was put aside as one of the curiosities of science.

Such curiosities arise whenever there is no comprehensive theoretical framework within which data can be understood. For example, for millennia people observed that the sun rises every morning in the East and disappears every evening in the West. But how does it get back to the East? Eventually, a good theory was developed that not only explains the path of the sun but also a large number of other phenomena that, for this reason, are no longer curiosities. The Copernican universe and Darwinian evolution are both good examples of ideas that integrated a great many otherwise unrelated or inexplicable data into a unifying common framework.

Similarly, contemporary neuroscience has provided a framework in which many different and otherwise unrelated data fall into place like the pieces of a large jigsaw puzzle. For example, Ira Cohen's (1994) proposed model of autism relates three otherwise inexplicable findings and observations: (1) the increased number of neurons in some memory-related cortical and subcortical brain sites; (2) the decreased capability for abstract thinking; and (3) the astonishing memory abilities of some autistic people. Within Cohen's neural network model of autism, these three features fall nicely into place.

Brains as Engines for the Estimation of Functions

As mentioned in the discussion of the Little Red Riding Hood network, there is a relationship between the number of neurons in hidden layers and the tendency of the network to come up with general, abstract representations. Let us focus a bit more on this relationship. Whenever an organism learns something, we can understand the process in terms of the estimation procedure of either the true value of a variable or the true relationship between two (or more) variables (cf. chapter 4). In contrast to programming, in which a rule or a function is put directly into the computer, learning works by example, that is, by observation of multiple instances of the function. In other words, during the process of learning, data points are acquired and the function underlying the data points is guessed from these points. We can assume no additional knowledge about the function to be approached.

For example, many organisms have to learn how much they need to eat in a given nutritional environment. For some foods, the relationship between the amount of food consumed and the optimum needed may be quite simple, in that the more the organism consumes, the better it fares. The relation may be different with other foodstuffs, however; there may be optimal quantities of certain foods or an even more complex relationship between the intake of a given food and, for example, the health of the organism. In any event, the organism must estimate this relation from individual experiences of eating a certain amount of such-and-such food—that is, from a limited number of data points. Biological systems, it follows, are confronted with the general task of approximating a function from some number of data points in an optimal way, making the best possible use of the limited available data.

When performing such estimates, it is important to take the golden mean between the function that is maximally descriptive of the particular data and the one that is most generalizable to many similar events. Notice that these two aspects are not identical and that the latter is at least as important as the former. When you learn, you want not merely to store what has happened but also to predict the future. You want to know the location of previously unknown data points in advance, which is why you do not want to store the raw data—a waste of resources anyway—but the general function that predicts all possible data. (See figure 6.9.)

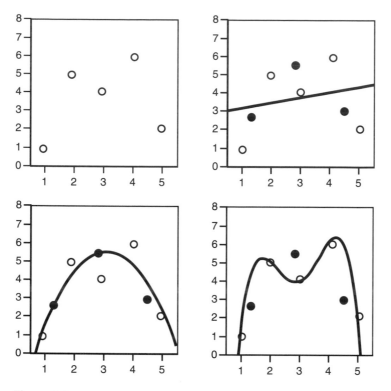

Figure 6.9
The problem of finding the true function describing the relation between two variables. The organism has five experiences (the five data points depicted as open circles in the upper left diagram) and needs to find the function that best predicts new experiences (represented by three black data points at the upper right). The upper right diagram and the two at the bottom display three possible solutions to this problem (i.e., three predictions of future experiences). In mathematical terms, this problem can be captured as follows: Every set of n data points can be completely characterized by a polynomial of the order n ™ 1. For example, *two* points are fully characterized by a straight line ($y = ax^1 + b$), three points are completely described by a parabola ($y = ax^2 + bx^1 + c$), and so on. If there is enough processing power (enough neurons in a network), any data set can be completely described by a function (polynomial). However, these functions may to be rather complicated, especially if the data set does not represent a simple mathematical function. If we assume that biological real world data are pretty noisy (cf. chapter 7)—because the organism, unlike the scientist, does not perform systematic measurements but rather gathers nonsystematic experiences—then it may be disadvantageous to fit the function too closely to the data. A too-close fit, therefore, not only requires more computational resources but also is not the best representation of the (noisy) data—that is, does not predict new experiences

Within this framework, generalization is nothing but an incomplete, approximative description of a data set. It requires only the limited computational resources of a system that is simply not capable of storing every single data point or of approximating every data point by a highly complex polynomial. To put it simply, a limited system does not get lost in large data sets but, rather, extracts the general features of the set.

This discussion provides a clue to the problem of why having too many neurons can be disadvantageous and may result in pathology. In the case of autistic people, difficulties in generalizing, as well as the ability to memorize a great many rote facts, can easily be related to the single fact that there are too many neurons in their memory-related brain structures. The excess of neurons both prevents generalization and allows for the storage of large amounts of data. In fact, these two features of the autistic syndrome appear to be just two sides of the same coin.

It should be noted that this model of autistic symptoms has therapeutic consequences, as pointed out by Cohen:

That is, behavior therapy may work, first, by focusing the child's attention on a larger and more varied data set than the child is used to attending. Then, through constant repetition of these many different patterns along with immediate feedback, higher-order recognition would emerge by weakening previously established, idiosyncratic connections that do not "pay off" and strengthening those that do. (Cohen 1994:18)

well. The figure displays this in a simplified way. At the top right, a linear relation is supposed to underlie the data. Such a relation is computationally not very intensive. At the lower right, a computationally intensive polynomial relation of the fourth order is supposed to underlie the data and in fact describes the data completely. At the lower left, the data set is approximated by a polynomial of second order (a rather simple curvilinear relation). The diagrams show how well the assumed relations predict the new data (black dots). It can be seen that neither the simple linear relation or the highly complex fourth-order polynomial predict future data very well; that is, as "models" they do not provide a good generalization of the data. (In a way, the first is too general, whereas the second is not general enough.) The second-order polynomial, in contrast, yields a good estimate of future data and therefore represents the most useful model (of intermediate complexity and computational intensity). It provides the best level of generality.

Recap

Neurons in hidden layers are capable of forming representations of the general features of inputs. It is obvious, therefore, that they play a major part in the formation of prototypes and abstract concepts from the fleeting experiences of mere instances and events. Such general representations of environmental features allow the organism to make highly adaptive predictions of new data and, hence, they are of great survival value. Therefore, over the course of evolution, organisms with increasingly complex nervous systems and an increasing number of hidden layers developed. These hidden layers were eventually integrated into a central nervous system. The brains of mammals are the most highly developed version of nervous systems containing these built-in hidden layers. In the human brain, for example, 99.9 percent of all neurons process input coming from other neurons within the brain, and likewise send virtually all their output to other neurons within the brain. Only a very small fraction of the processed information actually gets into or comes out of the brain.

Information processing in the cortex occurs by means of bottom-up processes from signals carrying low-level sensory information, as well as by top-down processes that transmit a gestalt (approximate generalization) of the input from information already in storage. Bottom-up processes and top-down processes happen simultaneously in different, but closely connected, cortical areas that work out among themselves an adaptive interpretation of the sensory input. Because the process is in principle interactive and involves information traveling back and forth between higher- and lower-level cortical areas, cognition has the well-known gestalt aspects.

The simulation of neural networks with hidden layers became feasible after new learning algorithms—most notably, the backpropagation algorithm—were worked out in the mid-1980s. The latter works by comparing the output produced by a given input to the desired output. The difference is then used to change the weights of the connections to bring the actual output a bit closer to the desired output. This comparison is reiterated for all layers of the network—backwards from the output layer to the hidden layer, and from the hidden layer to the input layer (or to other layers in between).

Neural networks with hidden layers are capable of providing solutions for problems that cannot, in principle, be solved by two-layer networks. When they have a suitable number of neurons in the hidden layer, these networks can spontaneously generalize and derive ideal types from input patterns. Networks with hidden layers, therefore, can go beyond the formation of simple relations between input and output patterns.

A network model of some features of the syndrome of autism provides the conceptual framework for integrating several otherwise unrelated and inexplicable features of the disorder: that is, the finding that autistic people have an abnormally high number of neurons in memory-related brain structures, the inability of these patients to form general concepts, and the phenomenon of astonishing idiot savant memory capabilities in many patients.

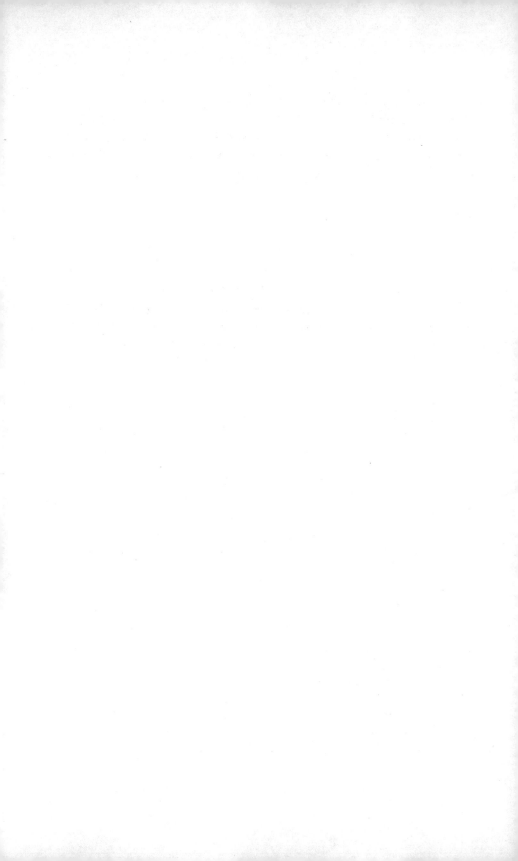

7

Neuroplasticity

The word *neuroplasticity* denotes the remarkable capacity of the brain to adapt continually to the demands placed on it by experience. Neuroplastic changes are not restricted to a certain stage of development but occur—rapidly at first and more slowly as the organism ages—throughout life. In this chapter, I explain the principle of neuroplasticity through examples that illustrate the uniquely adaptive and constantly self-optimizing structure of the cortex.

Artificial Ears

Scarcely more than ten years ago, many scientists held the view that the brain is basically complete and "done" at birth—notwithstanding some minor developmental processes—and then begins to die slowly, without much later change, let alone further growth.

Thanks to the work of California otologist Michael Merzenich and other researchers, we know that this rather pessimistic view of the brain is incorrect. Merzenich and his colleagues were treating patients suffering from hearing loss due to failure of the inner ear (the cochlea) by implanting an artificial inner ear. When they awakened from the operation, patients were highly irritated by a strange rumbling noise in their ears but reported no improvement in hearing. A year or so later, however, the majority of these patients could talk on the telephone; that is, they could hear well enough to understand spoken language without lipreading! While investigating the reasons for the delayed hearing gains, Merzenich discovered the highly general principle of neuroplasticity.

An artificial inner ear, or cochlea implant, works as follows: A microphone outside the body picks up sounds; these are fed to a signal processor, which dissects the signal into different frequency bands and transforms it into a stream of electrical impulses (cf. Moore 1995, Wilson et al. 1991). These impulses are transmitted through the skin to the implanted part of the system. The latter consists of a receiver and a device for distributing the electrical impulses to electrodes—small wires implanted into the patient's cochlea so that they stimulate the auditory nerve. In this way, the impulses reach the fibers that normally transmit signals from the cochlea to the brain.

When the auditory nerve is stimulated in this way, the person at first experiences nothing but unpleasant rumbling noises. What else should we expect? After all, the impulses coming from the "electrical inner ear" are completely different from the impulses sent by a biological inner ear. Whereas the natural cochlea stimulates each fiber of the auditory nerve with different information from a wide frequency band, the artificial cochlea provides—depending upon the type of device—only between four and twenty different signals. Therefore, after implantation of an artificial inner ear, neither the temporal nor the spatial order of the incoming signals is the same as before. This difference is what causes the patients' unpleasant experiences of rumbling chaos.

A year after the operation, however, the above-mentioned extraordinary changes in the patients' subjective experiences had occurred. Most of them were able to understand spoken language. This can only be possible if massive changes have taken place *in the brain*. Within about a year, the patients' brains had obviously learned to decode the messages they were receiving. They had adapted to the only thing the brain can use to drive reorganization—the spatiotemporal regularities in the incoming signal—even though they were completely different from signals received before the operation. The artificial inner ear had provided the brain with input of some regularity, which, it turns out, is enough for the cortex. As explained in chapter 5, the cortex works as a *rule-extraction machine* and produces maps of input according to the principles of frequency and similarity. The map in the primary auditory cortex, therefore, changes as input changes (cf. White et al. 1990).

Hearing, Too, Depends on Context

Understanding language, however, takes more than a tonotopic map of the perceived frequencies. The newly coded frequencies must be referred to the higher cortical areas that derive *phonemes* (the smallest sound units of spoken language) from the concatenation and sequence of frequencies. From these phonemes, they construct words and their meanings that, in the end, convey the messages of spoken language. The process is analogous to the operation of vision discussed in chapter 6 (figures 6.6 and 6.7). We do not hear sounds first, then extract phonemes, and then extract words from the phonemes. The analysis of the sounds is synthetic, in that auditory perception, like vision, happens within a meaningful context. This context guides top-down processes, which have a strong impact on what we in fact hear.

Like the previously described ambiguous figures that are disambiguated by appropriate context, auditory input becomes meaningful speech only by synthetic processes that put the input into context (figure 7.1).

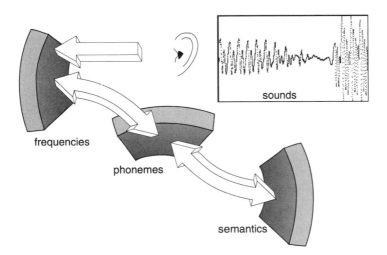

Figure 7.1
Auditory perception of spoken language. The spatiotemporal input patterns are processed through cortical areas specialized to extract the regularities of different abstraction levels. The cortical areas do this task in concert, as, for example, the higher-level semantic analysis influences lower-level phonetic analysis. During perception, information flows bottom-up as well as top-down. Hence, contextually generated expectations can influence what we hear.

There is no clear-cut relation between the acoustic input signal and the perceived speech, and single words or syllables do not correspond neatly to single acoustic signals (cf. Handel 1989:159). In brief, understanding auditory input is always at the same time both an analytic and a synthetic process.

This can be demonstrated experimentally by replacing parts of an acoustic signal with a brief burst of noise (e.g., the sound *sh-*, represented here by *). Depending on the context, this noise is perceived as different characters. For example, in "he took the spoon and ate the *oup," the noise is heard as an *s*, whereas in "come and sit with me at the *able," it is perceived as a *t*. Note that we do not hear the *sh-* first and then reinterpret it as something else. Instead, the process of hearing is concurrent with interpreting the input according to context and thereby fitting everything together.

If artificial input patterns that do not make sense are produced, perception runs into trouble. For example, when we speak we produce and understand about ten phonemes per second. By digitally manipulating the sound of speech, we can accelerate it without increasing the frequencies of the sounds and thereby producing higher pitch (thus avoiding the Chipmunks effect produced by playing an LP recording at forty-five instead of thirty-three rounds per minute (rpm). When researchers manipulated speech in this way, they found that we can understand language even when it is two or three times faster than normal. This finding implies that humans are able to decode sequences of sounds as short as thirty to fifty milliseconds (Bregman 1994:533). As we will see later, however, some people have trouble understanding such rapid sound signals.

In addition to the work with cochlear implants, the experiments demonstrating our ability to comprehend speech that is two or three times faster than normal suggest that auditory input is not *first* analyzed and *then* interpreted—this would take too long. Instead it is simultaneously processed at analytic and synthetic levels. Perception is thus much more than just passively forming an image of reality (cf. Gregory 1986 Gregory & Gombrich 1973).

Rewiring Maps

When implanting an artificial cochlea results in a regained ability to understand spoken language, we can be sure that the brain's primary-frequency map has been rewired. Such rewiring is driven by the new input patterns, but it must also comply with the structure of the maps to which the projections travel. In other words, the rewired map must be correctly connected to higher-level maps, which is only possible if the rewiring occurs with respect to these higher-level maps. The information needed to do so is guaranteed by the fact that the higher-level maps have dense projections to the lower-level maps.

The example of cochlea-implant patients thus clarifies what happens when input patterns are repeatedly presented to the cortex: New maps, whose structure is influenced by the input patterns as well as by higher-level maps, form.

Animal Studies on Neuroplasticity

A large number of animal studies have provided a detailed picture of how neurobiological processes and changes bring about neuroplasticity. For example, when monkeys are trained to discriminate between two slightly different tones, increases in the size of the area of their frequency map that codes for the frequency range of the tones (area A1) parallel the number of times the animal performs the task (Allard et al. 1991, Jenkins et al. 1990, Merzenich et al. 1983, Recanzone et al. 1993). In other words, as the animals learn to respond to a certain frequency range, the cortical area carrying out the computations increases in size. With training, the cortical representations of perceived frequencies change so that representations of frequencies important for task performance occupy larger areas. Thus an increased resolution of input signals is 'achieved; that is, the animal can discriminate more accurately between input signals that differ only slightly (Merzenich & Sameshima 1993).

A similar study was carried out on the sense of touch (cf. Jenkins et al. 1990). Training monkeys to discriminate different vibration frequencies with the tips of their index, middle, and ring fingers was found to increase the size of the cortical area representing the fingertips (figure 7.2). The study revealed that training not only influences the processing of spatial patterns (as in the case in the Braille-learning example discussed in chapter 1), but also affects temporal patterns (sounds and vibrations), which are processed more accurately after training (Merzenich 1996). At

sensory cortex before stimulation

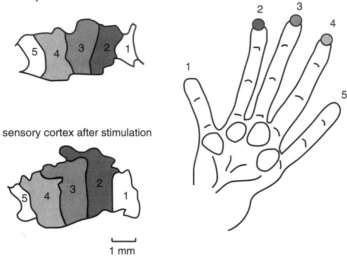

sensory cortex after stimulation

1 mm

Figure 7.2
The cortical areas that represent the tips of the index finger, middle finger, and ring finger. Areas are selectively increased in size when they are used. (Top left) The cortical areas that process sensations of touch from the tips of all five fingers before selective training of fingers 2, 3, and 4; (bottom left) the cortical areas after training. The drawing on the right shows the hand of the monkey and the areas that were selectively trained. The size of the cortical representations of the fingertips of fingers 2, 3, and 4 had clearly increased (modified from Jenkins et al. 1990).

the end of this chapter, I discuss a therapeutic application of these neurobiological findings.

It should be noted that the studies described above detected a large amount of variability of cortical representations in different animals. Even the seemingly low-level sensorium of the body surface is dependent upon the experiences of individual animals and is therefore differently represented in the cortex. For example, Recanzone and colleagues found individual differences in their vibration-frequency discrimination studies of the somatosensory cortex (Recanzone et al. 1992a,b,c,d). Pons and colleagues (1991) further demonstrated that completely depriving certain parts of the cortex of stimulation could reduce the somatosensory representations in the monkey cortex by more than a centimeter.

The cortical maps for the various aspects of sensory input described so far are not static. They are highly dynamic. Even in adult organisms they adapt to the input. It is as if the input signals have to constantly compete for cortical information-processing space: The more frequent and the more important the input, the larger the area and, hence, the more computational surface is assigned to it. (Or, to put it another way, the more space the input takes for itself.)

The driving forces of such experience-dependent self-organization of cortical representations are the spatiotemporal regularities in the (sensory) input. In the cortex, each finger has its own small processing area, because each finger of the hand receives different sensory signals. These different signals result in the formation of clear borders between the areas representing each finger. When two fingers are surgically sewn together, their inputs become quite similar and, accordingly, the fields representing the fingers merge until there is no longer a clear border between the fields (Clark et al. 1988).

The opposite happens in cases of *syndactyly,* the most common congenital anomaly of the hand. In this defect, the fetal webbing between adjacent fingers persists at birth, so that the fingers are more or less completely attached to each other. One week after the fingers are surgically separated, borders between their cortical representations emerge (Mogliner et al. 1993).

Such cortical changes are restricted to new input. As the researchers training monkeys in tonal discrimination note, "Psychophysical changes are largely, if not exclusively restricted to the neighborhood of the frequency range at which the monkey is behaviorally trained" (Merzenich & Sameshima 1993:187). If training is shifted to two slightly different tones in a different frequency range, the ability to distinguish between the originally presented tones deteriorates in the direction of the naive (i.e., untrained) condition.

Importance of the Input

For neuroplastic changes to occur, input has to be important. Animal studies have clearly demonstrated that merely presenting input patterns is not enough. They have to be processed as well. Unimportant events do not cause cortical changes, even if they occur with the same frequency as important ones (Ahissar et al. 1992). <u>Training has an effect only when animals pay attention to the stimuli.</u> In the vibration-frequency discrimination experiment, for example, control animals were stimulated just as often as the trained animals; the only difference between the two groups was that the control animals were not rewarded with juice when they made a correct discrimination. Even though they received the same stimulation as the trained animals, there was no learning and no changes of cortical representations in the control animals.

Selective Attention

How can we explain the role of *selective attention*—paying attention to very specific aspects of the environment—in terms of neural networks? Doesn't the importance of the input, as well as the fact that the organism has to pay attention to it, point to nonmechanistic influences on learning (in addition to the mechanistic influences of frequency and similarity)? Do the experiments described point to a function of the mind within the network that cannot be explained in purely mechanistic neurobiological and neurocomputational terms? The answer to this question is no.

Imagine that you are standing in the middle of a fairground. The colorful hustle and bustle provides you with a variety of different visual sensations: Here is a carrousel, there air balloons, music is everywhere, the smell of roasted peanuts wafts through the air. You are in an ocean of colors, forms, movements, sounds, and smells—fireworks for the senses. You can concentrate on every single aspect of what is around you; and in doing so you will perceive all these aspects more vividly and clearly. As we have known for some years, paying attention to something activates the cortical areas that specialize in processing specific kinds of information.

An important study of the effects of such selective attention on the brain was published by Corbetta and coworkers in 1991. The authors pursued the question of whether attending to a specific feature of the environment has a measurable effect on brain functioning. They used the imaging technique of positron emission tomography (PET), which allows researchers to distinguish between active and comparatively less active brain areas without opening the skull. Normal subjects watched a computer screen displaying up to thirty objects of a certain color and form moving at a certain speed; each object was seen twice for four hundred milliseconds per presentation. There was a pause of two hundred milliseconds between presentations of the complex stimuli. In half of the trials, the hustle and bustle of forms, colors and movements on the screen was identical for the two presentations, whereas in the other half of the trials the stimuli were different with respect to one or more features.

To investigate what happens in the brain when we attend to specific aspects of our environment, Corbetta and his colleagues registered the brain activity by means of PET under the condition of rest, as well as under the condition of attending to all features and of attending to specific features. The stimuli themselves were identical. During the resting condition, subjects merely had to watch the stimuli. Under the condition of divided attention, subjects had to look for changes in any of the features. Under three conditions of selective attention, they had to notice changes in color, form, or movement (figure 7.3). To determine whether subjects paid attention as they were requested to, they had to make yes/no decisions about whether the stimuli were the same or different. The speed and accuracy of these behavioral measurements decisions were evaluated to ensure that subjects paid attention and performed the task the way they were supposed to.

Subjects made fewer errors with respect to a specific aspect of the stimulus when asked to pay attention to that particular aspect, as compared to paying attention to all aspects. Obviously, it is easier to detect

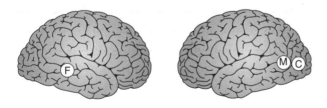

Figure 7.3
Summary of some of the results obtained by Corbetta and coworkers (1991). The drawing at the left depicts the right side of the brain; that and on the right, the left side. The circles indicate patches of activation (in subtraction images) caused by selectively attending to color (C), form (F), or motion (M).

differences when we focus our attention on a specific aspect in which the perceived items do in fact differ.

The PET scans provide images of the brain's activity at specific points in time. The human brain, however, is never at rest; it is highly active, even when you are doing nothing at all. In fact, although the brain's weighs only about 2 percent as much as the entire body, it consumes about 25 percent of the energy. Therefore, when the effects of a specific mental activity are under scrutiny, it is first necessary to take an image of the brain in the resting condition. Later, this image is subtracted from a second image taken under the condition of activation caused by performing a specific task. The subtraction image thus displays only the additional activity in the brain caused by the activity. Using this technique, researchers can compare any two conditions of activation. If, for example, words are shown to subjects who either have to read these words (condition 1) or find a second word associated with it (condition 2), then the subtraction of the image (condition 2 minus condition 1) reveals the brain activity caused by the mental activity of finding associations.

In the data from the Corbetta study, paying attention to all three features of the stimuli is equivalent to condition 1. If we assume that attending to a single feature (condition 2) of the stimuli causes activity in a specific brain area, the activity should show up in the PET subtraction image—selective attention to a specific condition minus divided attention (condition 1 subtracted from condition 2). This was the case. When subjects selectively attended to color *or* form *or* movement, the cortical areas that became active were either identical with, or close to, cortical areas known to process color, form, or motion during perception.

This study clearly demonstrates that attention has effects on the brain. When we attend to a specific aspect of the environment, we selectively increase the activity of the area that processes the relevant information. It is as though by selectively focusing on a specific feature—the color of an object, for example—we specifically turn on the processing device for that feature. Increased activity in a cortical area implies increased computational power and, therefore, increased synaptic transmission. As only active synapses can be strengthened by long-term potentiation (LTP; see chapters 2 and 4), the increased activation resulting from selective attention will cause more learning in activated areas. <u>The effect of attention, therefore, can be interpreted, at least in part, as an increase in the activity of respective cortical areas.</u> And this increased activity facilitates learning. Thus, the fact that the monkey who does not pay attention to the vibrations of his fingertips does not learn and does not show changes in cortical representations is demystified: Attention determines activity, and activity is a prerequisite for change.

The Higher the Level, the More Adaptive the Area
The higher a cortical area, the more plastic it seems to be. In monkeys it has been demonstrated that surgical ablation of the cortical area that codes the primary sensory representation of the entire hand has the immediate effect of rendering the higher, secondary sensory areas unresponsive to sensory stimuli. After two months, however, the entire secondary somatosensory cortex becomes responsive again—to the stimulation of the foot! The area has completely reorganized and rewired itself (cf. Kandel et al. 1991).

Researchers have also demonstrated that neurons in the motor cortex become selectively active even before they carry out a discrimination task (Mountcastle et al. 1992). According to Merzenich and Sameshima, these motor neurons may receive their decision-dependent input from sensory neurons that have learned to fire coherently—that is, in concert. We should also note that the concept of the population vector discussed in chapter 4 has proven fruitful in studies of decision processes. A decision is coded not by a single neuron but by a population of neurons spread out across an extended cortical area.

As discussed above, the spatiotemporal coherence of the input is the crucial variable leading to formation of internal representations. This fact is most obvious in the experiments in which the monkeys had to discriminate between vibration frequencies (Recanzone et al. 1992). Neurons distributed over a cortical area clearly learned to discriminate the frequencies that led to an increase in the number of action potentials fired in concert. This increase in coherent firing of the neurons correlated closely—at the extremely high correlation coefficient of 0.98—with the ability of the monkeys to actually discriminate (i.e., perform the task).

The researchers suggest that learning increased the connectivity between neurons, allowing them to respond uniformly to a stimulus. It may be added that whenever learning occurs, the connections between neurons change. In fact, I hope that while you read this book, or think and talk about it, synaptic weights in your brain are changing.

Phantoms and Amputated Networks

In the past few years, a number of studies on neuroplasticity in humans have appeared, and there are now quite a few neurobiological findings about neuroplasticity in our own species. Because human beings appear to be particularly adaptive animals capable of much learning, we would expect to find neuroplasticity in many realms of function. However, only recently has the development of noninvasive technologies enabled us to study cortical changes in the human brain that are due to learning at high spatial and temporal resolution.

In chapter 1 I described the remarkable example of increases in the size of the cortical area representing the tip of the right index finger that occur when blind people learn to read Braille (Pascual-Leone & Torres 1993). The neurocomputational counterpart of this finding has been documented for more than a hundred years in cases where the input has been decreased or even completely shut off. This happens when a limb is amputated. Clinically, the results are so-called *phantoms*. The research outlined in this section demonstrates how computer simulations of cortical-reorganization processes after amputation provide a model that parsimoniously explains many of the clinical symptoms of phantoms that are otherwise inexplicable, or at least unrelated.

Subjective Experience

The term *phantom limb* was introduced to the clinical literature in 1871 by the physician W. Mitchell, who used the term to denote the subjective experience of a lost body part as if it were still present. Such phantom limbs are experienced by almost all patients after amputation (Jensen & Rasmussen 1989), often as tingling sensations or as itching of the skin of the amputated body part. For example, after the amputation of a leg, patients still experience the presence of the leg, feel the foot in a certain position, and experience movements of the leg as well as tingling or itching sensations in its skin.

Phantom limbs have a number of peculiar clinical features (cf. Cronholm 1951; Jensen et al. 1984; Katz 1992). The more severe the trauma, the more likely and/or the more intense is the sensation of the phantom limb. Accordingly, elective amputations cause fewer and less pronounced phantoms than traumatic amputations. Changes in the phantoms—known as (a) *telescoping* and (b) *shrinking* also occur over time. (a) In approximately a third of the patients, the phantom limb becomes shorter (telescopes), so that an amputated hand, for example, eventually feels as if it were attached directly to the shoulder; or an amputated foot feels directly connected to the knee or hip. The patient may even experience the hand or foot as completely retracted into the stump but still feel it as a hand or foot. (b) Or, in addition to shrinking in length, the overall proportions of the phantom may shrink to, for example, the size of a child's hand or a postage stamp.

In addition to the continuing experience of the presence of the amputated limb, and sensations from the stump, patients have *referred sensations*.

Stimulation of the stump evokes sensations as if the phantom were a physical reality and were itself stimulated. The phantom hand is "represented" by the distal part of the stump, and the phantom-forearm merely by a narrow zone proximal on it. Conditions might be described by saying that the stump had "taken over" the sensory functions of the lost limb. (Cronholm 1951:183)

These referred sensations are topographically organized (figure 7.4) and maintain the quality of the original sensation. Touching the stump is experienced both as a touch to the stump and a touch to a specific point on the phantom limb; a breeze blowing on the stump is felt as two breezes, and water running down the stump is experienced as water running down the stump and down the amputated arm or leg.

Sensory acuity of the stump is increased. This can be shown by simultaneously touching the stump with two matches and, by repeating the process, finding the smallest distance between the matches that still evokes the experience of two touches. This *two-point-discrimination threshold* is a measure of accuracy of the sensitivity to touch. For example, the tips of our fingers can discriminate two points as close together

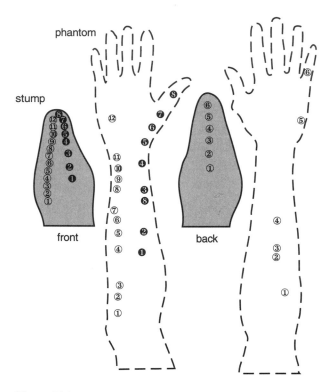

Figure 7.4
Localization of referred sensations in the phantom arm (broken line) of a patient with an amputated right arm when the front and back side of the stump (light gray) were touched with a pen. The patient indicated the site of his sensations by pointing to locations on a picture of an arm. Points of stimulation were marked with numbers on the stump; corresponding points on the graphically rendered phantom were marked by number as well, indicating a clear mapping between points of stimulation and sensation. (after Cronholm 1951:190).

as a few millimeters, whereas on our back two points as far apart as seven centimeters will still be sensed as one. We can understand the two-point discrimination threshold by considering the homunculus discussed in chapter 5 (cf. figure 5.11). The more cortex there is for analysis of sensory signals, the better information can be processed; therefore the finer the spatial resolution of the processing, the lower the two-point discrimination threshold. In amputees, two-point discrimination is better on the stump than it is on the contralateral healthy site (i.e., the intact limb). Moreover, the closer the skin area of the stump is to the amputation site, the more pronounced are these effects.

Finally, we should note that both the extent and the clarity of these sensations vary greatly from person to person. Clinicians have therefore stressed the importance of personality variables in the development of phantom limbs, although there is little data and only anecdotal evidence in support of this conjecture (cf. Katz 1992).

For decades, the origin and mechanism of phantom sensations puzzled neurologists. They questioned, in particular, whether a central (cortical) or a peripheral (sensory nerves–related) mechanism was the cause of phantoms. The puzzle is that there are convincing arguments for both hypotheses.

Cortical-Phantom Genesis
The clinical observations described are compatible with the view that the experience of phantom limbs is produced by a cortical mechanism. The recent findings on cortical neuroplasticity point strongly in this direction. According to a cortical model of phantom genesis, the cortex is a computational surface or map within which there is a constant competition of input patterns for processing capacity.

In a patient with an amputated hand, for example, the cortical "hand" area no longer receives any input. Because input fibers are referred to by neurologists as *afferents*, this state is called *cortical deafferentation*. After deafferentation, the representations of the body surface on the sensory map gradually change over time, such that the former "hand" area becomes responsible for some other part of the body (figure 7.5). Because of the principles of cortical reorganization, representations in adjacent cortical areas are most likely to "invade" the deafferented area. A quick look at figure 5.11 tells us, therefore, that the neurons in the cortical area that used to process information from the hand will—after deafferentation—start to represent the arm and the ipsilateral face (i.e., side of the face adjacent to the deafferented area) (Ramachandran et al. 1992, Yang et al. 1994).

Such cortical changes do not happen through the division or death of neurons. Instead, existing neurons form new connections, which either are already present but only now activated (*unmasking silent*

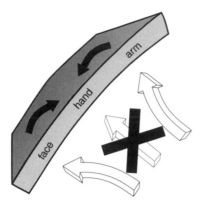

Figure 7.5
Cortical remapping caused by the deafferentation of the area that normally would receive input from the hand and lower arm. Because the sensory input from the face and the upper arm are still present, and because these areas are adjacent to the deafferented area, cortical reorganization involves both these areas. During reorganization, some neurons will represent both the former (lower arm and hand) and the new areas (face or upper arm). The patient therefore feels sensations from the upper arm (i.e., the amputation stump) in the arm as well as in the lower arm and the hand. Similarly, sensations from the face should be felt on both the face and on the lower arm and hand. Because of such reorganization at the border of the hand and the face area, a teardrop running down the face should be felt there and, in addition, as if it were running down the phantom lower arm (see figure 7.6). This double sensation of a tear is nothing but the consequence of cortical reorganization involving areas adjacent to the deafferented area.

connections) or are newly created connections (*neuronal sprouting*). In fact, there is evidence that both processes are involved in cortical reorganization (Killackey et al. 1995, Purves 1994).

The final proof of the cortical view of phantom genesis is the observation by Ramachandran (1992) of a referred sensation from the face to the lower arm. One of his patients with an amputated arm reported that stimulation of his face evoked localized and topographically mapped sensations in the phantom hand (figure 7.6). As the face is not adjacent to the arm, but the cortical representation of the face *is* adjacent to the cortical representation of the arm, this finding can only be explained by a cortical mechanism involving former "hand-neurons" starting to pick up input from the face and thereby becoming "face-neurons."

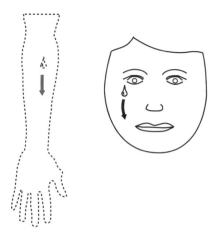

Figure 7.6
Schematic rendering of the subjective experience of a patient with a phantom arm. A teardrop running down the face is experienced simultaneously as if it were also running down the phantom arm.

The cortical view of phantom limb causation may be summarized as follows. The cortex, a two-dimensional computational maplike surface, changes according to the spatiotemporal characteristics of the input. If an area becomes deafferented (i.e., deprived of its input), reorganization takes place. Either during this process or as a result of this process, neurons representing input patterns that are no longer present become activated. This activation is subjectively experienced as the phantom sensation.

Peripheral Phantom Genesis

A number of authors have suggested that phantom limbs are caused by a peripheral mechanism or by a mechanism at the level of the spinal cord. According to this noncortical view, free nerve endings, neuromas, and axons proliferating into scar tissue are the cause of phantom pain that, in turn, leads to phantom sensations. Poeck (1963) quotes several authors who suggest that phantom limbs are caused by interactions between efferent autonomic fibers and afferent sensory fibers. This hypothesis was refined and put forward in a recent review by Katz (1992). He proposed that "a phantom limb, whether painful or not, is related to the sympathetic-efferent outflow of cutaneous vasoconstrictor fibers in the stump and stump neuromas" and that "the paresthetic or dysesthetic component of the phantom limb may be triggered by sympathetic-efferent activity" (Katz 1992:290).

In addition to peripheral nerves, the spinal cord has been implicated in the genesis of phantom limbs. For example, from his own detailed clinical observations, Cronholm (1951) concluded that hyperexcitability of the spinal cord was the mechanism by means of which phantom limbs come into existence.

The noncortical view of phantom-limb causation—whether at the level of the peripheral nerves or the spinal cord—is supported by one striking clinical finding: Patients with lesions of the spinal cord and the clinical condition of paraplegia rarely develop phantom sensations. If they do, the sensations are weak, lacking in detail, and occur months after the onset of paraplegia. Carlen and colleagues correctly point out the apparent consequence of this observation for the cortical view: "If phantoms were generated by the activity of brain cells rather than cord cells, the paraplegic should report an even more vivid phantom sensation since his brain has lost even more input than an amputee's" (1978:216).

In special support of this view are two cases of patients who suffered both thoracic spinal cord lesions and amputation of an arm (Bors 1951). These cases allowed investigators to compare the effects of amputation and spinal cord lesion within the same individual. In both cases, there was a pronounced and clearly experienced phantom of the arm but only a weak and hard to describe phantom of the lower body. This clinical observation makes it highly unlikely that individual differences account for the reported differences between the phantom experiences of amputees and patients with spinal cord lesions. The inevitable conclusion appears to be that the presence or absence of phantom sensations in these two patient groups are due to differences in their spinal cords or in their peripheral-nerve injuries.

The noncortical view of phantom-limb causation may therefore be summarized as follows. Amputees suffer from a lesion of the peripheral sensory nerve and experience phantom limbs; paraplegics, who have lesions of the spinal cord, do not experience phantom limbs, or do so only to a small degree. Because *both* conditions imply cortical deafferentation (loss of nerve input to the cortex), such deafferentation cannot explain the differences. Therefore, phantom sensations have to be caused by a mechanism that involves the peripheral nerve endings and/or the spinal cord.

Simulating Phantoms by Amputating Networks

In order to investigate further this conundrum of two incompatible hypotheses on phantom-limb causation, I and my colleagues simulated cortical deafferentation by using self-organizing feature maps (Spitzer et al. 1995). How do you amputate a neural network that is simulated in a computer? Not with a screwdriver and soldering iron but by simply altering the set of input patterns.

Let us briefly recap from chapter 5 the example of using characters of the alphabet as input to simulate cortical map formation. The set of input characters became represented on the map through self-organization according to the principles of similarity and frequency of the input patterns. Such a trained network can be "amputated" by removing the input represented by a part of the network. This can be done easily by examining the map, deciding which part should be deafferented, and deleting the input patterns that are represented by that part (figure 7.7). The deletion of input patterns thereby produces deafferentation of a part of the map. What happens then?

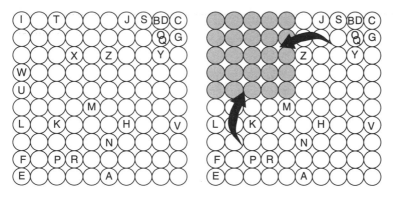

Figure 7.7
Expected and (under specific conditions) observed reorganization of representations within a Kohonen network after deafferentation. The deafferented area is shown in gray.

Nothing! This came as a surprise, as one might assume that the cortex would spontaneously reorganize the representations on its surface. However, when the input patterns were *degraded* (see below), reorganization phenomena were observed. In brief, degrading the input signals sometimes made them look like the missing input; these degraded input patterns, therefore, sometimes activated neurons in the deafferented area, setting reorganization processes in motion.

Noise

The reference to deformation of patterns can be specified more precisely by the use of the concept of *noise*. Noise disrupts the transmission of information. Most of us know about the concept from our last attempt to have a conversation from a telephone booth on a busy street. The concept of noise is derived from acoustics, where it can most easily be demonstrated. A pure tone can be visualized as a pattern on an oscilloscope, where it looks like a sinus wave function (see figure 7.8). If this tone is transmitted unreliably—for example when we play an old pho-

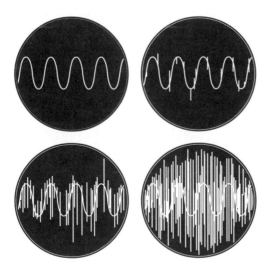

Figure 7.8
Oscilloscope displaying a signal as noise increases. (Upper left) pure tone; (upper right) pure tone with some audible and visible cracks; (lower left) noisy tone; (lower right) more noise than signal.

nograph record—cracks can be heard and seen as minor, spike-shaped deviations from the wavelike curve. If the signal is even more disturbed by unreliable transmission, single cracks are no longer heard; instead, we perceive less signal and more noise.

Figure 7.8 shows what we intuitively know from the sound systems in our living rooms. The quality of these systems is determined, among other features, by a parameter describing the ratio of the amplified signal to the internally generated noise: The higher this signal-to-noise ratio, the better the system.

The concept of noise, however, is by no means restricted to acoustic phenomena; it can be applied to any form of signal transmission and processing. We have already mentioned in chapter 1 that neurons are poor information processing hardware. In other words, because neurons have a low signal-to-noise ratio, they tend to produce random spontaneous activity. How does this factor affect the simulated neurons of neural network models?

The general answer to this question is that noise denotes an error in signal processing. For example, when a neuron fires spontaneously, or when signal conduction is disturbed randomly, the target neuron is less reliably influenced by the input signals. In simulated neural networks, noise can be provided in different ways. For example, a "noisy" activation pattern can be produced by simply adding and subtracting small random numbers (between 0 and 1) to and from the pattern of activation, as shown in figure 7.9.

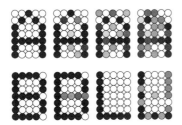

Figure 7.9
Examples of noisy activation patterns in the input layer of the character-recognition network. At the top, an increasingly noisy *A* is shown. The bottom row demonstrates that adding noise to an input pattern can make it similar to another pattern (*B* becomes similar to *D*, and *L* becomes similar to *U*).

Noise and Neuroplasticity

Equipped with the sharpened concept of deformation, which we can express as the amount of noise in an activation pattern or signal, let us return to the computer simulation of a deafferented Kohonen network. The concept of noise clarifies what we mean by a *deformed input.* Moreover, the degree of deformation can be specified by the amount of noise (i.e., random numbers) that is superimposed on (i.e., added to and subtracted from) the signal.

When noise is added to the input, it happens that input patterns that are not represented in the deafferented area are deformed in a way that renders them similar to a pattern that has been deleted from the input file to simulate deafferentation. Such a deformed input pattern will, therefore, activate a neuron in the deafferented area. In order to get a better sense of what happens under these circumstances, we ran a large number of computer simulations at various levels of input noise and counted how often a deformed input activated a neuron in the deafferented area. We found that the more noise we added to the input, the more often this activation occurred. In other words, the more deformed the input, the greater is its chance of activating a neuron that does not represent it (figure 7.10). As synapses change because of Hebbian learning, noise in the input accelerates the reorganization processes of the representational map.

We also demonstrated that—like the cortical face and arm representations located adjacent to the representation of amputated hands— the input patterns most likely to be picked up by the neurons in the deafferented area were those represented by neurons in parts of the map immediately adjacent to the deafferented area (figure 7.11). In other words, the neuronally coded representations adjacent to the deafferented area were most likely to "invade" it.

Turning a Conundrum into a Parsimonious Theory

How do the computer simulations fit with neurobiological and clinical reality? The simulation merely demonstrates that noisy input patterns may activate neurons that are deprived of their usual input. These neurons continue to code input patterns that no longer exist in the set of all possible inputs, because of the amputation. However, if these neurons

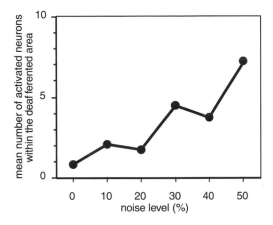

Figure 7.10
Number of activated neurons in the deafferented area as a function of the amount of noise superimposed on the input patterns (after Spitzer et al. 1995). The noise level indicates the percentage of deformation to the signal caused by noise. We found that increased noise in the input (i.e., increased deformation of the input patterns) increased the frequency of neuronal activation in the deafferented area.

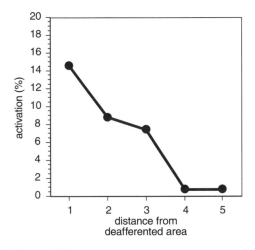

Figure 7.11
Distance of the "invading" representations from the deafferented part of the network (after Spitzer et al. 1995a). In a 10 × 10 network with one quadrant lesioned, the remaining neurons are one to five steps (i.e., changes in the x and/or y coordinates) away from the deafferented area. The closer to the deafferented area the representation of an input pattern was on the map, the more likely were its respective input patterns to activate a neuron in the deafferented area. Thus, representations that "invaded" the deafferented area of the network originated in adjacent areas.

are somehow activated, their firing is interpreted by higher cortical areas as tingling and itching sensations in the amputated part of the body.

For the model to apply to amputees, there must, then, be a mechanism that generates noise after the amputation. How, after all, is the noise that leads to the consequent activation of the deafferented area of the model generated? When a limb is amputated, nerve fibers, which are nothing but bundles of the axons of neurons, are severed. The sensory neurons innervating the hand or leg, for example, are located in sensory ganglia adjacent to the spinal cord. Lesions on these neurons occur when their axons are cut. Researchers have found that in about 30 percent of these neurons, the lesion causes spontaneous, random firing activity (Devor 1984, Welk et al. 1990). This is another way of saying that sensory neurons with lesioned axons generate noise. This random activity of the sensory neurons generates noise in amputees, and it is this noise that causes the tingling sensations of phantoms.

A crucial observation for the development of the model was that paraplegics seldom experience phantoms, and when they do, the phantoms are very different (i.e., they occur months after the lesion and are less pronounced and clear) from the amputees' phantoms, which are experienced sharply right after the amputation. This difference is a direct consequence of the lesion site, which in paraplegics is centrally located between the first sensory neuron and the central nervous system (CNS). If the fibers at this site are disrupted, no noise is transmitted to the CNS, and only "silence" comes through its information-carrying fiber connections to the periphery. In short, it is biologically plausible that the CNS receives noise in amputees and silence in paraplegics (see figure 7.12).

Are the assumptions regarding connectivity also biologically plausible? The computer simulation model implements full connectivity between input and output layers, whereas, neurobiologically speaking, it is highly unlikely that every fiber of every sensory nerve is connected to every sensory neuron. However, we know from our discussion of the mechanisms that can lead to rewiring of the brain that there are unused, silent connections that can be reactivated during the process of cortical reorganization (Bach y Rita 1990, Gilbert 1993). Moreover, neuroplasticity may involve the production of entirely new connections (Antonini & Stryker 1993).

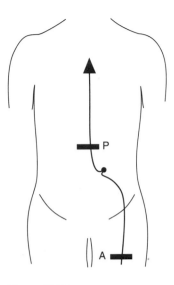

Figure 7.12
Site of the lesion in amputees (A) and in paraplegics (P). The main difference consists of the fact that in amputees the connection between the sensory neuron and the CNS is maintained, whereas in paraplegics, this connection no longer exists.

The model of reorganization of representations in a Kohonen network after deafferentation is not only biologically plausible but also provides a parsimonious account of the following clinical and experimental observations that otherwise appear unrelated or puzzling.

1. Phantom limbs are experienced immediately after amputation. This may be explained by the fact that the very mechanism of amputation produces "sensory input noise" (i.e., random activity of the dorsal root ganglion sensory neurons), which leads to random activation in the deafferented area. Subjectively, this corresponds to the tingling and itching sensations in the nonexistent limb immediately after amputation.

2. Compared to planned amputations, amputations occurring after traumatic events are more likely to produce phantom sensations and, indeed, to do so more rapidly. This can easily be explained as a result of the extra incoherent input (i.e., noise) provided by the traumatic event and the time that elapses before the operation is carried out.

3. Recent studies reveal that the amount of cortical reorganization occurring after amputation is strongly correlated with the severity of phantom pain (Flohr et al. 1995). This suggests a possible common mechanism

of pain and reorganization; for example, that massive, noncorrelated neuronal activity may cause pain and lead to cortical reorganization.

4. Telescoping and shrinking sensations of the phantom are likely to correspond to decreases in the size of the cortical area that codes for the amputated limb. These decreases occur over a long period of time, during which the neurons of the deafferented area must "unlearn" previous representations. It is likely that this process is facilitated by input noise.

5. Stimulation of body surfaces corresponding to cortical areas adjacent to the deafferented area gives rise to "referred sensations" in the phantom limb. According to our model, the extra noise provided by the random firing of sensory neurons leads to activation of cortical cells within the deafferented area. This happens almost immediately after amputation. It is important to note that the representations "invade" from areas adjacent to the deafferented area. The somatotopical organization of the referred sensations corresponds to the fact that the redistribution in feature maps is governed by the internal structure of the map.

6. According to the model, amputation leads to an unused (deafferented) cortical area, which is taken over by adjacent areas. In other words, the deafferented cortical surface takes over computational functions from adjacent areas, which thereby increase their computational capacity. This increased capacity can be demonstrated by the reduced size of the receptive fields of sensory neurons on the stump; that is, the processing of sensory information from the stump's sensory neurons is improved as a result of the increased cortical computational surface devoted to them.

7. When the computer simulations were run with rather high noise levels, we observed some wobbling of the representations of input located within the nondeafferented areas. Presentation of a given input did not always lead to activation of its representing neuron. Instead, the added noise caused the input to activate neurons that used to code other input patterns. This led us to predict that clinical cases in which similar "misplacements" of sensory input, caused by processes that can be expected to lead to extra noise, might occur. Such extra noise may be expected to arise in particularly severe injuries and/or in cases of additional injuries. In such patients, touching an arm, for example, might result in the sensation of touch in a (nonamputated) leg. A search through the older, and usually more descriptive, literature revealed two such cases. In his monograph, Cronholm (1951) described a patient with multiple leg fractures that led to amputation four months after the injury and another patient with one leg amputated who sustained injury to the other leg. Both patients reported referred sensations of the kind just described: that is, when parts of their bodies were touched, they felt the touch at that location and, in addition, at another location on the body (but not on

the phantom). In both cases, a high level of sensory noise could be expected, caused—in the first case—by the severity of the injury and the delay of the amputation and—in the second case—by the additional injury. Our model provides a straightforward explanation of these clinical observations. In our view, it is likely that such experiential phenomena occur with some frequency but are rarely scrutinized by a physician.

8. Finally, the model does not rule out the possibility that personality traits may influence the subjective features of phantoms, a suggestion that has been subject to considerable debate in the past (cf. Katz 1992, Schilder 1923, Spitzer 1988, Zuk 1956). In chapter 12, I discuss the hypothesis that an individual's genetic makeup may include, among other things, the amount of the different neuromodulatory agents present in the brain. Because these neuromodulators may affect the signal-to-noise ratio in the brain, they seem likely to affect phantom experiences.

In sum, the model of cortical reorganization proposed can account for a large number of empirical and clinical observations and findings in a very simple and parsimonious way. It not only exemplifies an important principle of neural-network functioning—that is, that noise facilitates neuroplasticity—but it also rejects the argument that computer simulations are of no use when it comes to understanding purely subjective phenomena. What could be more subjective than the sensations of something that is not present?

The Cortex Plays the First Violin

An important example of the cortex's ability to adapt to the conditions of its use was published by Elbert and coworkers in 1995. The authors started by considering that professional guitar and violin players very frequently have to process with very high accuracy sensations of touch coming from the fingers of the left hand. The researchers assumed that, like the blind people who learned Braille and developed larger than normal cortical areas representing the tip of the right index finger, violinists and guitarists would have unusually large cortical areas representing the fingers of the left hand.

To test this hypothesis experimentally, Elbert and coworkers used a guitarist and nine violinists. They employed magnetoencephalography (MEG) to measure the distance between the cortical representations of the thumb and pinkie finger in the right and the left cortex (i.e., the areas corresponding to the fingers of the left and the right hands). Because the map of the body surface extends in only one dimension (see figure 5.1), this distance can be used to detect increases in the cortical surface area. Moreover, comparing the left and the right sides of the same person's brain assured researchers that the results were not due to individual differences. Instead, the differences between the right and the left brain could be readily interpreted as a result of practicing an instrument that depends more on the work of the left hand (i.e., the computational power of the right sensory cortex) than of the right hand.

The results show that the cortical area representing the left hand is indeed larger in players of stringed instruments such as violins and guitars (figure 7.13). It was further demonstrated that this effect was most pronounced in those persons who had begun practicing the instrument

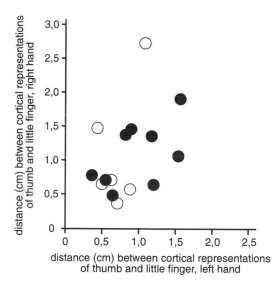

Figure 7.13
Distance of the cortical representations of thumb and fifth finger (in centimeters) of the left and the right hand of violinists and guitar players (black circles) and of control subjects (white circles). In right-handed control subjects, the right hand is represented by a larger cortical area than the left hand, as indicated by the larger distance between the cortical representations of the thumb and fifth finger. This asymmetry is virtually absent in the stringed-instrument musicians tested; their left hands are cortically represented by areas about as large as, or even larger than those of the right hands (after Elbert et al. 1995).

before the age of twelve. Thus the study demonstrates, first, that the cortex remodels itself according to the input it has to process during the lifetime of the organism. Second, this remodeling is more pronounced in younger than in older organisms. An observation made by my daughter's violin teacher nicely fits these data: People who start learning to play the violin after the age of twelve never learn vibrato technique as well as those who begin early.

Therapeutic Application: Plastic Understanding of Spoken Language

The final example in this chapter demonstrates once more that nothing is more practical than a good theory. Insights into the neurobiology of learning can, at present, guide the development of new therapeutic strategies—not only in pharmacotherapy but also in the realm of purely psychological interventions.

It has been estimated that 5 to 8 percent of all children suffer from auditory deficits relating to the understanding of spoken language and that 85 percent of these children develop reading difficulties (Barinaga 1996). Paula Tallal and coworkers (1985) were able to show by clever experiments that many of these children suffer from a deficit in the early stages of auditory signal processing. In fact, they were found to suffer from slow cortical sound processing. This condition often goes unnoticed but causes problems whenever rapid changes of sounds have to be processed; for example, the processing of rapidly changing sounds is highly important in the perception of speech. The syllables of *ba-* and *pa-*, for example, differ only with respect to their beginning consonants, whose sound patterns differ by only a few milliseconds. If rapid changes cannot be processed correctly, these consonants cannot be properly distinguished. The net result for the child is difficulty in understanding spoken language.

It is easy to imagine what happens if this problem is not detected. Because the child is not deaf, and in fact has perfect hearing in standard tests using pure tones, caregivers may suppose negligence or disobedience on the child's part. (I leave it to the reader to imagine all the possible consequences of this assumption.) In fact, the child suffers from defective sound processing at a relatively low level of input processing. The level is low because the defect does not affect semantics, pragmatics, or other high-level language processing. It rather affects the analysis of temporal input patterns. Because of spoken language's special requirements for processing speed, the defect is noticed almost exclusively in speech comprehension.

Investigators also found that these children had difficulties processing rapidly changing nonlanguage sound-input patterns and, even, rapidly changing sensory and visual input. Whenever the processing of rapidly changing sequences was required, the children were at a loss. Again, in everyday life, such a disorder hardly shows up, except in the understanding of spoken language.

Tallal's findings cleared the unfortunate children of disobedience, but she believed that there wasn't anything to be done about their disorder. However, she was able to show that the children could distinguish *ba*- from *pa*- if the crucial consonants were artificially extended in time, which can be done digitally in a speech laboratory. Thus, it was clear that the children were able to decode the relevant input when given more time. They were just too slow to do it in real time.

We have already discussed the results of Michael Merzenich and his group, which show that the cortex can be trained with temporal patterns (tones and vibrations). Tallal and Merzenich teamed up to study whether children afflicted with slow sound processing could be trained by using the correct temporally stretched input (Merzenich et al. 1996, Tallal et al. 1996). They trained the children by providing them with temporally slowed input, then gradually speeding up the input until each child was always able to process it. The children learned to process rapid input patterns with increasing speed, with highly encouraging results. After only four weeks of training, they had not only learned to process the training patterns but had increased their ability to understand normal speech as well.

This example supports my view that neurobiological understanding of cortical reorganization processes can motivate new forms of purely psychological therapy. Hence, it clearly demonstrates how useless and conceptually wrong are the old dogmas of biological versus psychological treatment methods. These squabbles between different schools of thought are beside the point. Brain and mind are woven together more densely than we ever imagined before. I discuss further examples of this intricate interaction in later chapters.

Neuroplasticity and Thought

When discussing learning and neuroplasticity, why did we refer only to simple functions and capabilities and, hence, to the primary sensory cortex and to low-level auditory processing? Are complex functions and the respective higher cortical areas not also plastic? The answer to these questions is based on certain systematic as well as methodological considerations about human neuroplasticity.

1. First, it should be noted that studies of neuroplasticity in humans are relatively new. Therefore, we can discuss only the tip of the iceberg in research that is currently being done and will be done. There is a lot more to learn in the future.

2. Systematically speaking, the investigation of sensory areas is easiest, because their maplike structure was worked out decades ago and is well known. This does not imply that higher cortical functions are not also built up of maplike representations. It merely points to the fact that we do not know the structure of higher-level maps and therefore cannot (yet) refer to these structures as maps. Nor can we investigate changes in these "maps." However, in the coming years the situation may change (cf. the evidence for semantic maps discussed in chapter 10).

3. Furthermore, methodological considerations have to be taken into account when discussing neuroplasticity in the higher cognitive functions. The sensitivity of currently available noninvasive methods for the study of cortical representations increases every year. However, even the studies of simple processes and low-level representations operate close to their limit of resolution and threshold of detection. This is one reason why neuroplasticity has been difficult to demonstrate in cortical areas performing high-level mental functions. However, we know that the human brain shows its unique capacities not in low-level sensory motor performances but rather with respect to the rapid acquisition of complex skills and knowledge. Hence, we must assume that plasticity plays a major role in high-level cognition. We just cannot yet detect it. But I am quite optimistic that this will change in the next few years.

Recap

Neuroplasticity has been confirmed in animals and in the human cortex. When a blind person learns Braille, the cortical area processing signals from the tip of his or her right index finger grows larger; and if you learn to play the violin or guitar, the cortical area representing the fingers of the left hand enlarges. If deaf people receive an artificial inner ear (cochlea implant) and regain the capability to understand spoken language (even over the telephone), massive reorganization must have taken place in the cortical areas that process sounds.

The changes in cortical sensory representations observed in animals after deafferentation are analogous to the reshuffling of cortical sensory representations of the body surface that occur in patients with amputated limbs—because a part of the amputee's cortex no longer receives input. These processes can be simulated with neural networks of the self-organizing feature-maps type. Such simulations are the core of a neurocomputational model of phantom limbs that can resolve the puzzle of central versus peripheral genesis and parsimoniously explain several otherwise unrelated or inexplicable clinical features of phantoms. The model described accounts for the effects of noise (unreliability in neuronal information processing) and demonstrates the importance of such noise for neuroplasticity.

Animal studies have shown that neuroplasticity further depends not only on new input but also on the relevance of the new input to the organism. Irrelevant events do not cause neuroplastic changes, even when they occur with the same frequency as relevant events (Ahissar et al. 1992). <u>Whether an event is relevant or not depends upon the motivation of the organism, and the extent to which an event is further processed depends upon attention.</u> Since we know from functional-imaging studies in human beings that attention leads to the activation of cortical areas carrying out the corresponding computation, it is easy to see why the motivated child learns and why the daydreaming pupil doesn't.

Because of the uniformity of the structure of the neocortex, it is unlikely that neuroplasticity happens only in low-level areas. Just the opposite should be the case. It is not the sensory cortex, but rather a number of higher cortical areas that are the substrate of the higher mental functions specific to human beings. We therefore need to assume that plasticity is at work whenever we learn something new.

8

Feedback

As mentioned before, the brain is mainly concerned with itself. In human beings, only about 0.1 percent of all connections between cortical pyramidal calls conduct signals into and out of the brain; the remaining 99.9 percent are internal connections.

Taking into account that cortical pyramidal cells receive their inputs from up to ten thousand other cells and send their outputs to just as many cells, a simple calculation suggests that feedback has to be a general feature of cortical architecture. If one neuron sends fibers to ten thousand other neurons, and these neurons, in turn, send fibers to ten thousand neurons, then the output of all these neurons has to return to the original neuron: $10^4 \times 10^4 \times 10^4 = 10^{12}$, which is more neurons than the about twenty billion (2×10^{10}) that make up the human cortex. In short, after just three synaptic transmissions, on average, a signal is back to where it started. A similar calculation for the mouse cortex, which has between ten and twenty million neurons, shows that a signal is back to its point of origin after traveling across just two synaptic clefts (cf. Braitenberg & Schütz 1989). What are the consequences of such massive feedback for the way the brain works?

That question is the subject of this chapter, and, again, the answers are neurocomputational in nature. One of the interesting features of feedback, it turns out, is its role in the representation of time in neural networks. Of course, I refer to a very basic notion of time. A network in a given state at time, t_0, has an effect upon itself at a later stage, time t_1. This implies that a network responds not only to similarities of single input patterns but also to sequences of input patterns. Such sequences are nothing but temporal patterns, the importance of which we discussed in chapter 7; there we also demonstrated that changes in temporal patterns can cause neuroplastic changes in the cortex. In this chapter we expand on our discussion of networks that can process temporal patterns.

Connectivity across the Board: Hopfield Networks

Neural networks in which every neuron is connected to every other neuron are termed *autoassociative networks*. They were first comprehensively described by the American physicist John Hopfield and so are also called *Hopfield networks* (figure 8.1). They consist of a single layer in which every neuron is connected to every other neuron. If the Hebbian learning rule is implemented in a Hopfield network, it takes on a number of properties:

1. An input signal (i.e., a spatially distributed pattern of activation) can be stored in the network simply as a pattern of activated and nonactivated neurons. Under Hebbian learning, when a new input is presented, the synaptic weights within the network change, which takes some time. Some neurons are excited by the input and signal their excitation to all the other neurons in the network; these neurons, in turn, receive both the new input and the input from all the other neurons. To put it simply, the internal connections of the network ensure that when a new input is presented there is much more going on in the network than just the activation of the neurons receiving that input. It has been demonstrated that reception of an input changes the activation state of the network for some time before it reaches a stable state. This stable state is the memory

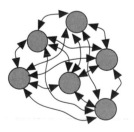

Figure 8.1
Structure of a Hopfield network. Each neuron is connected to every other neuron but not with itself. In addition, the network has input and output connections (not shown) for the reception of patterns and for sending out the activation pattern of the network as output.

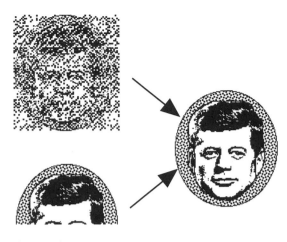

Figure 8.2
Pattern recognition in a Hopfield network. Input patterns like the two depicted
on the left (top: face with added noise; bottom: partially presented face) are
correctly recognized by a Hopfield network after appropriate training. That is,
when presented with one of the input patterns on the left, the network produced
the activational state shown on the right.

of the input pattern and is also called an *attractor*. Hopfield networks
are therefore sometimes referred to as *attractor networks*.

2. A network can store more than one pattern in this way and can
therefore produce more than one attractor. Other input patterns can be
stored in the same way as the first signal. However, the maximum
number of patterns that can be stored in this way is equal to about 13
percent of the total number of neurons in the network (Anderson 1995).

3. A stored activation pattern can be recalled by the presentation of
partial or deformed versions of the stored pattern (figure 8.2). If the
network receives a part of the stored pattern, the internal connections
make sure that the entire pattern is reproduced. The network completes
the incomplete input pattern by using the stored information. For example, a Hopfield network containing ten thousand neurons may be used
for the storage of faces. Presenting just a part of a particular face stored
in the past may be enough for the network to reproduce the pattern of
the entire face.

4. Even if the input is only somewhat similar to a stored input, the
activation pattern of a network will converge on the closest attractor. In
other words, the network will spontaneously "judge" similarity and
thereby generalize across a set of input patterns. In marked contrast to

conventional computers trained to recognize patterns, the network recognizes input patterns even if they are only partially present, similar to the stored input, or partially degraded (as in figure 8.2, top). These features of Hopfield networks for storing and processing patterns are also found in biological systems (i.e., brains).

Attractors

We can summarize the way Hopfield networks perform by saying that upon presentation of a given input, the pattern of activation of the network's neurons converges toward a specific output state. The stored output states (or attractors) are stable activation patterns, which Hopfield first likened to the energy states of physical systems in 1982 (see Hopfield 1982, 1984).

If we scrutinize closely the sequence of neuronal states when activated by an input, we can observe that the pattern of activation changes to become increasingly similar to the stable state that most closely resembles the input pattern. The network thus converges on the attractor that is closest to the input pattern. All the possible states of a network can be metaphorically described as a landscape of energy (figure 8.3) where the attractors form valleys between mountains of unstable network states (Amit 1989). Or, similarly, we can compare the temporal behavior of the

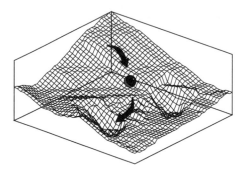

Figure 8.3
Topological surface of an "energy landscape." The height of "mountains" and the depth of "valleys" illustrate the energy states of the system, which strives to reach an energy minimum. This can be illustrated by a sphere rolling downhill into a valley. Hopfield networks minimize their energy level and hence gravitate toward such minimal energy states, which are also called *attractors*.

network upon activation to the movement of a sphere rolling downhill from a point in the energy landscape until it reaches a stable position in the deepest point of a valley (i.e., an attractor).

The metaphor of a landscape with stable minima and unstable maxima has been used by a number of psychologists and psychiatrists to explain cognitive processes. As Anderson comments on Hopfield networks and the landscape metaphor,

This idea has an agreeable feel. Certainly, subjectively we believe that meaningful mental states somehow are solid, coherent, and long lasting. Something like this behavior has been suggested by a number of modelers. Psychological measurements suggest that most significant mental operations take a hundred milliseconds or more, suggesting a time course involving network operations with significant temporal integration and relatively long-term stability. (1995:402)

In short, Hopfield networks have features that resemble, and can be related to, some features of mental processes.

Auditory Hallucinations

About two-thirds of all schizophrenic patients suffer from auditory hallucinations (see chapter 11). They often hear voices that talk about them or "put them down." The content of the voices is often stereotyped, always saying the same thing, or at least rambling on about the same subject.

Ralph Hoffman of Yale University, the first psychiatrist to employ neural network models to understand this psychopathology, used Hopfield networks to simulate what goes on when schizophrenic patients hear voices (Hoffman 1987; see also Hoffman & Dobscha 1989, Hoffman 1992, Hoffman et al. 1995). According to his simulations, hallucinations may result from an information overload of the network used to store memories. Hoffman argues that if such networks are diminished in size and storage capacity, they can no longer handle the individual's experiences. Eventually, information overload leads to deformation of the landscape: "Memory overload . . . causes distortions of energy contours of the system so that gestalts no longer have a one-to-one correspondence with distinct, well delineated energy minima" (Hoffman 1987:180).

The overload, in addition to deforming the structure of the network, causes formation of new attractors, which Hoffman characterizes as parasitic. Such parasitic attractors are produced by the amalgamation of many normal attractors, which creates particularly stable attractors (i.e., "deep valleys") in the energy landscape. These deep valleys are the end state of the system that began with a large number of positions. Thus parasitic attractors are formed almost regardless of the input presented to the system. According to Hoffman, these attractors are the basis of the voices and other major symptoms of schizophrenia.

These parasitic states are the information processing equivalents of "black holes in space" and can markedly disrupt the integrity of neural network functioning by inducing "alien forces" that distort and control the flow of mentation. If a similar reorganization of the schizophrenic's memory capabilities has taken place, it would not be at all surprising for him to report one or more schneiderian symptoms, namely, that he no longer has control of his thoughts, or that his mind is possessed by alien forces. (Hoffman 1987:180)

In simulations with other networks types, Hoffman and coworkers (1995) proposed another model of schizophrenic hallucinations that incorporates findings on the specific effects of neuronal loss in the frontal lobes and the effects of dopamine (see chapter 11). This model has reached a level of sophistication that allows it to be tested empirically.

Elman Networks

Elman networks are a type of neural network especially developed to represent time (Elman 1991, Mozer 1993). In these networks, the problem of representing a series of patterns in time is solved by a so-called *context layer*. The neurons in this layer are connected to the neurons in the hidden layer of what is otherwise a perfectly normal three-layer network (figure 8.4). The number of neurons in the context layer is identical to the number in the hidden layer; and the connections from the hidden layer to the context layer are unusual in that they are one-to-one connections, which provide the context layer with an image of the activation pattern identical to the image in the hidden layer. This is why Elman networks are also called *recurrent networks*.

Because of this architecture, the input that the context layer receives is the activation pattern of the hidden layer. The context layer then feeds this first pattern back to the hidden layer when the latter receives the *next* input pattern. The hidden layer thereby receives two inputs: new

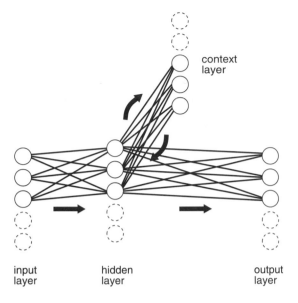

context
layer

input
layer

hidden
layer

output
layer

Figure 8.4
Architecture of an Elman network. An additional context layer is connected to the hidden layer with one-to-one connections. These connections provide the context layer with a perfect copy of the activation state of the hidden layer. When the subsequent pattern from the input layer is transmitted to the hidden layer, this copy of the previous state of the hidden layer is fed back to it through distributed connections whose weights can change. Thus, each pattern influences the processing of the subsequent pattern. (The arrows indicate the flow of information in the network.)

input from the input layer and a copy of its own previous state from the context layer.

As the connections from the context layer to the hidden layer are modifiable, patterns can have different effects on the processing of subsequent patterns, making it possible for a pattern to have an effect across time. This influence is not restricted to one computational step, because a subsequent new input can also be affected by the earlier input through the latter's effect on an intervening input. In fact, such effects across time can extend over quite a few computational steps. Thus, during training, the hidden layer of an Elman network not only forms internal representations of the input patterns, which enable it to produce the correct output patterns, but also comes to represent the temporal order of the input patterns.

In an Elman network, representation of the context of an input is therefore possible. A word, for example, is not processed by itself, but in the context of previously presented words. The word *bank,* for example, is processed differently in the context of words like *money, interest,* and *Wall Street* than it is in the context of *river* and *sand.* The effects of context can only be simulated in neural networks if the relevant context is in fact represented in the network, which it is in neural networks of the Elman type.

Working Memory

In psychological terms, the extra layer of an Elman network can be interpreted as a working memory, because it keeps the immediate context of an item on line for the system (Baddeley 1986, 1992, 1995). The same thing happens when you decide to call a friend, look up his or her number in the telephone book, dial the number—and then forget it. During this brief behavioral sequence you have used your working memory to keep the number on line.

Whenever we produce and understand language, we use working memory to a greater or lesser degree, simply because we have to keep several words in mind in order to understand the entire sentence (Just & Carpenter 1992, Just et al. 1994, Petrides et al. 1993). The characteristic features of working memory are its short time span and its limited capacity. You can easily overload it. Everyone has probably had the experience of realizing that the span of what he or she can keep in mind—even with full concentration, and even in the absence of distracters, such as the thoughts, images, and fantasies that the mind may conjure up—when reading a somewhat longer than usual sentence in a highly awake state, or when tired, let alone under the influence of beer, wine, hard liquor, or maybe even so-called recreational psychoactive drugs (which have little to do with the re-creation of anything and let your mind go down the tubes anyway), is rather limited.

What you may have just experienced, you can experience even with short sentences when you are tired, sick, drugged, or under the influence of any combination of the above. You are able to read every single word, but you simply do not "get it"; that is, you cannot put the words together into a meaningful whole.

Animal studies on the neurobiological basis of working memory have demonstrated that this ability is located in the frontal lobes. It has been demonstrated that if activity from single cells in the frontal cortex of a monkey is recorded, neurons fire selectively under working-memory conditions. In one study, the monkey is shown a stimulus that is not immediately relevant for behavior but becomes relevant after a brief interval. After the monkey has been appropriately trained, it memorizes the stimulus until it uses it to generate a correct response. During the period of memorization—that is, from the time the stimulus vanishes to the time it produces a response—neurons in the frontal lobe are selectively active. They start to become active when the stimulus disappears, and they cease to be active when the response is carried out. We may assume, then, that these neurons temporarily store information relevant to the subsequent behavior (Funahashi et al. 1989, Goldman-Rakic 1990, Goldman-Rakic et al. 1990, Goldman-Rakic & Friedman 1991). Selectively cooling the dorsolateral prefrontal cortex until its neurons no longer function properly (cooling induces reversible lesions) brings about a reversible loss of working memory (Fuster 1991, 1993, 1995). A study by Wilson and coworkers (1993) suggests that there are neurons in the frontal lobes that are specific to working memory of different aspects of the environment, which become active whenever that aspect or function has to be kept in mind.

Even in human beings, functional imaging methods have revealed activation of parts of the frontal lobes under conditions of working memory (figure 8.5)—that is, when information has to be kept in mind for brief periods of time (Cohen et al. 1994, Jonides et al. 1993, McCarthy et al. 1994, Petrides et al. 1993).

Patients who suffer from damage to the frontal lobes often show deficits in their working memory. Some psychiatric patients, most notably schizophrenic patients, have been found to suffer from a selective deficit of the working memory (Goldman-Rakic 1991, 1994, Park & Holzman 1992, Spitzer 1993). These studies show that the frontal lobes of schizophrenic patients are less activated under conditions that strongly activate the frontal lobes in normal subjects (for a review, see Andreasen 1994).

If you are used to working at a computer, you may think of working memory as something like your computer's random access memory

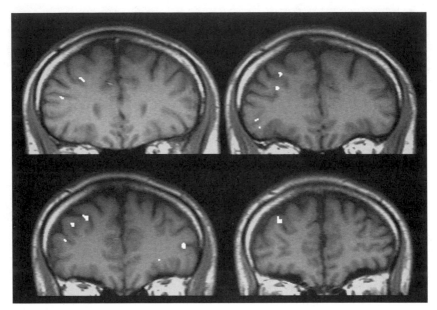

a

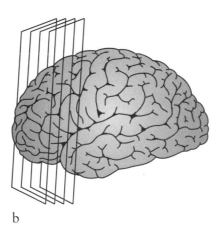

b

Figure 8.5
(a) Activation (shown in white) of small areas in the frontal lobes (bottom) while a subject in an MRI scanner carries out a working-memory task. (b) The drawing shows the orientation of the planes seen in the scanner images below (cf. Spitzer et al. 1996).

(RAM). The computer only loads into RAM from the hard drive (its long-term memory) what it needs to carry out the specific task at hand. Similarly, whenever we speak, we activate only a tiny fraction of the words stored in our long-term memory. The few active words are used and then vanish from our stream of consciousness. Working memory, as stated above, plays a role in keeping the relevant information on line for a short period of time.

Development of the Frontal Lobes

Like the electric wires in your house, nerve fibers are insulated. This insulation helps nerve fibers to carry signals at speeds of up to a hundred meters per second. Without insulation, the speed of signals is less than three meters per second. The insulation around nerve fibers, which consists of sheets of a substance called *myelin,* are important because they increase the speed of signal conduction by a factor of between thirty and forty.

At birth, all the neurons a person will ever have are already present in the brain, as are most of the connections. However, many of the connecting fibers still lack insulation. In fact, the brain of an adult is larger than the brain of a newborn baby mainly because of the insulation that is added in the years after birth. We know from neuroanatomy that the connecting fibers of different areas of the brain are myelinated at different

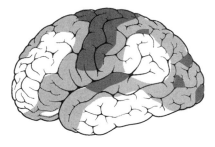

Figure 8.6
Order of myelinization of the brain (after Flechsig 1920). Areas that are myelinated early are drawn in dark gray; the light gray areas become myelinated later; and the white areas latest (at about the time of puberty).

ages after birth (figure 8.6). The neuropsychiatrist Paul Flechsig drew detailed maps of the cortex that indicated at which point in time after birth the various areas were fully developed, that is, connected to other areas by myelinated fibers (Flechsig 1929). These maps, although based on microanatomical data, are highly informative about brain function, as a nonmyelinated fiber is something like a telephone line that is not yet connected; it is there, but it has no function. Only when the fibers get their insulation and are able carry information quickly does a given area go on line and begin working with other areas.

We know that the primary sensory-motor areas are hooked up with myelinated fibers at birth. The baby comes complete with the basic hardware it needs to move, see, hear, and feel. Subsequently, secondary areas receive insulation, and the developmental process ends with the myelinization of fibers connecting the highest cortical areas, most notably the frontal lobes. Some parts of the frontal lobes are fully functionally connected to the brain as late as at puberty (Fuster 1995).

Compared to other primates, the development of the human brain proceeds slowly. This has long been regarded as a major drawback that needs an explanation, as the "unfinished" baby is, from an evolutionary point of view, highly vulnerable. Such slow brain development would appear to be maladaptive.

One suggested explanation for the particularly slow postnatal brain development is that a fully developed human brain would not fit through the birth channel. Because of our upright posture, which puts static constraints upon the width of the pelvis, this opening is unusually narrow. The female human pelvis was thought to result from conflicting evolutionary pressures: the advantages of upright posture (hence its narrowness) and the necessity to allow passage of the baby's head (hence, its need to be wide). Upright posture, which frees the hands for tasks other than locomotion (for example, manufacturing and using tools), in turn requires more complex means of guiding fine movements, planning the uses of tools, and thinking things through. Therefore, a large brain is needed to harvest the benefits of upright posture, even though only a small brain can pass through the female pelvis, whose very static construction allows upright posture in the first place. As a corollary, we note that there are no complicated births in monkeys (the babies fall out of their mothers quickly and without much to-do), because they do not walk upright and need no big head to house a big brain. This is, in brief, the view of contemporary anthropology about why human babies—unlike the offspring of other species—are so immature at birth and have to go through years of development. One prominent anthropologist discussed this state of affairs by characterizing the newborn human being as a defective and incomplete creature (*ein Mängelwesen;* see Gehlen 1978) and as an altricial animal (*Nesthocker*). The basis of this claim is, of course, the incomplete connections, at birth, between certain cortical areas, most notably the frontal lobes.

Interaction of Brain Development and Learning

Computer simulations of neural networks are usually performed with models that do not change grossly; that is, during learning they change only with respect to synaptic weights. The number of neurons and connecting fibers is established at the beginning, and this architecture remains constant throughout the simulation. Only recently have modelers started to study what happens in neural networks that are not static but are subject to developmental change (Elman 1991, 1994, 1995). The results are fascinating and throw a completely new light on the above discussion of infant development in humans and, especially, the role of the immature frontal cortex.

Elman set out to study the ability of the network type he had developed to learn about the complex input-output relations that must be at work whenever we understand complex sentences. Because Elman networks take into account the sequence of patterns, he reasoned that they should be able to process not just single words, but also complex sentences. In brief, Elman networks should be able to learn grammar. After training, they should, for example, be able to predict the part of speech of the next word in an incomplete sentence. Being able to make such predictions implies a knowledge of grammar rules. Elman believed that these networks should be able to learn grammar because they take sequential (temporal) patterns into account.

At first, the results of simulations were disappointing. When sentences of varying complexity were used as input patterns, the network only learned to "understand" simple sentences—that is, to make correct grammatical predictions for them. Complex sentences, such as sentences with embedded clauses, seemed to be beyond the reach of its comprehension. It appeared unable to extract the complex rules that structure the sequence of such sentences.

Further simulations, however, proved that the network *was* able to digest complex sentences and to learn complex grammar. It did so when researchers first used simple sentences as input. Once the network had successfully learned these simple sentences, they added complex sentences to the set of input patterns. Complexity was thereby able to piggyback upon simplicity. We can compare this method with the way we learn a foreign language—by first learning simple structures and then more complicated ones. We would not get very far by starting out with the most complicated structures in the new and unknown language. We learn complex structure on top of simple structures.

Although this finding makes perfect sense in the context of our school systems and institutions of higher learning, it creates problems when applied to biological reality. The complex environment of organisms does not come with a teacher to provide a carefully controlled sequence of inputs (i.e., learning experiences), with simple ones given first and more complicated ones introduced once simple tasks have been successfully learned. The difficulty is quite obvious when we look at how children learn their first language. Although studies have shown that caretakers usually engage in some kind of baby babble during about the child's first year of life, most children are subject to all kinds of language input. We do not take much care to ensure that we give children only language input that they can process. If language acquisition were dependent upon such carefully orchestrated, increasingly complex sets of input, few of us—quite possibly none—would actually learn our first language. In brief, we cannot assume that in real-world learning anyone is taking care to provide the input in the most effective way. With respect to language, children are bathed in all kinds of inputs from the very beginning.

It is of interest, therefore, that in further simulations Elman demonstrated another condition that leads to the successful learning of complex input patterns. When the capacity of the context layer was set at a low level and then increased during learning, the network learned complex grammatical structures. This was the case even if complex input was given to the network from the very beginning of training. Obviously, the network was able to extract simple rules of grammar first and then increasingly complicated ones because it was itself developing its processing capacity from low to high as it learned.

To a network with low-context processing power, input sequences governed by complex rules (sentences with embedded clauses) are just like input sequences without any rules. Hence, no rules are learned, and the complicated input is processed as if it were nothing but computational noise. To such a network, natural language, with its mixture of simple and complex structures, is nothing but a mixture of simple structures and no structure at all. Because of its limited capacity, the network extracts only simple structures from the input, and hence, learns only those simple structures. Once the simple structures have been learned, and once an increase in the processing power of the context layer has taken place, it can process somewhat more complicated input structures. It can do so because it has become capable of holding more information together on line (increased capacity) and because it can piggyback its learning, that is, use the already-learned simple structure to process the more complex input.

The increased capacity of the system, therefore, automatically takes care of what a good teacher does: it provides the system with digestible input. Generally speaking, a system whose capacity increases during learning can learn complex structures better than a system working at full capacity from the start.

These results from computer simulations with Elman networks shed new light on frontal lobe development. In contrast to animals that possess a fully developed brain at birth, the postnatally developing brain of the human infant permits it to learn more complex structures. The process of extrauterine maturation takes place mainly in the frontal cortex—that is, the area in which the highest and most complex mental functions, including language, are localized. In addition, the frontal cortex is the part of the brain connected to other parts of the brain in a kind of extra feedback loop, just as the context layer in an Elman network is connected to the hidden layer. The frontal lobes are the site of working memory, where immediately relevant information is kept on line to be applied to the here and now. In children this part of the brain comes on line during nursery school and the very early grades.

With respect to language acquisition, this developmental scenario implies that the not fully developed frontal lobes of the newborn baby are not an obstacle but rather a prerequisite for learning the complexities of language.

Pidgin and Creole Languages

The computer simulations performed by Elman not only explain why there is a critical period for language acquisition, but also why children are able to invent new languages and adults cannot (see Pinker 1994).

Pidgin and creole languages are forms of communication that come into being whenever people speaking different languages have to communicate with each other without really learning each other's language. *Pidgin languages* have highly reduced repertoires of only seven hundred to fifteen hundred words and are structurally extremely simple. Pidgin languages are, by definition, not anyone's mother tongue. When a mixture of languages actually becomes the mother tongue of someone, it is called a *creole language* (see Katzner 1995; Todd 1990).

It used to be assumed that the transition from a pidgin language into a creole happens slowly and gradually. Detailed linguistic studies, however, have shown that all it takes to bring about a creole language is children growing up under certain conditions. If during the period of language acquisition children are exposed to a pidgin language only, their speech will spontaneously develop complex structures and all the features that characterize a true language. This formation of a creole language is driven by the subtle use of pidgin and by the ability of children to produce complex grammatical structures from any kind of input. As the philosopher Ludwig Wittgenstein reminds us in his *Logical Investigations* (1969:241), a language is a form of life and so includes our environmental responses, including social behavior. These interactions with the environment and other people will always be complex, even if the language used is not, as in the case of pidgin. This complexity of life and action is obviously enough to drive the development of a new language, as long as *children* are exposed to it.

Pinker (1994) describes linguistic studies of children working and growing up at the turn of the century in sugar plantations in Hawaii. Some of these children were looked after by overseers who spoke only Pidgin English to them. The children spontaneously developed a language that was more complex than Pidgin English, not only with respect to wording but also in its grammatical structures. Adults, however, are not capable of developing a language in the same way; they remain pidgin speakers, because they have lost the capacity to extract complex structure from the hodgepodge of input patterns without a teacher.

The acquisition of the first language (the mother tongue), we may infer, necessarily presupposes a brain under development. This can explain why so-called feral children, like Caspar Hauser and others not exposed to language at a young age, never master language properly. One of the best described cases is the American girl Genie, who was kept in isolation by her father until the age of 13, and who never learned English properly despite intensive teaching by teachers and linguists (see Mestel 1995, Rymer 1992). As the simulations performed by Elman show, the reason appears to be neurocomputational in nature.

Linguistic observations in Nicaragua may serve as yet a further example. Until the reform of the education system in 1979 by the Sandinista regime, there was no official sign language for the deaf. Contrary to widely held prejudices and opinions, sign language is not a set of convoluted gestures and pantomimes devised by well-meaning hearing caregivers. Instead, a sign language comes into existence in communities of deaf people in which children grow up. A sign language is a complete language, with its own words and grammar and everything else that belongs to a language. Just as there is no single language on earth, there is no single sign language for deaf people, but rather many. American Sign Language (ASL), for example, is completely different from British Sign Language and contains elements of Native American languages (Pinker 1994).

Until the end of the 1970s, deaf children in Nicaragua were drilled in lipreading, without much success. The children, however, used signs to communicate—signs that were determined by the circumstances of their individual environment and community. However, the children lacked adequate language input and their sign language, with its highly restricted vocabulary and grammatical structure, was only a pidgin language. Because of the education reforms of the Sandinista government, deaf children were schooled together, and deaf young children began growing up in an environment rich in the use of the signs the older children employed for communication (sign pidgin). Like the children in Hawaii exposed to Pidgin English who formed their own creole speech, the children in Nicaragua spontaneously produced their own rich, full-blown sign language. At present, deaf children in Nicaragua use this sign language, which is similar to other creole languages (see Pinker 1994). Most researchers currently hold that deaf children should learn sign language as early as possible in order to train their language capabilities as much as possible (Mestel 1995). Observations of feral children like Genie demonstrate that normal acquisition of a mother tongue is no longer possible after the age of 12 or 13.

It is unlikely that the insights gained from Elman's simulations apply only to language acquisition. The acquisition of any complex aptitude, it seems, is likely to be dependent on the interaction of brain development and learning. As mentioned above, language is not acquired in isolation from our social circumstances, but instead comes out of the life-world. Other complex structures in this world, such as social relations, facts and relations in the physical and biological sphere, as well as the complexities of art and music are, like language, acquired by children under development.

The developing brain takes care of the fact that the input (i.e., what is to be learned) is filtered in such a way that simple and basic things are learned first, while more complex learning is piggybacked on earlier, basic learning. A developing brain, therefore, does not need a teacher. It needs only experiences, which it can use and process without a teacher.

From an evolutionary point of view, the postnatally developing brain must represent a compromise. This compromise, however, is not between brain size and the size of the female pelvis, but is, instead, neurocomputational in nature. Surely there is evolutionary pressure for organisms to be born as "ready made" as possible. The human newborn, in 'this respect, does pretty badly, and we may ask (just as earlier anthropologists did) about the advantage of long postnatal brain development. This advantage, we may say now, lies in the capability to learn and process much more complex input patterns, that is information about environmental structures. The better an organism is at this task, the better it will perform in the world (which we assume to be highly complex), and, hence, the more likely it is to survive. The human baby, it follows, is the result of the compromise between being fit and ready from the start, on the one hand, and becoming even fitter later, on the other. Unlike other species, the human emphasis is on the latter aspect—potential for the future.

You need not fantasize much to imagine the consequences of the issue under discussion. Children are different from one another. Evolution always brings about both a mean and a variance of a feature. The single individual, however, is special in that it has a specific genetic makeup and its own unique history of learning. This implies that not everything is good for everybody. Although developing brains take care of their own input somewhat automatically, we may still assume that the better learning is synchronized with development, the more effective it will be. Because of these mechanisms, people will be quite different once they reach adulthood.

This also means we should no longer take our methods of educating our children from outdated and old-fashioned dogmatic theories but, rather, should base them on real knowledge about learning and memory! Neural network simulations can contribute to such dearly needed knowledge.

Recap

Our brain is full of feedback loops. Cortical neurons receive most of their information from other cortical neurons and, hence, indirectly from themselves. Researchers can use Hopfield networks to simulate the behavior of biological networks characterized by massive feedback.

A crucial feature of such feedback networks consists of the fact that their behavior—that is, changes of their activational state over time—is dependent not only on changing inputs but also on the previous activation state, which itself is part of the input (because of the massive number of built-in feedback connections). Therefore, such networks can represent the temporal sequences of activation states they undergo when they receive input.

Hopfield networks have the remarkable ability to recognize input patterns that were previously learned, even when they are presented in a degraded or only partial form. The behavior of the network during recognition has been likened to the response of a system drawn by gravity toward an attractor.

In addition to the input, hidden, and output layers, Elman networks are characterized by a context layer, which is hooked up to the hidden layer. This context layer provides the hidden layer with the pattern of its own previous activation state. In Elman networks, therefore, single patterns are not processed in isolation but in their temporal sequence. Thus Elman networks are capable of representing structures—grammar is a good example—for which sequential order is important. Computer simulations of language processing have revealed that the processing of complex sentences (those containing embedded clauses) can only be learned if the capacity of the context layer is increased during learning. Neurobiologically, the context layer is analogous to the frontal lobes, the site of the psychological function of working memory.

Simulations demonstrate that a developing brain can learn more complex things than a brain that comes ready made at birth. From Flechsig's maps of the cortex we learned that the brain of the newborn child is immature at birth and develops gradually. Compared to other species, the period of postnatal brain maturation is extremely long. Furthermore, we now know that the frontal lobes—which are responsible for planning, goal-directed thinking, working memory, and (especially) keeping on line the immediately relevant (language) context—are the subject of the longest postnatal maturation. Only at puberty do the fibers connecting the frontal lobes become completely myelinated and, therefore, integrated into the brain's information-processing system.

With respect to language acquisition in children, this sequence of development implies that an immature brain at birth is not an obstacle but rather a prerequisite for learning complex grammatical structures. It explains why there is a critical period for language learning (and, very likely, for other complex cognitive abilities) after which a child is unable to acquire these abilities. To a system with limited information-processing capacity, complex input is nothing but noise and leaves no traces in the system. The developing brain can thus filter inputs and learn simple, basic things first, making it possible to process increasingly complex materials subsequently.

The neural network simulations also cast new light on older anthropological explanations of why there is an extended period of postnatal development in human beings. These ideas characterized the infant's immaturity as a nuisance that, although necessary for birth, was detrimental to cognitive functioning. The simulations, however, demonstrate that only a brain in the process of development can extract complex structures from the environment. In short, a fully functioning frontal lobe at birth would be detrimental for our ability to learn the complexities of our life-world, including language. Historically, these conclusions are quite unusual. The thinker who came closest to anticipating them may have been the eighteenth-century German philosopher Johann Gottlieb Herder, who, in his *Treatise on the Origin of Language* (1772), speculated that human language acquisition is related to specifically human instincts.

III

Applications

Neural networks can form ideal types and create abstract representations of the general features of input data. Self-organizing feature maps extract any kind of regularities from input patterns and map them onto a two-dimensional surface according to similarity, frequency, and importance. Additional layers in networks hold relevant context on line. We can apply these ideas and principles of functioning to a great many questions and problems concerning human experience and behavior. The possible areas of research range from creativity to delusional states, from developmental psychology to memory processes and disorders of thinking.

9

Representing Knowledge

Until a few years ago there was little reason to doubt that the concepts of psychology would someday be able to explain everything that happens in the brain. We spoke of thoughts, intentions, emotions, memories, and so on, and assumed that these phenomena have equivalents in the brain that somehow resemble these thoughts, intentions, emotions, and memories. For example, some psychologists sought to explain the structure of thoughts, which we subjectively perceive as inner speech, in terms of formal symbolic logic operating upon internally stored knowledge. These attempts employed computer programs that mimic mental functions by manipulating symbols and, often, complicated algorithms represented on flow charts. As we saw in chapter 1, however, brains and computers are very different. A brain is not programmed the way computers are, and does not clearly distinguish between the storage and processing of data. But if they don't do it the way computers do, how *is* knowledge stored in our brains?

Static Rules versus Dynamic Processes

Within the past decades psychologists have often postulated that memories are stable and related to one another during thought through the application of rules. These ideas therefore characterized memory as *static* and *rule-based*. It was conceived in this way because no one really knew how the brain brings about the higher mental functions. In other words, we knew that there were thoughts, on the one hand, and brain structures, on the other, but we did not have the slightest idea how their respective realms come together. This problem has often been referred to as the mind-body problem (or the brain-mind problem) and has been viewed by empirical scientists as intractable.

This situation has changed. In current psychology, network models of mental functions play a major role. They allow us to simulate with computer models all kinds of psychological phenomena—from objective behavior to the most subjective fleeting thoughts and sensations—and so achieve a deeper understanding of the processes and principles that govern them. Like James Watt—who did not ask, "How could heat bring about motion" but instead investigated the principles by which various forms of energy are transformed and then applied them to the real world—psychologists now recognize that general questions (such as "How does the brain produce consciousness") are ill founded. This way of thinking is new to psychology. In the past, psychological theories were often characterized by a large degree of vagueness, so that almost any observation could be made to fit a theory. Because this made theories immune to falsification, it rendered them practically useless. Any theory that is indifferent to empirical data is useless! Human beings (*all* human beings, not just scientists) theorize, in order to gain a better understanding of their experiences, organize them in meaningful ways, and predict future experiences.

The advantage of psychological theories based on neural network models lies in the ability to test their predictions by means of simulations. Moreover, such simulations often produce new phenomena and unexpected functional characteristics that might never have been discovered by data collection, statistical analysis, and clever thinking alone. In short, psychological theories based on neural network models are not only more applicable and testable but also more fruitful than earlier theories. Simulations not only provide better answers, but also new questions!

A decade on neural network research has changed our view of mental processes as static and rule-based to dynamic and process-based. Mental functions are not rule-based operations acting on static symbols; instead, they more closely resemble processes that can be only approximately described by rules and that involve the constant change of internal representations. Rules, for example the rules that govern our use of language, are not *in the head* as such; nor are they *used* to produce language. The rules of grammar merely provide a parsimonious post hoc description of the production and understanding of language, which actually happen in a completely different way (see Bechtel & Abrahamson 1991, Churchland & Sejnowski 1992, Clark 1993). This different way consists of vector transformations within neural networks.

In this chapter I present several examples of the new view, then, in the subsequent chapter, focus on one of the highest human cognitive functions—language.

Piaget and Stages of Development

Neural network models, because of their emphasis on learning and the self-organization of internal representations of environmental features, have a systematic affinity with developmental psychology (Karmiloff-Smith 1995). Moreover, when formulating plans for simulation experiments that included recording network performance (e.g., errors produced over a training period), modelers often focused on problems and data important in developmental psychology. In the terms of the landscape metaphor described in chapter 8 (see figure 8.3), we can view learning as a slow descent from an error mountain into a relatively error-free valley within a multidimensional error landscape. As long as the descending vehicle itself does not change, its path depends entirely upon the topography of the landscape, as McClelland and Plunkett point out:

It is, therefore, appropriate to conceive of learning in these networks as a process of gradient descent on a multidimensional error landscape. Although the device that drives learning (the learning algorithm) usually only promotes gradual change in the weight matrix, the uneven surface of the error landscape can result in relatively sudden, dramatic qualitative shifts in network performance. Conversely, the error surface may be relatively flat at a particular configuration of the weight matrix, and the behavioral consequences of weight changes may be comparatively minor. Learning in networks can easily result in periods of stable behavior interrupted by sudden discontinuities, even though the basic mechanism for learning is one of small continuous change. (McClelland & Plunkett 1995:193)

We have already discussed the model simulating the acquisition of the past tense. One of the most striking features of this model was its spontaneous generation of phases of performance that are similar to those seen in children. It should therefore come as no surprise to learn that psychologist Jean Piaget's ideas about the stages of cognitive development have inspired neural network modelers. Piagetian notions of assimilation and accommodation are of particular interest. Although conceptually distinct, these two processes are nothing but two sides of the same coin: the organism's adaptation to its environment. *Assimilation* means that an organism can only take in those parts of the environment that it somehow already knows. Every organism interprets the world according to its senses, perceptions, and cognitive structures. The small child, for example, only perceives short sentences as sentences. When the processing power of its brain increases, however, it recognizes an increasing number of longer strings of what was earlier perceived as babble (noise) as sentences. *Accommodation,* according to Piaget, is the process of change that occurs in the organism's knowledge base through new experience. Structures in the environment (spatiotemporal input patterns) are taken in by the organism and—because these input patterns guide development of internal structures—cause changes in the organism's knowledge base.

Almost by definition, assimilation and accommodation are present in any neural network model. In most cases, it is necessary to preprocess the input (i.e., to transform the input into a vectorized representation) so that it can be presented to the network (assimilation). The input then causes changes in the network it is incorporated into (accommodation).

We have already discussed two simulations in which phases in the learning process become spontaneously apparent, either because of the structure of the input or because of features inherent in the network. In the simulation of past-tense learning, we can distinguish three phases of network performance. At first the model can generate the past tenses of irregular verbs; then it can apply the rule for the regular verbs; and then it can do both—just like children (see chapter 2). Note too that the Elman networks discussed in chapter 8 could learn complex grammar only after they had learned simple grammar.

We can demonstrate the spontaneous generation of phases of development as a feature of a system that learns slowly and gradually by citing yet another example. It is based on an observation by Bärbel Inhelder and Jean Piaget published in 1958 (cited in McClelland 1989). If coun-

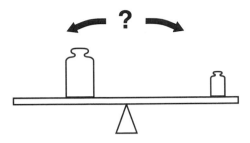

Figure 9.1
Task presented to children by Inhelder and Piaget (1958; cited in McClelland 1989).

terweights of different sizes are positioned at various distances from the vertical axle of a beam scale, children asked which side the scale will tip toward give different answers depending on their ages (figure 9.1).

1. At the age of five (phase 1), the children's answers take only the size of the weight into account. (Note that children under the age of four years old cannot fully understand the task.)
2. In phase 2 the children take into account the distance of the weight from the axle of the scale but only in cases where the same weight is sitting on both sides of the scale.
3. In phase 3 the children take into account both the weight and the distance, but inconsistently so.
4. Only in phase 4 do the children appear to have formed a rule with respect to the weight and the fulcrum of the scales, thereby giving consistent answers for various weights and distances.

McClelland was able to demonstrate that these phases, which had been empirically observed in children, also occur in a network model of the task. A network was trained with sets of two weights and two points on the beam scales to produce the correct output: prediction of the direction toward which the scale would tip. At first, the network performed rather badly (like children under the age of four). Then there was a rapid transition to phase 1, after which the network went through the same stages as children do.

The crucial point of this simulation consists in the fact that during the entire simulation the synaptic weights were changed gradually. Moreover, the processes involved were always the same. Nonetheless, the overt behavior of the model displayed distinct phases! Hence, it was demonstrated that developmental phases may occur spontaneously as a systems feature of neural network learning.

Memory

Learning and memory are essential features of both the cortex and the hippocampus, a structure located deep within the temporal lobes (figure 9.2). On the basis of a large number of animal experiments, researchers long assumed that the hippocampus stores only spatial information (as in the rat experiment reported in chapter 4, which demonstrated that the animals stored the spatial coordinates of their environment in the hippocampus). However, we now know that even the rat's hippocampus does more than merely store spatial coordinates (Bunsey & Eichenbaum 1996).

Living without the Hippocampus

The hippocampus must play a major role in the short-term (and medium-term) storage of memories, for if the hippocampus is damaged in both hemispheres, *anterograde amnesia* results. This condition is characterized clinically by the inability to form new memories. The most widely known patient with this condition is H.M., who in the mid-1950s underwent surgical ablation of both hippocampuses and of other structures in the temporal lobes for treatment of severe seizures (Scoville & Milner 1957, Corkin 1984, Hilts 1995). Since his operation, this man, who lives without new memories, has been unable to live on his own, thereby demonstrating the importance of memory for almost every aspect of our lives. He can read the same newspaper every morning, and the investigators who tested him had to introduce themselves every time they came—even when they had visited only the day before. Anything that H.M. had to remember for more than a few minutes was gone.

In most cases, when both sides of the hippocampus are damaged, patients also suffer from *retrograde amnesia*, in which memory loss is most complete for events that occurred in the weeks, and even months, just before the injury and tapers off for events in the more distant past.

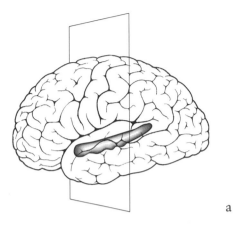

a

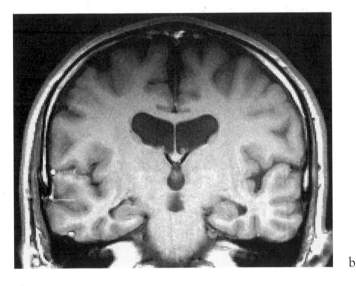

b

Figure 9.2
Location of the hippocampus in the human brain (top). A magnetic-resonance image of the cross section depicted at the top is shown at the bottom. The hippocampus is located at the lower inner part of the temporal lobes (the black arrows point to it).

That is, events that took place a week before the damage occurred are remembered less well than events that took placed a month before then.

A number of studies has demonstrated that the loss of memory found with hippocampal damage mainly involves memory for events—facts, and relations between facts. The memory for skills, such as riding a bicycle or writing in mirror script, is largely spared. H.M., for example, was trained to write mirror script after his operation, and he attained this ability about as quickly as most people do.

Because of these and other findings, two types of learning and memory have been distinguished by psychologists:

1. *Explicit learning,* also referred to as *episodic* and *declarative memory* (memory for events; knowing that . . .)
2. *Implicit learning,* also called *nondeclarative* and *procedural memory* (memory for *motor skills* and *capabilities;* knowing how to . . .).

Patients with lesions on both sides of the hippocampus suffer from a massive impairment of explicit memory, whereas implicit learning remains intact. This has led to the assumption that the hippocampus is involved only in explicit learning.

Memory in the Network

Why does it take both the cortex and the hippocampus (i.e., two modules) to form memories? McClelland and coworkers (1995) proposed a neural network model of the cortex and the hippocampus that clarifies the role of each structure and the teamwork necessary to the formation of memories. To fully grasp the significance of the model, we have to understand, in general, how the function of memory is implemented in simulated neural networks. As we have seen before, the following points are important:

1. Knowledge is represented by the strengths of the synaptic connections between neurons. The very same neurons that store information also carry out its processing.
2. Whenever information is processed, the strengths of the synaptic connections between neurons change a little. The changes have to be small in order to avoid oscillations in the system.
3. The long-term effect of learning is adaptation of the network to the input patterns and the extraction of their general structure.

In preceding chapters, we encountered examples of these features of network functioning. Furthermore, we can all think of skills that illustrate them, like riding a bicycle or playing the piano, which often require rather a long period of repetitive training that leads, gradually, to an increase in skill.

Applying these characteristics of network functioning to our understanding of the cortex can explain a number of the characteristic features of learning and memory. However, such a model still fails to capture two essential features of memory: our ability, first, to memorize single events and, second, to avoid rather easily the *interference effects* between already-learned patterns and new patterns the model has to learn. Let us look at these features in more detail.

Single Events versus Generality

If neural networks form representations of general structures from a great many examples, the changes in the synaptic weights that occur during the processing of any given single input pattern must be very small. This implies that single events are not learned as such.

Because synaptic weights in the cortex appear to change slowly, it seems that the cortex cannot be used for the memory of single events (episodes, facts). For a neuronal structure to store single events, its synaptic weights have to change rapidly and in large increments. In other words, there is a trade-off between the level of generality that can be attained by the representations in a network and the network's ability to represent single events. You cannot have it both ways; the goals of representing the general structure of the environment and single events are mutually exclusive, if they are to be realized within a single network structure.

Catastrophic Interference

A good gymnastics coach knows that you must not teach the somersault and the flip-flop (backward handspring) during the same lesson, because their movement patterns are opposite to each other. They interfere with one another; that is, each one hinders the learning of the other. Similarly, if you try to study two foreign languages at the same time, you may experience the same effect; you may mix them up and end up learning very little.

Such interference phenomena can be readily observed in neural network simulations of learning. If a network has learned a general rule from a lot of input patterns, new and incompatible patterns can lead to interference. This is called *catastrophic interference,* because the learning of new information may completely wipe out whatever has been previously learned. McClelland and coworkers. (1995) provide an example to illustrate this point.

As we will explain in chapter 10, we can present combinations of words and their meanings (i.e., a vectorized list of attributes) to a network as input, whereupon the network will come up with an orderly representation of the input. In such a network, the word *swallow* may become associated with *can fly* and with *is a bird.* Likewise, the word *herring* may be associated with *can swim* and with *is a fish.* If a network that has learned these associations is then presented with the new input pattern of *penguin*—associated with the features *can swim* and *is a bird* but not with the feature *can fly*—catastrophic interference may result. The network may associate *bird* with *can fly* and with *can swim* and generalizes this new pattern over other patterns it has already learned.

In computer simulations of neural networks, catastrophic interference can be prevented by alternating the new input with the old input, a procedure called *interleaved learning.* This method allows the network to learn the new pattern and at the same time keep the old ones. McClelland and coworkers explain this phenomenon as follows: "Interleaved learning allows the network to carve out a place for the penguin, adjusting its representation of other similar concepts and adjusting its connection weights to incorporate the penguin into its structured knowledge system" (McClelland et al. 1995:434).

Thus an ideal memory network should meet the following demands:

1. It must be able to store general structures; therefore its learning should be slow.

2. It must be able to learn new facts that are presented only once.

3. It must not forget what has been learned whenever something new is learned. This can only happen if new information is learned together with old information in an interleaved way.

Race Against Decay

It is quite obvious that a single-module network cannot meet the all these demands. A network may learn either slowly or quickly but never both at the same time. Furthermore, how can a single network learn new information and keep what it has already learned?

McClelland and coworkers propose that this problem is solved by the systematic teamwork of the hippocampus and the cortex. Their arguments are important and interesting, because they are based on neurobiological and psychological grounds as well as on computational considerations and simulations. By thus drawing on data and theory from different fields, the authors present an impressive model of memory.

Let us start with what we already know. In chapter 4 we described the experiments of Wilson and McNaughton (1993), which convincingly demonstrate that neurons in the hippocampus can learn—that is, can form new representations of locations in the environment—within minutes.

The Hippocampus as the Trainer of the Cortex

More recent studies performed by the same group of researchers provide further, highly interesting results. The researchers allowed the rats to check out their new environment and then put them to sleep. Recordings from the hippocampus taken during the nap showed that the connections newly formed during the preceding learning session were activated (Wilson & McNaughton 1994). In other words, the new experience-driven patterns of activity were processed again while the animals were sleeping (i.e., while they were *off line*).

Because of the dense connections between the hippocampus and the cortex, it can be assumed that this activation during sleep provided the cortex with some sort of a replay of the input acquired during the learning episode. In other words, whenever a certain pattern becomes active in the hippocampus, this pattern is "downloaded" to the cortex, which—in contrast to the hippocampus—learns very slowly. When we learn to ride a bike, or ski, or dance, we directly experience the slow speed of the cortex, in that we have to repeat the skill over and over again in order to gradually become proficient. This type of learning occurs in the cortical areas that control movement, which are not affected by the hippocampus. The slowness of our learning provides us with a clue to how slow the cortex really is.

In contrast, when we experience something new and interesting (i.e., a new fact, not a new skill), it is first stored in the hippocampus. This structure then serves as the *trainer of the cortex,* by repeatedly presenting the newly learned input patterns to the cortex. The hippocampus therefore does exactly what we do with conscious effort when we train ourselves in a new motor skill: It repeats the patterns to be stored over and over again.

This model of the functioning of the hippocampus and the cortex has the following consequences for our understanding of memory.

1. There are not two different systems for implicit and explicit learning. Instead, the function of memory is performed by an integrated system composed of the hippocampus and the cortex. The cortex always learns the same way, by the repetitive processing of signals. The apparent distinction between implicit and explicit learning is due to the fact that experiences (new associations, new facts) can be stored rapidly in the hippocampus and then referred to the cortex (explicit learning). In contrast, during the implicit learning of skills, the repetitive presentation is performed not by the hippocampus but by the repetitive experiences. The person acquiring the skill has to take care of repeating the input.

2. When new facts are learned, there appears to be a race between decay of the information in the hippocampus and storage of this information in the cortex (see McClelland et al. 1995:31). The storage capacity of the relatively small hippocampus is limited, in contrast to the capacity of the relatively large cortex. It therefore makes sense for the hippocampus to present the content of its temporary storage to the cortex as quickly and as often as possible.

Anyone who has ever tried very hard to learn a skill and who remembers the experience of doing so, knows that frequent short periods of practice work better than infrequent long ones. (Practicing the piano six times for ten minutes is better than practicing once for an hour!) The reason is very simply that neural networks digest the new input with every repetition, thereby changing the weights of the synaptic connections—that is learning. Because the hippocampus takes over the repetitive training once the facts are learned, it must not be disturbed as it teaches the information to the cortex. If you do not sleep well, or you disturb your night's sleep by consuming too much caffeine or alcohol, your memory of the new fact will get worse.

3. The long-known fact that new memories take time to become fixed within memory is referred to as the *consolidation* of memory. McClelland's model explains clearly why it takes time for new information to become permanent. Consolidation is simply the changes in the cortex that take place during repetitive training by the hippocampus.

4. The model further provides a parsimonious explanation of the clinical picture presented by patients with bilateral hippocampal lesions: The anterograde amnesia results from the lack of a temporary storage area for new material. Without the hippocampus, new associations can neither be formed nor presented to the cortex. These patients' graded retrograde amnesia can be explained just as easily, in that facts are more firmly fixed in cortical long-term memory when there has been more time for them to be repetitively downloaded from the hippocampus. The salvaged ability to acquire new skills (implicit learning) is due simply to the fact that the hippocampus is not needed for their acquisition. Even without a hippocampus, the cortex can still learn, as long as training is repetitive.

It is evident that insights from network simulations have practical therapeutic consequences—but not just for the treatment of patients with hippocampal lesions. Such therapeutic implications of neural network research are discussed further below and in chapter 12.

A Neural Network Model of Alzheimer's Disease

In 1906 the neuropathologist Alois Alzheimer described pathological changes in the brain of a deceased fifty-six-year-old woman who had suffered from progressively severe dementia in the years before her death. Later it became clear that similar microscopic changes can be found in the brains of many elderly demented patients. At the beginning of such dementia processes, the memory for new facts is particularly impaired, while other mental functions remain intact. Later, long-term memory is also impaired and, during the final stage, the person becomes completely incapacitated, is no longer able to recognize close relatives, and requires permanent physical care.

In the recent past, the senile and presenile dementia of the Alzheimer type, as this disorder is currently called, has been the subject of intensive research. The reason for this is simply the frighteningly high frequency of the disorder, which strikes from 2 to 4 percent of all people over the age of sixty. Moreover, after that age, the relative frequency of the disorder doubles every five years (Cummings 1993). Even though we do not yet fully comprehend the cause of the disorder, recently impressive progress has been made in understanding certain aspects of it. One such aspect is captured by the model of Alzheimer's disease proposed by Michael Hasselmo (1994). This model, like other neural network models, puts together a number of otherwise inexplicable or unrelated characteristics of the disorder.

Hasselmo starts from the fact that in neural network simulations we often have to distinguish the learning phase from the retrieval phase. During learning, the spreading of activation throughout the network must be prevented to some degree; otherwise, synaptic activation and change spread through the entire network like an avalanche, and no information is learned. This phenomenon is called *runaway synaptic modification*. Let us look at an example of it.

In a small neural network three input patterns have to be learned by three neurons of the output layer. The function to be learned is depicted in figure 9.3. The network (like the simple network for pattern recognition discussed in chapter 2) has to learn an association between the activation patterns on the left and the activation patterns on the right.

As figure 9.4 shows, the learning of the first pattern occurs without any problems. Neurons A and B, as well as neuron 1, are activated by some process external to the network, strengthening the connection between neurons A and 1 and between B and 1. This process causes the first input pattern to become correctly associated with the desired output.

When the second pattern is learned, however, an undesired association is formed as well. Neurons B and C, as well as neuron 2, are externally activated to strengthen the associations between B and 2 and between C

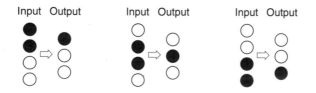

Figure 9.3
Relations between input and output patterns to be learned by the network (active neurons in black; inactive neurons in white).

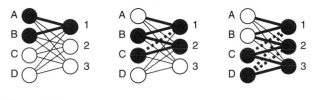

Figure 9.4
Two-layer network learning the input-output function depicted in figure 9.3.

and 2. As the connection between B and 1, however, has already been strengthened, neuron 1 may become active during learning of the second pattern. Because neurons B and C, as well as neurons 1 and 2, are now simultaneously active, not only are the connections between B and 2 and C and 2 strengthened, but (because of the already-strengthened association between B and 1), the connection between C and 1 (the dotted line in the center of figure 9.4) is also strengthened. The same thing happens again when the third pattern is learned. In this case, in addition to the desired connection, two undesired associations between neurons D and 2, and between neurons D and 1 are formed.

In most computer-simulated network models, runaway synaptic modification is prevented by inhibiting the spread of activation within the network during learning, because such spread, as we just have seen, interferes with learning. Only during the process of retrieval (i.e., whenever the network carries out what it has previously learned) does the spread of activation through the network become essential. This change in the spread of activation within computer simulations of networks can be regulated in various ways by mathematical procedures. The question, however, is how runaway synaptic modification is prevented in biological systems—for example, in our brain.

Again, the problem is that during learning the network must be sensitive to activation from outside, while the spread of activation through internal connections must be suppressed. When information is recalled, by contrast, activation has to be able to spread throughout the network. Recent neurobiological findings on the role of *acetylcholine* in the dynamics of cortical activation are of special importance for this framework of requirements. For a long time, researchers have known that acetylcholine is related to processes of learning and memory. The substance is produced by a small number of neurons clustered together in a so-called nucleus (the *nucleus basalis Meynert*). From there, acetylcholine is distributed through almost the entire brain by means of tiny fibers that head toward the cortex.

Experiments using slices of the entorhinal cortex (the part of the cortex that processes information from the sense of smell) have demonstrated that acetylcholine selectively suppresses excitatory synaptic connections between neurons in the same cortical region. In contrast, signals from other cortical areas can pass through synapses unimpaired. In short, acetylcholine has the very function needed in neuronal networks to prevent runaway synaptic modification so that learning from new and overlapping patterns can occur. In order to be effective, acetylcholine must be liberated during learning but not during retrieval. This demand, in turn, presupposes the existence of a fast-acting mechanism that evaluates and detects the novelty of an incoming stimulus pattern and sends that evaluation to the nucleus basalis Meynert. The existence of such a mechanism in the brain is conceivable and has, in fact, been assumed for other reasons, even though researchers have not as yet produced a detailed explanation of how it works (see Hasselmo 1994:22).

For many years, researchers have known that the amount of acetylcholine in the brains of Alzheimer's patients is lower than normal. However, before Hasselmo's model it was not clear how the lack of this substance affects learning. Within the framework of the model, however, we can begin to see what happens when the brain is deficient in acetylcholine.

1. The model explains why the learning of new information is severely affected at an early stage of Alzheimer's disease.

2. We know that overly active neurons using the transmitter glutamate may be damaged by their own excessive activity. This phenomenon, referred to as *excitotoxicity,* has been well observed in glutamatergic neurons and has long been implicated in the neuronal loss seen in the brains of Alzheimer's sufferers. The functional role of acetylcholine in the prevention of runaway synaptic modification explains how lack of that substance can lead to excitotoxicity and neuronal loss.

If acetylcholine is decreased or lacking, the number of associations that form within neural networks increases (as shown in figure 9.4), which causes increased neuronal activation when a new input is presented. In short, acetylcholine puts the brakes on cortical excitation that occurs during encoding; lack of acetylcholine, therefore, increases cortical excitation. In these circumstances, any new learning causes changes in undesired as well as desired synaptic connections; the undesired changes not only interfere with learning but also lead to the increased activation of glutamatergic neurons, which, as mentioned above, can be toxic for the neurons themselves.

Hasselmo's model predicts that the pathological changes observable under the microscope in the brains of deceased patients with Alzheimer's disease would occur in the brain areas, like the hippocampus, that are highly involved in associative learning. Thus the model predicts that the hippocampus should be particularly affected in Alzheimer's disease, which is exactly what has been found. The typical pathological changes of Alzheimer's disease—most importantly the Alzheimer tangles—become visible first and most frequently in the hippocampus. Even within the hippocampus, the Alzheimer's-related pathology occurs in regions known to have the most easily modifiable synaptic connections, notably those in which the long-term potentiation discussed in chapter 3 was first discovered.

Hasselmo discusses a number of other neuropathological changes that can be easily explained by the model (1994:22–37). With the guidance of this detailed and neurobiologically highly explicit computational model, researchers may even be able to envision new therapeutic strategies for Alzheimer's and other disorders.

Recap

Neural network models represent a new way to approach a central issue in psychology, the question of how knowledge is stored in the brain. Contemporary views on learning and memory are therefore subject to rapid advances and change.

The examples we have considered in this chapter each shed some light upon the storage of knowledge. Neural network models of developmental stages, of the function of memory, and of a severe mental disorder of elderly people make it clear that neural network models can be put to work in the fields of developmental psychology as well as the psychology of learning and memory. Such models can explain how gradual uniform development can nonetheless bring about distinct stages of child development. They help us understand features of neural systems that cannot be grasped at other levels of description and analysis.

From the computational point of view provided by considering issues at the network level, we can clarify why and how the hippocampus and the cortex work together when new facts are learned (with the former functioning as the teacher of the latter). The network perspective also allows us to see why the lack of acetylcholine in the entire brain first causes pathology in the hippocampus—because when the brake on formation of new associations permanently fails, the structure that forms new associations most quickly burns out first.

These considerations demonstrate that the psychological harvest from the seeds of network models is not yet over. In fact it has only just started, as the next chapters show.

10

Semantic Networks

There are about eight thousand languages in this world. The exact number is unknown and hard to determine. By definition, a language is different from a dialect in that an interpreter is needed for the former but not for the latter. However, if you travel from Innsbruck, Austria, to Amsterdam in the Netherlands, you will notice a continuous change of the language, which is called *German* at the start of your journey, and *Dutch* at the end. Any two locals from villages and cities thirty miles apart will have no trouble communicating, but any two native speakers, one from Innsbruck and one from Amsterdam, will definitely need an interpreter (Comrie 1990).

There are marked differences in the number of people speaking any particular language. More than half the world's population speaks one of the following five languages: Chinese, English, Spanish, Russian, and Hindi. Ninety-five percent of the world's population speak the one hundred most common languages. At the other end of the scale, fewer than a thousand people speak about a third of the world's languages (Kleiner 1995). In Ethiopia, for example, the Ongota language is spoken by nineteen people, while there are only six speakers of Elmolo. A few years ago, the last two people who spoke Gafat died after a linguist brought them out of the jungle into the highlands, where they caught deadly colds. The Aore language is spoken by a single inhabitant of the Pacific island-nation of Vanuatu (Vines 1995).

Wouldn't it be nice if all human beings spoke the same language? Yes and no! Of course, all of us could then communicate easily, but there would be much less to talk about! The reason for this will become obvious in this chapter.

Understanding and Speaking

Differences in ways of coding information, as discussed in chapter 4, are most obvious in language, which can be spoken and heard (i.e., an acoustic phenomenon), written (i.e., a visual system), or implemented in some other way (as in the tactile code of Braille and the body-gestalt-motion code of a sign language).

Different codes are at work when we are producing or understanding language. Immediately upon hearing or reading a word, we recode its temporal or spatial patterns into strings of specific sounds (phonemes) or graphic elements (graphemes); from these elements, we then produce the entire heard or read word (again by recoding), only to recode it once again in order to get at its meaning. There is good evidence that meanings of words are stored "in the head" differently from the sounds of words. For example, we may have a word at the tip of our tongue—which by definition means that we know what we want to say (i.e., we know the meaning), but we do not know the "name" (i.e., the sound) of the word. In 60 to 70 percent of these cases, we even know the first letter of the word, and in 60 to 80 percent we know the number of syllables (cf. Levelt 1989). If we are tired, we are more likely to encounter difficulty finding the right words, which clearly indicates that sounds and meanings are stored separately. The problem we have when tired is obviously one of recoding.

The meaning of words depends on the context in which they occur. Take, for example, the two sentences "Time flies like an arrow" and "Fruit flies like a banana." Here the words *flies* and *like* can have completely different meanings and completely different grammatical functions. How do we ever understand such sentences, if sentence comprehension depends on understanding the words, but understanding the words depends on the comprehending the entire sentence? This problem may appear familiar to you, since we have already encountered a lower-level variant of it (see figures 6.7 and 7.1). In the right context, we are able to "hear" an unknown sound correctly, as in "Standing at the river bank, the man took his net and caught a little #ish." Cases like this make it obvious that you need the whole to understand the parts, and you need the parts to understand the whole. No wonder psychological experiments suggest that we recognize words even before we recognize the single characters they are composed of (cf. Posner & Raichle 1994:chs.5, 6, Posner et al. 1996).

The solution to these apparent puzzles, or even paradoxes, is found in the way our brains process information. Cortical areas especially do not perform tasks in a serial fashion—with a higher-level operation starting after another at a lower level has finished—but operate simultaneously at various levels of complexity and coding. Areas at higher and lower levels of processing inform each other about the status of their analyses. Moreover, the analysis itself consists of feeding information back and forth between areas at several levels.

Each single step of language processing is performed by a particular cortical area that, as we have seen, has a structure able to spontaneously form maps of information presented to it (cf. chapter 5). We know that when we hear spoken language, the impulses from the inner ear are first analyzed by a frequency map, a so-called tonotopic map (figure 10.1). As all human beings perceive more or less the same sound frequencies, we may suppose that this map is quite similar in all individuals.

At the next level of processing, the incoming patterns of frequencies in time are coded as phonemes (the smallest identifiable units of sound in language). Languages differ with respect to the phonemes they use. It is well known that English speakers have trouble understanding the German word *Gemütlichkeit*. This is not so much because there are no cozy homes and restaurants in Britain and North America, but because the people living in those countries have never learned to distinguish *u* from *ü*, as this phonetic distinction does not occur in English. For a while, the German car maker Volkswagen advertised its cars in the United States by saying that they bring about the (to Americans) unpronounceable *Fahrvergnügen* (driving pleasure). Likewise, the Japanese proverbially have trouble with the distinction between "*la,*" and "*ra,*" because it does not exist in their mother tongue. It is these very differences in the use of phonemes that drive the development of cortical phonetic repre- sentations. What you do not hear, you do not learn to distinguish; such sounds do not, therefore, become represented and so cannot be used when needed.

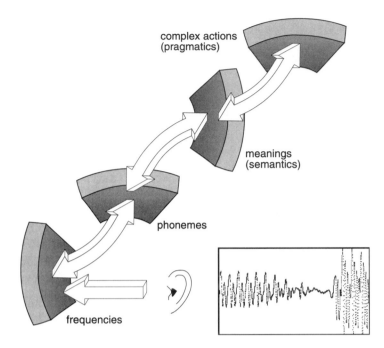

Figure 10.1
Processes of analysis during understanding of spoken language. Cortical areas
work interactively at different levels of coding and recoding information. The
spatiotemporal patterns coming in through the auditory nerve are first coded by
a frequency map, then further analyzed phonetically, semantically, and contextually. At each level, the analysis is at the same time a synthesis of what is
expected by higher-level representations and what is already there (i.e., the results
of previous analytic-synthetic processing). Hence, at each "higher" level the most
probable input pattern supposedly present at the "lower" level is synthesized and
fed back to the lower level. This is why the sound of a word can actually depend
upon its meaning and why the meaning can depend upon the context.

Among the many interesting consequences of such a cortical design is
the fact that newborn babies must be able to detect all the possible
phonemes in order to specialize gradually in the ones they actually hear.
This is exactly what recent research suggests. Any one of the world's
languages can be constructed out of a subset of the existing seventy
phonemes. (This is not a typographical error; there are in fact only about
seventy.) The English language, for example, consists of forty-four phonemes. By six months old, children are already able to distinguish be-

tween phonemes of their mother tongue and foreign phonemes, according to recordings of their electrophysiological responses to each class of phonemes (Dehaene-Lambertz & Dehaene 1994). Obviously, experience with the input patterns of speech sounds in their mother tongue causes children's language-comprehension system to develop *phonetic maps* on which only the phonemes that have become represented are actually heard. Once the map has been formed, it becomes increasingly difficult to change it. Accordingly, we know that when we learn a foreign language after puberty, we almost always speak it with a noticeable accent. Obviously, the brains of adult speakers of different languages are wired somewhat differently, at least with respect to the phonetic maps formed by experience.

The ability to understand (and utter) speech sounds may be characterized as follows: The newborn infant is potentially able to do everything but can actually do nothing. The more the infant learns about and deals with its concrete environment, the more its potential turns into capability. The flip side of the increasing capability, however, is the reduction of potential.

Now that we have dealt with a general model of language comprehension, in particular with the perception of phonemes, we can proceed to the main subject of this chapter, the representation of meaning.

Associations: What Comes to Mind, and Why

All of us have stored the meanings of several tens of thousand of words, as well as their spelling, grammatical features, categorical types, contextual relations, and pronunciations (cf. Aitchison 1994, Miller 1993). How are these meanings organized? How are they coded? How can we find out? Isn't this organization, if there is any, different in each human being?

More than two thousand years ago, Aristotle asserted that meanings are not unrelated within memory. He knew from his own experience that words come to mind in a succession determined by meaningful relations of similarity or contrast and, hence, that words must be stored in a similarly connected way. He gave the following example: Associations may go "for instance from milk to white, from white to air, from air to damp" (1975: 305)—that is, in various ways according to similarity, opposition, and contiguity.

In the eighteenth and nineteenth century, these ideas were further developed into *associationist psychology* by philosophers John Locke and David Hume, as well as by the physicians and psychologists David Hartley, Thomas Brown, and James and John Stuart Mill. They formulated the *laws of associations,* according to which similar as well as opposite ideas are closely associated in the mind. Ideas that are temporally and/or spatially contingent are associated as well.

The English scientist Sir Francis Galton (figure 10.2) was the first person to conduct experimental research on associations. He clearly saw the problems involved in introspective observations and tried to solve them by extremely careful and detailed description.

When we attempt to trace the first steps in each operation of our minds, we are usually baulked by the difficulty of keeping watch, without embarrassing the freedom of its action. The difficulty is . . . especially due to the fact that the elementary operations of the mind are exceedingly faint and evanescent, and that it requires the utmost painstaking care to watch them properly. It would seem

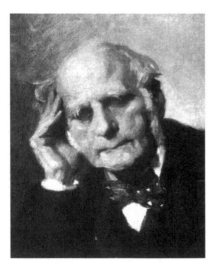

Figure 10.2
Sir Francis Galton (1822–1911), founder of the method of free association for the study of thought processes (portrait from Galton 1910).

impossible to give the required attention to the processes of thought, and yet to think as freely as if the mind had been in no way preoccupied. The peculiarity of the experiment I am about to describe is that I have succeeded in evading this difficulty. My method consists in allowing the mind to play freely for a very brief period, until a couple or so of ideas have passed through it, and then, while the traces or echoes of those ideas are still lingering in the brain, to turn the attention upon them with a sudden and complete awakening; to arrest, to scrutinize them, and to record their exact appearance. (Galton 1883:185)

Galton conducted a large number of introspective experiments in order to investigate even the most remote and smallest units of thought. He was interested in how thoughts occur, how they are motivated, how they are strung together, and so forth. He used a list of words, which he covered with a book so that he could see only one new word at a time. In this way, he presented these words to himself and wrote down the first word that came to his mind. Sometimes he used a stop watch to measure the time he took to respond. He summarizes the results of these experiments as follows:

I have desired to show how whole strata of mental operations that have lapsed out of ordinary consciousness, admit of being dragged into light, recorded and treated statistically, and how the obscurity that attends the initial steps of our thoughts can thus be pierced and dissipated. . . . Perhaps the strongest of the impressions left by these experiments regards the multifariousness of the work done by the mind in a state of half-unconsciousness, and the valid reason they afford for believing in the existence of still deeper strata of mental operations, sunk wholly below the level of consciousness, which may account for such mental phenomena as cannot otherwise be explained. (Galton 1879:162; see also Galton 1883: 202–203).

The quotation clearly demonstrates that Sigmund Freud and Carl-Gustav Jung were following Galton when they introduced the method of free association for the diagnosis and treatment of mental disorders. By the turn of the century, associations of thoughts and ideas were being investigated on a rather large scale by many investigators, particularly after Wilhelm Wundt founded the world's first psychological laboratory in Leipzig, Germany, in 1879. Emil Kraepelin, the founder of modern psychiatry, worked in this laboratory for two years and learned the experimental method of word association.

The method used is actually very simple. The investigator presents the subject with a spoken or written word, and the subject has to say (or

write down) the first word that comes to mind. Before you continue
reading, you should try this out for yourself! Please say, as quickly as
possible, the first word that comes to mind when you read the following
ten words:

white
mother
table
cold
brother
song
knife
hammer
sun
good

There is a good chance (with high probability), that you came up with
the following associations:

black
father
chair
hot
sister
sing
fork
nail
moon
bad

Maybe one or two of your associations were different. Nonetheless,
you are likely to admit that the century-old finding that most people make
strikingly similar associations is quite correct (cf. Spitzer 1992). The
investigation of hundreds of subjects have established word-association
norms for a number of languages. The books in which they are published
look something like telephone books; their columns of words, each with
a number to the right, allow one to look up what comes to most people's
minds when presented with a given word.

Rhymes, Fatigue, and Attention

The kinds of questions tackled with the method of free associations over a hundred years ago is amazing (cf. Spitzer 1992). For example, Gustav Aschaffenburg, one of Kraepelin's residents, was interested in the effects of fatigue on thought processes. He therefore had his colleagues on night shifts perform the word-association task four times: at about 9:00 P.M., midnight, 3:00 A.M., and 6:00 A.M. The colleagues had to write down the first word that came to mind for each of a hundred words presented. Aschaffenburg analyzed the resulting four hundred words—a hundred from each run—one by one to determine the kind of relationship between the stimulus word and the response word.

Ordinarily, these relations were conceptual in nature, that is, determined by the meaning of the words and by meaningful thoughts. Conceptual associations are similar to those generated by the list above: e.g., *sun–moon, white–black,* and so on. They are conceptual because they are determined by the meaning of the words. When presented with *white,* you could come up with *fight,* but only if your conceptual thinking is somewhat disturbed. In such a state, the flow of thoughts may be determined less by concepts and more by low-level information relating to the sound of the word (its *clang*).

As Aschaffenburg found out, this is exactly what happens when you are tired. In this state, the frequency of conceptually driven ("deeply related") associations decreases, and the frequency of clang and rhyme ("superficially related") associations increases.

What is the effect of fatigue upon association processes? The general finding of the experiments is that the quality of associations decreases at night. Conceptual relations are replaced by loose associations to the clang of the stimulus word, whose meaning seems to have no influence on the response. We found no exception to this rule, although the size of the phenomenon's effect varied to a considerable extent. (Aschaffenburg 1899:48, my translation)

Besides counting the various kinds of associations made each night, Aschaffenburg could do no more than "eyeball" his results. He was not able, as we now are, to provide a measure of the possible error of his conclusions; that is, he was unable to state that clang associations were *significantly* more frequent when subjects were under the influence of fatigue than when in a fresh waking state. As a matter of fact, the concept of statistical significance was not developed by Ronald Fisher until a quarter of a century after Aschaffenburg published his results. And even then, it took another few decades for this concept to became a standard procedure for the evaluation of results in medicine. However, because Aschaffenburg published his raw data on the frequency of different types of associations per night (in the form of very detailed tables), we can use the currently available statistical methods to process his data. For example, as shown in figure 10.3, the increase in the number of clang associations at three o'clock in the morning turns out to be significant, while the even larger increase of such associations at six o'clock in the morning is highly significant (cf. Spitzer 1992).

These results can be easily interpreted in the light of the ideas depicted in figure 10.1. The word-association test reveals the structure of the *semantic map* and, possibly, the *concept-level maps*. As certain words

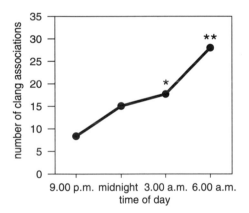

Figure 10.3
Effect of increasing fatigue on the frequency of clang-related associations, defined as rhyming words, meaningless rhyming syllables, and completions of words according to clang characteristics. Word associations were obtained from nine subjects four times during the night at specified times. Five of the subjects produced associations to four blocks of 50 monosyllable words; and; four subjects produced associations to four blocks of 100 two-syllable words on the same time schedule. The difference between the 9:00 P.M. results, and the 3:00 A.M. results were significant (*); at 6:00 A.M., this difference was highly significant (**) (Aschaffenburg 1899, reanalyzed data from tables 3, 5, 7, 9, 11, 13, 15, 17, and 19).

occur together within sentences and certain contexts, they become associated with each other. During the wide-awake state characterized by conceptually driven (i.e., meaningful) thinking, structure-generating processes in high-level cortical areas are at work producing coherent, adaptive, and well-structured output—for example, meaningful actions and meaningful speech. As fatigue increases, these processes become progressively weaker, causing thought processes to be increasingly determined by such lower-level structures as the phonological map (which codes the sound aspects of words). In short, when the flow of thoughts is no longer (or to a smaller degree) driven by concepts, the influence of simpler structures increases. In these circumstances, thought is less driven by meaningful relations and more by clang relations. This principle—that the decreased influence of "higher" areas permits the increased influence of "lower" areas—was formulated in the last century by the neurologist John Hughlings Jackson.

Aschaffenburg discussed his own findings within the framework of everyday experiences. He claimed, for example, that a tired audience appreciates jokes employing rhymes more than a fully awake audience does. I quote the following observation by Aschaffenburg in some detail to encourage readers to conduct their own empirical research.

When I was climbing mountains in Switzerland a few years ago, I tried to determine my companions' forms of associations by shouting words at them at the beginning and at the end of the tour. Although circumstances prevented me from taking extensive notes, I can assure you that almost always a large number of clang-related associations and rhymes occurred at the end. Simple close observation of utterances under such circumstances reveals to the attentive observer the role of clang associations for the form of rhymes and, particularly, for the typical jokes with words (puns). (Aschaffenburg 1899:51, my translation)

Another observation of Aschaffenburg's is also worth quoting.

A direct confirmation of the tight connection between rhyme and—though almost entirely somatic—fatigue can be obtained from looking at the visitor's book on a mountain top or in a mountain hut. Of course, I disregard those products obviously written under the influence of alcohol. I think everyone would probably have to admit that only rarely is a poem really rich in content found in such visitor's books. Nor are all of these poems written by uneducated people but in many cases are by those who, in the quiet of their studies, would be ashamed of penning such thoughtless rhymes. (Aschaffenburg 1899:51–52, my translation)

Before Carl-Gustav Jung turned to the worlds of mythology and fairy tales, he was an excellent experimental psychologist. From 1902 until 1909 he worked as a resident under Chairman Eugen Bleuler at the famous Burghölzli Hospital near Zürich. During this time, he carried out extensive studies on word associations in normal subjects and mentally ill patients. In his inaugural lecture, he described the association experiment as follows.

The experiment is similar to any experiment in physiology in which we stimulate a living object to test the effects of a stimulus, such as an electrical stimulus at various locations in the nervous system, or light stimuli at the eye, or auditory stimuli at the ear. Similarly, by means of a stimulus word, we bring a mental stimulus to the mental organ. Introducing an idea into the consciousness of the subject lets us observe what further idea has thereby been produced in the brain of the subject. This way we can obtain a large number of relations between ideas, or associations, respectively, within a relatively short period of time. From this material, and by comparisons between subjects, we are able to state that a given stimulus in most cases leads to a particular reaction. Hence, we possess a means to study the "laws of the associations of ideas." (Jung & Riklin 1906/1979:431, my translation)

Jung's 1906 paper (with Franz Riklin), analyzed more than thirty-five thousand associations from about a hundred and fifty normal subjects. Jung wanted to demonstrate that, contrary to Aschaffenburg's conclusions, it was not so much fatigue as a decrease in selective attention that caused the reduction in conceptual associations, as well as the increase in associations with words of similar sounds. For his experiments, Jung used a method that in Anglo-American experimental psychology became known in later decades as the *dual-task method.*

Jung had his subjects draw short lines with a pencil on a piece of paper according to the rhythm of a metronome, which could be set to various speeds. Subjects had to make either one or two strokes a second. While subjects were performing this task (the *distractor task,* in current terminology), Jung and Riklin administered the word-association task; that is, they read out words and asked the subjects to say the first words that came to mind. By having subjects perform two tasks at the same time, they could investigate the influence of cognitive function A (drawing lines at different speeds) upon cognitive function B (word associations). The effect of this "experimental manipulation of the independent variable, attention" (as experimental psychologists would today describe the pro-

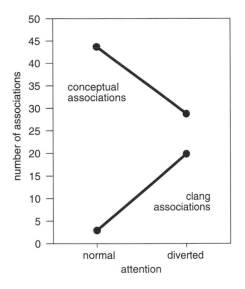

Figure 10.4
Frequency of conceptually related and clang-related word associations under normal conditions as well as under conditions of diverted attention. (The figures graphed are the means from three subjects.) The decrease in conceptual and the increase in clang associations is clearly visible (data from Jung 1903/1978:180–181).

cedure) was determined by analyzing the associations produced under the two conditions (figure 10.4).

Like Aschaffenburg, Jung published his raw data in tabulated form, which allows us to analyze them statistically. The bottom line of the experiments is that Jung was able to show that clang associations are not caused by the peculiar state of fatigue but, rather, by the diversion of attention from association processes. This diversion occurs during fatigue, but other states of decreased selective attention have the same effect.

Aschaffenburg's and Jung's studies of the conditions under which clang associations occur are not merely of historical interest. Rather, they point to the important organizational principle of cortical information processing discussed above. This principle of the *interactive hierarchy* of cortical areas plays a major role in higher cognitive functions. We discuss these functions, traditionally cast in terms such as *meaning, context,* and *use of language,* in the following sections.

Associative Networks

A large number of studies on the meaningful relations between psychologically associated words, as well as other studies in the field of psycholinguistics, have produced data that were interpreted some decades ago as evidence for a network structure of semantic memory. Words and their meanings are not stored alphabetically in the mind; nor are they stored in a totally disordered way. Instead, they are stored in a networklike structure (cf. Collins & Loftus 1975, Neely 1977). Within such a network, the meaning of a word is represented by *nodes* as well as by the relations of these nodes with other nearby nodes.

We can get an impression of how these networks may work by looking at them in the context of the word-association norms. These norms can be used to construct a cartoon version, as it were, of a semantic network (figure 10.5). Brendan Maher provides the following examples (I have italicized the related words).

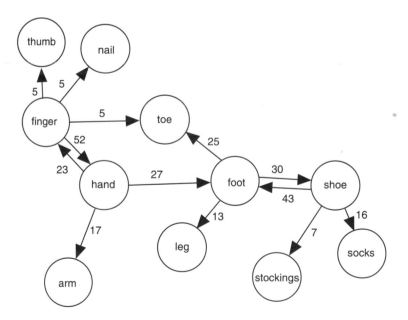

Figure 10.5
Semantic network drawn by using data from the norms published by Palermo and Jenkins in 1963. The numbers represent the relative frequency (in percent) of the word associations of a thousand male and female college students.

- Intended: A career in art has problems; said: A career in *art* has *draw*backs.
- Intended: This book, written by a man awaiting execution in Sing Sing prison, is quite amazing; said: This book, written by a man awaiting *execution* in Sing Sing prison, is quite *electrifying*.
- Intended: China is a giant looking cautiously at the world; said: *China* is a giant *peeking* cautiously at the world. (Maher 1988:117)

As these examples demonstrate, words that are already activated may be built into a subsequent utterance if they fit, sometimes distorting or even completely destroying the meaning of the utterance in the process. Examples such as these are more frequent than you might think; once you have learned to look or listen for them, you will notice quite a few. Furthermore, the actual wording of utterances often reveals more about the true intentions of the speaker than what the statements appear to mean on a superficial level.

To sum up, a network theory of semantic memory fits well with what has been termed the *spreading-activation model*. According to this model, the activation of a node spreads through the adjacent nodes for several hundred milliseconds, then either decreases passively or is actively inhibited. The spreading activation triggered by a single word causes words of related meanings to become somewhat active as well. Because of this activation, subjects are not only increasingly likely to use the associated words in subsequent utterances, but also to detect them more easily when asked to perform an experiment, such as the lexical-decision task illustrated in figure 10.11. If you see the word *white*, activation spreads to some extent to *black*; and hence, the word *black* is recognized comparatively faster (figure 10.6).

Why would our mental lexicon be organized like this? Why would we store similar (*table–chair*) as well as opposite (*black–white*) items close to each other so that whenever one of these items is activated the other becomes somewhat active as well?

Self-Organizing Semantic Networks

We should not confuse semantic networks with neural networks. They are different concepts, with a different history and different systematic features. However, we need not view them as completely different:

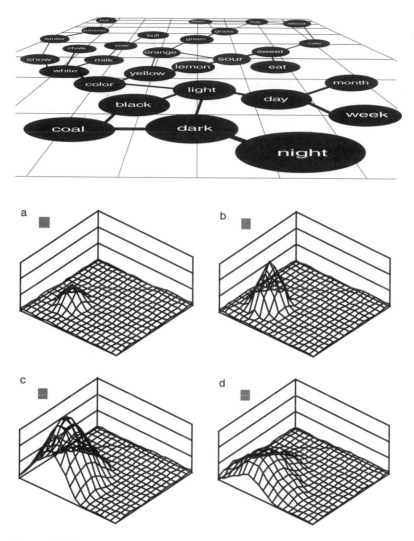

Figure 10.6
Schematic rendering of a semantic network (top) and time course of activation
in such a network upon activation of a node (bottom). The amount of activation
is shown on the vertical axis of the coordinate system. Activation starts about
200 to 300 milliseconds after a stimulus word is flashed on a screen in front of
the subject (a); it increases (b), and spreads to adjacent nodes (c), only to decrease
again (d).

"Neural networks and semantic networks have much in common and should be regarded as two points in a rich, quasi-continuous space of computational architectures rather than as radically different types of network" (Barnden 1995:857).

By the end of the 1980s, research had demonstrated for the first time that neural networks of the self-organizing feature-map type can not only create maps of simple features of input signals, such as sound pitch or graphemic similarity (as discussed in chapter 5), but can also produce maps of meaningful input. Because of the special significance of these simulations for the current discussion, we need to discuss in some detail how self-organizing networks form ordered maps of abstract semantic and grammatical input (cf. Ritter & Kohonen 1989).

When we teach character recognition to a self-organizing feature map, we assume that the features of the characters can be presented clearly. That is, the way in which any two characters are similar or dissimilar has to be clear. In the case of graphic representations of characters in a 5 × 7 dot grid, this is an easy task. We only need to count the number of dissimilar dots to get a quantitative measure of similarity (cf. figure 5.10). But how can we do this for words and meanings?

Because the objects or ideas that words denote have features, these features create order in the representations of words in neural networks. Let's have a detailed look at a computer simulation of this phenomenon.

Ritter and Kohonen used sixteen names for animals, which were characterized by thirteen features, as indicated in table 10.1. When the characteristic features of animals are brought into such a scheme, they can be represented by thirteen-dimensional vectors, in which a 1 (one) represents the presence and a 0 (zero) the absence of a given feature. In this scheme, "catness" is represented by the vector 1,0,0,0,1,1,0,0,0,1,0,0,0, as the numbers in the table indicate.

Whenever we learn words, we learn not only combinations of features but also their names, which in most cases are arbitrary sequences of phonemes (i.e., words). In computer simulations, names can be represented by vectors as well; that is, by arbitrary sequences of zeros and ones, which are linked to the feature vectors by simply stringing the two vectors together. Such combinations of features and names are used as

Table 10.1
Representing animals with feature vectors

		dove	hen	duck	goose	owl	hawk	eagle	fox	dog	wolf	cat	tiger	lion	horse	zebra	cow
is	small	1	1	1	1	1	1	0	0	0	0	1	0	0	0	0	0
	medium	0	0	0	0	0	0	1	1	1	1	0	0	0	0	0	0
	large	0	0	0	0	0	0	0	0	0	0	0	1	1	1	1	1
has	2 legs	1	1	1	1	1	1	1	0	0	0	0	0	0	0	0	0
	4 legs	0	0	0	0	0	0	0	1	1	1	1	1	1	1	1	1
	hair	0	0	0	0	0	0	0	1	1	1	1	1	1	1	1	1
	hoofs	0	0	0	0	0	0	0	0	0	0	0	0	0	1	1	1
	mane	0	0	0	0	0	0	0	0	0	1	0	0	1	1	1	0
	feathers	1	1	1	1	1	1	1	0	0	0	0	0	0	0	0	0
can	hunt	0	0	0	0	1	1	1	1	0	1	1	1	1	0	0	0
	run	0	0	0	0	0	0	0	0	1	1	0	1	1	1	1	0
	fly	1	0	0	1	1	1	1	0	0	0	0	0	0	0	0	0
	swim	0	0	1	1	0	0	0	0	0	0	0	0	0	0	0	0

input vectors in self-organizing feature-map simulations. As we saw in chapter 5, this type of neural network simulates features of the cortex and does not need a teacher to learn. Instead, self-organizing feature maps form maplike representations of the regularities across the input patterns according to the principles of similarity and frequency. In the simulation performed by Ritter and Kohonen, this had happened after two thousand presentations of the input patterns (figure 10.7).

In figure 10.8, each neuron is labeled with the animal that corresponds to the input vector causing the highest activation. As can be seen, the neurons around a winning neuron also represent the same word. In other words, for every input, there is a small population of neurons in the network that becomes specialized in this input. It follows, therefore, that the map works even when some of its neurons are no longer functioning. The representations created by the network are therefore not only ordered and specific but also quite robust.

In sum, the computer simulation—notwithstanding its simplifications—has created a highly informative scheme for ordering repre-

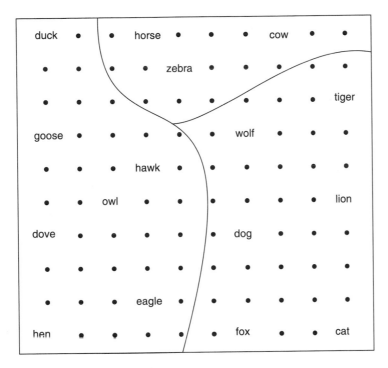

Figure 10.7
Self-organizing feature map after 2,000 learning trials (after Ritter and Kohonen 1989). Vectors consisting of feature strings and name strings of zeros and ones were used as input. Black dots mark neurons that became somewhat weakly activated, whereas neurons with names denote "winning" neurons. It is clear that the names of the animals became represented on the map in a meaningful way. To the left the birds, at the top the hoofed animals, and on the right the wild predators established their places on the map. Moreover, within the groups, similar animals are proximal, while dissimilar animals are located at greater distances from each other. Notice that birds of prey are closer to the wild animals than, for example, the duck and the dove. This order developed spontaneously during training, just because of the features of the animals and without any feedback from outside.

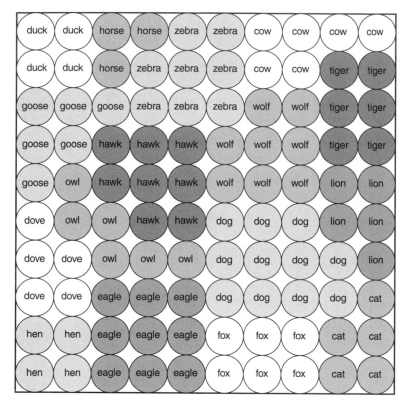

Figure 10.8
The same network as in figure 10.7, with every neuron labeled by the name that corresponds to the input causing the highest activation (after Ritter & Kohonen 1989).

sentations in a two-dimensional space. As Ritter and Kohonen comment on these orderly memory traces, "Although highly idealized, this result is very suggestive of how a self-organizing system can learn to spatially guide the formation of memory traces in such a way that its final physical layout forms a direct image of the hierarchy of the most important concept relationships" (Ritter & Kohonen 1989:248).

This example should not be misunderstood. It does not suggest that we learn language by simply combining clusters of features while simultaneously perceiving sound patterns. Once we learn a few words, these words form a large part of the context (features) of other words; that is, we can learn words by piggybacking them on other words; the simulation just described is therefore most similar to what occurs to a human child during an early stage of language acquisition. In contrast, the next simulation demonstrates the feasibility of the piggybacking approach at later stages of language acquisition, when we learn by processing sentences. In the second example, therefore, short sentences were used as input for a self-organizing feature map.

The sentence input was constructed in the following way. Words (again, only a few) were categorized by their grammatical features. These categories were numbered, and a sentence construction scheme was devised such that only certain sequences of numbers were allowed. This provided a set of rules for the order of words—that is, a very simple grammar that the input sentences had to obey. Table 10.2 contains some examples of the vocabulary, the grammar, and exemplary sentences of the entire set of 498 sentences produced in this way and used as input.

In this second simulation, Ritter and Kohonen wanted to show that contextual information can be used by self-organizing networks to

Table 10.2
Self-organization of semantic and grammatical features in a neural network, showing words, types of sentences, and examples of sentences formed (see also figure 10.9)

Word	Grammar			Example
1 Bob, Jim, Mary	5-12	1-9-2	2-5-14	Mary likes meat
2 horse, dog, eat	1-5-13	1-9-3	2-9-1	Jim speaks well
3 beer, water	1-5-14	1-9-4	2-9-2	Mary likes Jim
4 meat, bread	1-6-12	1-10-3	2-9-3	Jim eats often
5 runs, walks	1-6-13	1-11-4	2-9-4	Mary buys meat
6 works, speaks	1-6-14	1-10-12	2-10-3	dogs drink fast
7 visits, phones	1-6-15	1-10-13	2-10-12	horse hates meat
8 buys, sells	1-7-14	1-10-14	2-10-13	Jim eats rarely
9 likes, hates	1-8-12	1-11-12	2-10-14	Bob buys meat
10 drinks, eats	1-8-2	1-11-13	1-11-4	cat walks slowly
11 much, little	1-8-3	1-11-14	1-11-12	Jim eats bread
12 fast, slowly	1-8-4	2-5-12	2-11-13	cat hates Jim
13 often, rarely	1-9-1	2-5-13	2-11-14	Bob sells beer
14 well, poorly				etc.

produce maps in which the semantic and grammatical features of the words become spontaneously represented in a meaningful, orderly way. As in the first example, every word was represented as a vector. The context of a word was represented by combining the vectors of two words into one, so that the context of a word became its set of characteristic features. The simulations were performed by using a 10×15–node output layer. After two thousand training trials, the layer had formed the map shown in figure 10.9.

The words were distributed on the map according to semantic and grammatical characteristics. Words of a common grammatical type

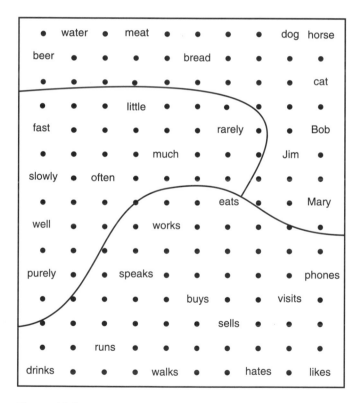

Figure 10.9
Results of a computer simulation with sentences of the type given in table 10.2. Nodes are labeled with the name of the input that activated it the most (after Ritter and Kohonen 1989). It is obvious that the network ordered the words according to grammatical and semantic features, producing a two-dimensional map of complex grammatical and semantic relations.

(nouns, adverbs, and verbs) each occupy their own regions of the map, in which meaningfully related words are located closely together. For example, antonyms, such as *well–poorly* are located next to each other, because they occur in the same context (as in *the dog is big/small*). Notice that the map is strikingly similar to the one derived from word-association norms depicted in figure 10.5.

In this work we have now shown that the principle of self-organizing maps can also be extended to higher levels of processing, where the relationships between items are more subtle and less apparent from their intrinsic features, a property that is characteristic of *symbolic expressions*. Symbols, in general, do not contain metrically relatable components. Consequently, meaningful topographic maps of symbols must no longer display intrinsic features, but instead the *logical similarities* of their inputs. It turns out, however, that organized mappings of symbolic data may still ensue from the same basic adaptation laws, provided that the symbolic input data are presented together *with a sufficient amount of context, that then defines the similarity relationships between them.* (Ritter & Kohonen 1989:251, italics in original).

Needless to say, the simulation had to simplify matters considerably to render the task manageable, given the computational limits of existing hardware. Nonetheless, the model clearly demonstrates that self-organizing feature maps can, in principle, be the engine of the formation of complex semantic feature maps. As the authors put it, "Any realistic semantic brain map would need a much more complicated, probably hierarchical model. The purpose of the simple artificial model in this work was only to demonstrate the *potential* of a self-organizing process to form abstract maps" (Ritter & Kohonen 1989:251; italics in original).

Language Is Used

The philosopher Ludwig Wittgenstein emphasized in many of his writings that language comes to life by being used; the meaning of a word is determined by its use. Neural network research sheds new light on this view. Ritter and Kohonen's first simulation clearly demonstrates how orderly representations of meanings can result from merely presenting the proper input—a word together with clusters of features—to a network. Under the influence of this "experience" the network spontaneously generates simple ordering structures, the way a child lumps together anything that moves in a certain way under the term "woof-woof." For the small child, "woof-woof" denotes not so much a specific dog, but rather something like the "manifestation of dogginess." Later, memory traces distinct enough to allow the child to sort out dogs from cats and cows—and to distinguish between different individual dogs such as Fido, Max, and Spot—are formed.

Just as the sound environment of a six-month-old child has already guided the proper development of the phonological map in a way that enables it to process the sounds of the mother tongue better than other sounds, the child's cultural environment—which is in large part mediated by language—brings about the development of semantic maps in the cortex. The experiences of the child are represented in these maps according to the principles of similarity and frequency, very crudely at first but with increased detail as the child grows older. The use of language and interactions with the environment make up the sum of every person's experience and, throughout his or her entire life, provide the momentum for the formation and changing of high-level, maplike representations of meaning.

We have emphasized a number of times that neural networks store the general features of the input (rather than complete single instances) through slow incremental learning. In chapter 8, in addition, we learned about the ability of Elman networks to process temporal sequences and, thereby, derive grammatical structures from strings of words. Very generally speaking, our brain treats language just as it does other input patterns—by extracting regularities from it.

What is special about language is that these regularities of experience can be uttered as such and directly referred to other members of the language community. In contrast to capabilities like playing the violin or riding a bicycle, which have to be acquired by every individual from scratch, language allows us to communicate the regularities extracted from the input. Moreover, language itself is not fixed, but adapts to changes in our experiences and is adapted by us to our experiences. Language is thus continually developed and invented by creative speakers; Shakespeare, for example, invented about 10 percent of the words he used in his plays.

Language can be conceived of as the collective memory of a given culture. Although Edward Sapir and his student Benjamin Lee Whorf were wrong in hypothesizing that the Hopi Indians have no concept of time because they cannot express time in their language, there is no doubt that language shapes our thoughts. The relationship goes both ways, however, and our thoughts shape language as well. The experience and the knowledge of *many* people is what shapes our language, making it a unique system of related concepts and rules that captures a part of the world, our existence in it, and our relationship to it.

The unification of communication brought about by the mass media has potentially positive effects upon our society. It brings about more mutual understanding among people and, therefore, has the potential to bring peace and liberty. "The fax shall make you free" was the title of a newspaper article that appeared in the early 1990s. It dealt with the political situation in Eastern European countries and clearly demonstrated the power of unimpaired communication in modern society. On the other hand, as no language and no culture is omniscient, the dying out of languages also brings about cultural impoverishment and the loss of perspectives on the world that distill ages-old interpretative schemes about human experience.

Semantic Maps in the Head

Do we really carry semantic maps in our heads, as psychological studies of word association and network simulations suggest? Again, the answer to this question is "yes and no"! First of all, it is important to note that, in addition to the psychological and neurocomputational evidence discussed above, there are neurobiological data that support this idea. The cortex forms maps of the input patterns that reach it. The machinery that produces these maps does not care what these patterns represent—frequencies, phonemes, semantic content, the context of actions, aims, or values. Whenever there are regularities in the input, they are extracted and the input patterns are represented in a topographic manner according to these regularities. Since we know that there are, for example, somatosensory, retinotopic, and tonotopic maps, we may conclude, by analogy, that there are also maps of higher-order information, such as semantic maps. There is no doubt that we have semantic representations stored in our brains; so (the argument runs in brief) they are no doubt stored in the cortex. And, if the cortex forms maps (which it does), then there must be cortical semantic maps. Notwithstanding this logic, it would be nice to have direct evidence of cortical semantic maps, since the opposite position—that storage in the brain is completely distributed—has also been proposed.

In fact, both positions are rather old (cf. Finger 1994). About two hundred years ago, the Viennese physician Franz-Joseph Gall proposed that an individual's abilities are manifested in the shape of his or her skull. He argued that because every feature and capability is strictly localized in the brain, we can infer a person's strengths and weaknesses from the observable and measurable shape of the head. This idea, later baptized *phrenology,* was controversial from the very beginning, but it gained wide attention when Paul Broca and Carl Wernicke discovered the motor and sensory language areas, in 1861 and 1874, respectively. Nonetheless, since about the middle of the last century, many respected scientists have opposed *localizationism* and proposed instead a *holistic* theory. The most prominent representative of this view, that every brain function is the product of the entire intact brain, was Karl Lashley.

Even though it seems that neuroscientists still adhere to one or the other view, controversy between the views waned for a time. When network models of brain function became widely known, however, the controversy regained momentum. Network models, it appeared, clearly suggest that mental representations are distributed over large numbers of neurons and even larger numbers of connection weights (cf. chapter 2). As we have shown, however, this view simplifies matters too much, because it assumes that the entire brain acts as a single neural network. This view is wrong; the brain is better conceived of as a network of modules that are, in turn, composed of neural networks of possibly different kinds. Moreover, the discussion of self-organizing feature maps clearly demonstrates that parallel-distributed processing (PDP) models and localized representations are by no means mutually exclusive. In fact, feature maps are both: They are PDP models, and they employ localized representations.

In the following sections, we discuss two sets of data that provide direct evidence for the existence of local representations of high-level (supposedly semantic) information in the cortex.

Missing Vegetables Only

The naming of objects is part of the standard neuropsychological examination used with patients who have had strokes or other brain disorders. If there is a language problem (aphasia), the person may encounter problems in naming objects. As early as 1966, Goodglass and coworkers reported in a study of 135 aphasic patients that quite a few of them suffered from a selective naming deficit. The patients were able to name most objects but had great difficulty in naming certain others.

In addition, case studies have described individual patients who could name anything but, for example, animals, or anything but furniture, or anything but fruits and vegetables. This condition is called a *category-specific naming deficit*. Table 10.3 provides an overview of the literature on such cases.

The simplest explanation for category-specific naming deficits is the assumption that there is a localized memory of these categories. A single category need not, however, be represented in a single, small spot on the brain. On the contrary, it is much more likely that any given category is represented within several maps of different degrees of complexity or that represent different aspects of the category. For example, tools may be represented on a map that codes the use of things and on another map that codes moving things or on a map of action-related objects. Other maps may represent the entertaining aspects of tools, or their shapes. In other words, it is unlikely that there is a single semantic map for a given object. It is much more likely that there are multiple interconnected maps coding various aspects of the outside world, just as the visual system is composed of more than a dozen retinotopic maps that work together in a complex way to produce visual perception.

If several parts of several maps are destroyed by a stroke or an infection, a certain category could be completely (or almost completely) knocked out. In these cases, we would see the selective deficits described in the case studies.

Category-Specific Activation in Functional Magnetic Resonance Imaging

The method of functional magnetic resonance imaging (fMRI) allows researchers to study brain activation while a subject is carrying out a

Table 10.3
Research literature on category-specific naming deficits

What cannot be named?	Reference
Living or nonliving things	Warrington & McCarthy 1983 Warrington & Shallice 1984 Basso et al. 1988 Pietrini et al. 1988 Silveri et al. 1988 Sartori & Job 1988 Sirigu et al. 1991 Mehta et al. 1992 De Renzi & Lucchelli 1994
Animals	Hart & Gordon 1992 Hillis & Caramazza 1991 Caramazza et al. 1994
Objects inside the house, furniture	Yamadori & Albert 1973
Fruits and vegetables	Hart et al. 1989 Farah & Wallace 1992
Tools and kitchen utensils	Warrington & McCarthy 1987
Body parts	Dennis 1976 Sacchett & Humphreys 1992 Semenza 1988
Artificial objects	Sacchett & Humphreys 1992 Caramazza et al. 1994

certain task. This noninvasive method was developed in the early 1990s and is now one of the most important tools for researchers in the field of cognitive neuroscience.

The method depends on the fact that the magnetic properties of blood differ according to oxygen levels. Oxygen in the blood is bound to the molecules of the substance called *hemoglobin,* which gives blood its red color. *Oxyhemoglobin* is diamagnetic, whereas *deoxyhemoglobin* is paramagnetic; that is, hemoglobin is magnetically different depending upon its oxygenation. If neurons in a certain brain area are particularly active because they are involved in the computations needed to carry out a specific task, they will use up more oxygen. Within half a second, the small blood vessels respond to this increased demand by widening their diameter, thereby allowing more blood rich in oxygen to flow in. The net effect of this is the presence of more oxygenated hemoglobin in brain areas that are especially active. By applying different magnetic fields, we can detect the resulting changes in the magnetic properties of the brain and use the information to compute an image of brain activity with a resolution of about a square millimeter (cf. Bellemann et al. 1995, Brix et al. 1994, Cohen et al. 1994).

In the fall of 1994, my colleagues and I, motivated by studies of patients with category-specific naming deficits, began to look directly at categories in the cortex—that is, to look for category-specific activation of cortical areas while subjects were asked to name pictures of objects from various categories (Spitzer et al. 1995b).

While lying in the MRI scanner, subjects saw through a mirror a series of pictures projected by a computer-controlled video projector. Subjects were asked to name the objects to themselves as soon as they saw them. Each of the pictures, which had been scanned from a visual dictionary, was displayed for 1.5 seconds. Guided by what we already knew from earlier neuropsychological studies (cf. table 10.3), we used eighty pictures of objects, twenty from each of the following four categories: animals (A), furniture (Fu), fruit (Fr), and tools (T). As each of the twenty pictures in each category was displayed for 1.5 seconds, display of objects in the first category consumed thirty seconds. Then the category changed, and the second category with its twenty pictures was presented for thirty seconds, followed by the third and the fourth categories. After two minutes, the pictures were shown again, in the same succession, and, after four minutes, the procedure was repeated a third time. The subject thus saw the four categories three times within six minutes in the succession A-Fu-Fr-T-A-Fu-Fr-T-A-Fu-Fr-T. At the end of the six minutes, we paused for several minutes, then repeated the entire procedure. After another pause, there were two more repetitions.

We did so many repetitions because, like other researchers, we realized that if you take multiple measurements and average across all the results, the accuracy of the results is increased (cf. chapter 3). The MRI machine at the Massachusetts General Hospital in Boston is capable of producing one image every four hundred milliseconds. As we scanned for twenty-four minutes, we obtained thousands of images we could then analyze statistically.

Our analysis focused on the question of differential activation caused by the naming of different categories. When you see and name an image, your visual system becomes active, as do the brain areas that further process the image, access and generate meaning, select a name, and generate the motor programs needed to guide the orchestrated action of the speech muscles. (This happens even if you do not say anything out loud.) All this brain activity—and there was a good deal of it—was not of interest to us. In fact, it obstructed the view of the tiny increases of activity that occurred when areas became involved in processing an image of, for example, an animal or a piece of furniture.

In order to get rid of the obvious but uninteresting activity, we used a trick that dates back more than a hundred years. We didn't compare the brain's activity during a resting condition with the activity that occurred during picture naming but, instead, compared the brain's activity while the subject was naming pictures from one category with the activity generated by naming the pictures in each of the three other categories (figure 10.10). Because the pictures had been chosen and graphically processed to be very similar with respect to brightness and color, the differences in brain activity should be caused solely by the semantic categories of the objects. In several subjects, in fact, the method made it possible to locate small areas of the brain that were activated only when they named objects of a specific category.

A note of caution is in order. These data should not be taken as indicating that there is a "tool center" or a "fruit center" in the human brain. All that can be said is that in a particular subject we can locate a cortical area representing some high-level feature of tools that becomes active whenever the subject names tools. Another subject may have stored this information, or even some slightly different kind of information (e.g., tools involved in other activities and contexts), in a different location. We have to assume a high degree of variability across subjects. After all, people are different, and the higher the representations we investigate, the more these representations are likely to be shaped by experience.

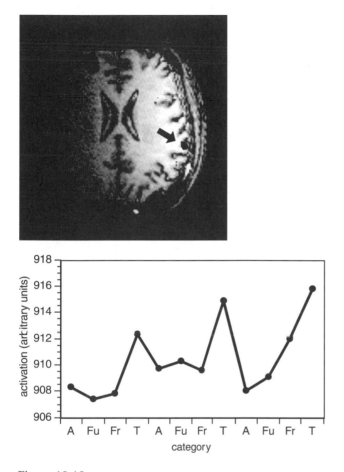

Figure 10.10
Category-specific activation of a small cortical area in the left temporal lobe.
MRI images, like x-ray images, are in reverse (i.e., left is right and right is left).
The arrow points to the small black area, which became active whenever the
subject was naming tools. The graph below shows the time course of the activation. As the average of all four runs were taken, every point on the curve
represents sixty measurements. Only by averaging the results could we detect the
weak signal caused by naming items from different categories (after Spitzer et al.
1995b).

Therefore, the higher the cognitive function under study, the more variability between subjects we should expect. In other words, although the left big toe is represented at about the same location on the somatosensory cortex in all of us—because we have roughly the same body surface sending input to form the body-surface map on the somatosensory cortex—we differ much more with respect to the objects we come across in our individual lives. Some of us have had a lot of experience with animals, while others know them only from books or television. Others like to do crafts, sell furniture for a living, or work in the fresh fruit department of a supermarket. Given these differences in experience, it appears to make little sense, in humans, to refer to a "brain center" for animals, furniture, fruits, or tools.

The experiment, which pushed the current technology to its limits, is in agreement with data from other researchers using other methods. Martin and coworkers (1996) used positron emission tomography (PET) to compare brain activity in sixteen normal subjects naming animals or tools. Likewise, Damasio et al. (1996) presented evidence for a somewhat localized representation of animals and tools in a neuropsychological study, as well as in a PET study. Both these studies, however, suffer from the fact that, for methodological reasons, group averages had to be taken. In these averages (that is, *across* individuals), certain cortical areas were shown to be active during the processing of different categories. Does this finding imply that there is in fact an animal center or a tool center in the human brain? In my view, this is not the case. All that can be shown by studies involving group averages are tendencies to prefer using certain processing strategies for certain stimuli. For example, animals may be most readily distinguished through their appearance (and, hence, may activate a subject's visual brain areas more than, for example, tools do). Tools, on the other hand, may be perceived in terms of movement and action-directed processing (and hence, might activate those cortical areas). This is what the studies of Martin et al. and Damasio et al. have actually demonstrated. However, at the level of the individual subject, we can look not just at processing strategies (although the latter may be among the guides for map formation) but, instead, at localized representations as well. Further studies are clearly needed to clarify this point.

We should note that electrophysiological evidence, too, points to the localized representation of different categories. Dehaene et al. (1995)

recorded electrical brain activity with electroencephalography (EEG) while subjects were classifying verbs, proper names, names of animals, and numbers. The researchers found that the electrical activity involved in performing these tasks was localized in different cortical areas, depending on the category of input. The drawback of the EEG method is that its resolution is only within the range of a few centimeters, in contrast to the one-millimeter resolution of fMRI. However, EEG can resolve time with an accuracy of one millisecond; therefore, its resolution in the time domain is between a hundred to a thousand times better than that of fMRI. Future studies of higher cognitive functions will, to an increasing degree, employ a combination of methods and make use of the spatiotemporal advantages of each one.

The activation of single nodes in semantic networks cannot be directly probed at the present time. It can be inferred, however, from experiments that rely on reaction times and error rates, the standard variables in psychological experiments. In the next section, we discuss these experiments and their results as they pertain to semantic activation.

Measuring Associations within Networks

At the beginning of this chapter, we showed that the word-association method employed by Francis Galton, Gustav Aschaffenburg, and Carl-Gustav Jung revealed interesting features of human thought processes. However, there are problems connected with the evaluation of associations spontaneously produced by giving subjects stimulus words. This was pointed out as early as 1910 by two American researchers in a seminal paper on word associations (Kent and Rosanoff 1910) The authors made their point by using the association between the words *health* and *wealth* as an example. Is this a relation of semantic content (especially in the United States), or is it merely an association based on sound similarity (perhaps for a person of Scandinavian background)? It would not be helpful to ask the subject how he or she arrived at the association, since even if the subject were able to provide an answer, it would be one derived from introspection and might not represent the associative process that actually occurred. In short, the word-association method is compromised by the fact that associations must be evaluated on a post hoc basis. Wouldn't it be nice if we could specify associations in advance and then measure their relationship? In other words, we are looking for a method that does not rely on the production of associations, which are interpreted *later*, but that allows us to measure previously selected associations.

While such a method sounds too good to be true, it actually has been used on a large scale in experimental psychology since its invention in the early 1970s. In order to measure the associative strength between two words, one word (the *prime*) is visually presented on a computer screen for about a fifth of a second (about the time it takes to read a word). Then the second word is displayed and the subject has to decide whether it is in fact a word. The subject has to work through a number of such trials, in half of which (in random order) the second item presented is in fact not a word but a meaningless string of characters (a nonword, like *tuble* or *safo*). So the subject has to make a lexical decision about the second string of characters presented in any given trial, responding by pressing one of two keys of a computer keyboard, which records the response time as well as the response itself.

In a typical experiment of this sort, the subject has to make eighty such lexical decisions (figure 10.11). When, in half the cases, the subject sees first a word, then, briefly thereafter, a nonword, the decision should be "no." These cases (i.e., all the word–nonword trials) are not analyzed; they are used merely to force subjects to make decisions. The word–word trials, on the other hand, are the focus of interest. (Note that *any two words* can be used in these trials.)

It has been shown in a large number of these lexical-decision experiments that the second word (for example, *black*) is recognized as a word faster when it is preceded by a meaningfully related word (such as *white*). The close semantic relationship between the two words causes the second word to be rapidly detected as a word. In contrast, if subjects have to detect an unrelated word (e.g., *cheese*) as a word after seeing *cloud,* they take a little longer to make the lexical decision.

As a single response in any one trial can be influenced by many factors, researchers use various types of associations and present at least a dozen or so trials of each type. This allows them to compute response times and error rates for each type of association. For example, if the experiment contains eighty pairs altogether, it may contain, in addition to the forty word–nonword pairs, twenty pairs of related words (e.g., *black–white*) and twenty pairs of unrelated words (e.g., *cloud–cheese*). With normal subjects, the result is almost always faster reaction times for the related words than for the unrelated words. The mean difference, called the *semantic priming effect,* ranges between thirty and fifty milliseconds.

Priming effects can be calculated and expressed as (1) either the difference between the mean of the reaction times to the unrelated words minus the mean of the reaction times to the related words (in milliseconds), or (2) as a percentage increase in the speed of responding to related over unrelated words (Spitzer et al. 1993). Semantic priming, in other words, provides information about how much faster (in milliseconds or in percentage) a word is detected as a word when it is preceded by a related word. Experimental measurements of the semantic priming effect can thus provide information about the degree and timing of node activation in a semantic network. We discuss this topic in more detail in chapter 11.

Recap

We use language every day. It is an important part of the world in which we live, and of our experience of this world. Language experience is processed by our brains in the same way as other experiences; that is, it influences cortical representations at different levels of analysis and processing. By the age of six months, the infant has already learned to distinguish between the phonemes of its mother tongue and other phonemes and is able to process input from the mother tongue better than input from another language. At the same time, the child has lost some of its potential responsiveness to other languages.

The child learns the meaning of words by using language in appropriate interactions with the environment and by storing experiences on the cortex in a maplike way. We may assume that even the highest human capabilities—such as the representation of context, planning, and decision making—are based on maps of high-level representations of general structures of experience.

During further development of the child, higher cortical areas become involved in language processing (see chapter 8), making possible the

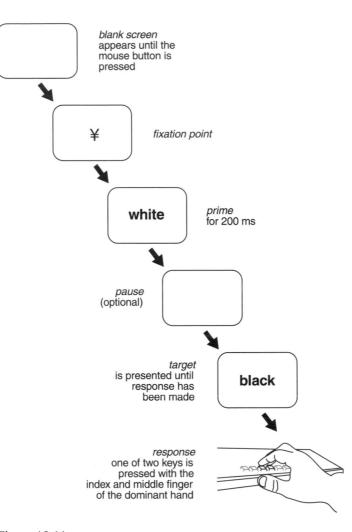

Figure 10.11
Sequence of events in a single trial of a lexical-decision experiment. At first the screen is blank. When the subject is ready, he or she presses the mouse button of the computer with the nondominant (usually the left) hand, thereby initiating the trial. A fixation point appears for 700 milliseconds to direct the gaze and attention of the subject to the location on the screen where subsequent stimuli appear. After the fixation point, the first stimulus (which is always a word) appears for 200 milliseconds. The first stimulus is called the *prime*. After the prime, there is either a pause of a certain length or the next string of characters—the *target*—is presented immediately. The target is either a word or a meaningless string of characters (a nonword). The subject has to press one of two buttons (a "yes"-

processing of increasingly complex language input. After just a few years, the child can use and understand rather complex grammatical structures.

Neural network simulations with self-organizing feature maps have demonstrated that representations of semantic features can become spontaneously organized topographically according to the principles of input similarity and input frequency. Such simulated self-organizing semantic maps bear a close resemblance to the associative networks inferred from experiments on people's free associations. That representation of high-level (meaningful) representations is localized topographically is further suggested by clinical data and by the results of recent neuroimaging and electrophysiological studies.

Associations within networks can be measured by cleverly designed psychological experiments, such as the lexical-decision task, that allow researchers to measure and compare different prime-target relations. The priming effects found in these experiments indicate the degree and timing of node activation in human semantic networks.

Postscript on Aschaffenburg and Jung
or, Whether Rhyming Is Priming Depends upon Timing

We can demonstrate the power of the lexical-decision method by looking again at the word-association results of Jung and Aschaffenburg. Both found that the frequency of clang- and rhyme-related associations increases under conditions of fatigue or diverted attention. Moreover, both authors postulated that there must be an inhibitory mechanism that is active under normal conditions to prevent these kinds of associations from intruding into thought- and goal-directed speech. In other words, they believed that there must be a mechanism to keep us from talking in nonsense rhymes all the time.

button and a "no"-button) as quickly and as accurately as possible to indicate his or her decision about whether the target is a word. When the subject has responded, the screen goes blank and the next lexical-decision trial can be initiated by the subject. The computer records which button the subject pressed and the time elapsed between the beginning of the second stimulus and the response (reaction time).

Jung, as well as Aschaffenburg, later published studies on the associations of mentally ill patients, some of whom showed an increased frequency of clang and rhyme associations in their spontaneous speech. (Within the framework of current diagnostic systems, most of these patients would probably be diagnosed as schizophrenic; we know that 5 to 10 percent of these patients show an increased number of clang and rhyme associations.) Given the limitations of the word-association method, Jung and Aschaffenburg could do little more than describe the phenomenon and speculate about its possible underlying mechanisms.

Clang-related associations, like meaningful associations between words, can be studied with the lexical-decision method. To do so, we divided the word–word pairs into those that are similar in sound—for example, rhyming words like *house–mouse* and those—like *cloud–cheese*—that are dissimilar (Spitzer et al. 1994b).

Preliminary experiments had further suggested that the timing of the stimulus is crucial in that the effect of a rhyming prime on target recognition is different when the target immediately follows the prime than when there is a pause of half a second between them. Half a second is a long time in experimental psychology. It is therefore conceivable that subjects consciously start to think of rhymes during that interval, especially when the task has sometimes involved rhyming stimuli.

Because of these considerations, we set up a lexical-decision task using nonwords, rhyming word–word pairs, and word pairs that were unrelated in either meaning or clang. We also prepared three blocks of stimuli such that the target either followed the prime immediately or was followed by either a brief pause of two hundred milliseconds or a longer pause of half a second. In normal control subjects, we found that the priming effect of a rhyming stimulus depended on the exact timing of the stimulus. If the target followed the prime without a pause, there was an inhibitory effect upon recognition of a rhyming word. In other words, if you read *mouse* and have to decide immediately afterwards whether or not *house* is a word, you are actually slower compared to reading *cloud* first and then making a decision about *cheese*. This inhibitory effect of rhyming stimuli is in sharp contrast with the facilitatory effect of meaningfully related stimuli. However, if there is a five-hundred-millisecond pause between rhyming prime and target, a facilitatory effect is also obtained. So it appears that half a second is enough time for a subject to start to make rhymes.

We obtained the inhibitory effect in two studies, one performed in German and one performed in the English language, which is infamous for its low spelling-to-sound correlation and, hence, allows for the visual presentation of rhyming stimuli that are graphemically dissimilar (e.g., *mile–aisle*). In this experiment, the drawback of English spelling turned into a virtue, since we were able to exclude effects related to graphemic similarity, which were an issue when we did the experiment in German. (German may have some disadvantages, but it also has the virtue of a pretty good spelling-to-sound correlation.) The effects, however, were similar in both the German and English studies.

The inhibitory effect obtained in these experiments relates directly to the inhibitory mechanisms posited by Jung and Aschaffenburg. It makes little sense for rhyming words to come to mind immediately when we hear or see any thought-directed sequence of words. In fact, goal-directed, clear thinking would hardly be possible if rhymes constantly guided what comes to mind and is said.

We also performed this study with schizophrenic patients, as described in the next chapter. They showed the same pattern as the normal subjects, with one important exception: They lacked the inhibitory effect (see figure 10.12). From that experiment, we may conclude that a mechanism functioning automatically in normal subjects to prevent them from talking rhyming nonsense all the time is disordered in schizophrenic patients. This mechanism may obviously be disturbed, for example, under conditions of extreme fatigue or diverted attention, or in the disordered states of mind that occur in schizophrenic patients. The experiments demonstrate that schizophrenic patients do not consciously rhyme, but rather are disturbed by rhyming words not inhibited by an automatic mechanism.

Experiments like this one may contribute to a better understanding of mentally ill patients, as we explain in more detail in the next chapter.

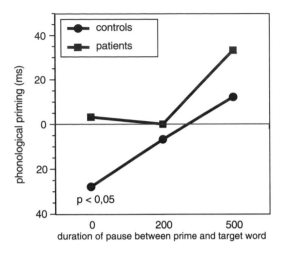

Figure 10.12
Phonological priming in 84 normal subjects and 70 schizophrenic patients (after
Spitzer 1994b). The phonological priming effect (i.e., the difference in reaction
time to the unrelated words minus the words related by rhyme) is shown under
three different conditions relating to the timing of the target: (1) no pause
between prime and target (the 0-millisecond condition); a 200-millisecond pause;
and a 500-millisecond pause. Normal subjects shown an inhibitory effect in the
no-pause condition that is absent in schizophrenic patients.

11

The Disordered Mind

How can the mind become ill? We have little trouble understanding how the mind can shut off completely, as for example during a coma. But how are we to understand the mind changing in a way that causes our experiences to become strange, weird, foreign, mad? Is there, after all, anything to be understood about madness? Are madness and genius related? Could neural networks provide a way to understand, and maybe even find some answers to these questions?

The latter question is already settled. We have demonstrated that neural network models can enhance our understanding of a variety of mental disorders and syndromes, such as autism, Alzheimer's dementia, and hallucinations. However, this chapter is about *schizophrenia,* arguably the most severe of all mental disorders. At some point in their lifetime, about one in a hundred people is stricken with the illness, which causes disordered or altered thoughts, sensations, affect, and behavior.

Schizophrenia is unlike any other malady. If a leg cannot be moved. or if speech is no longer under the command of the patient, or even if the patient is in a comatose state, it is clear that movement, speech, or the entire mental apparatus is no longer functioning. Yet the functions of schizophrenic patients, in contrast to such cases, are not completely gone but are in some peculiar way different from everyone else's. So, while it is relatively simple (at least on a conceptual level) to relate the lack of function generally to a brain structure that is no longer working properly, it is much more difficult to envision exactly *how* mental disorders such as madness and delusions are related to the brain's normal functioning.

This difficulty has led many to believe that schizophrenia does not have a neurobiological cause at all but is related wholly to such psychological factors as harmful life experiences and stress. Yet, even though the cause of schizophrenia is still unknown, we know that it must involve some dysfunction and pathology of the brain that, combined with psychosocial factors, plays a role in its inception and course. In short, schizophrenia is a disorder of mind *and* brain, and it will only be understood by understanding the interface between them. This is exactly where neural network models enter the picture.

The Birth of Schizophrenia

In all cultures and at all times, people have suffered from the disorder we now call schizophrenia. However, it has only been in the past two hundred years that such people have been regarded as ill. Before then, they were burned as witches, imprisoned, or exiled from the community. Further, it is only in the last hundred years that their illness has been the subject of scientific research.

At the turn of the century, psychiatrists Eugen Bleuler (figure 11.1) and Carl-Gustav Jung undertook detailed investigations of the obviously disturbed thought processes of schizophrenic patients. Along with other tools, they used the word-association test described in chapter 10 and found that many of the mentally ill patients had strange associations. Schizophrenic patients did show normal associations such as *table–chair,* but they did so less frequently than other patients and normal people. They often spontaneously produced weird associations.

The peculiar association disturbance is always present. . . . In this malady the associations lose their continuity. Of the thousands of associative threads which guide our thinking, this disease seems to interrupt, quite haphazardly, sometimes such single threads, sometimes a whole group, and sometimes even large segments of them. In this way, thinking becomes illogical and often bizarre. Furthermore, associations tend to proceed along new lines. G254
. . . During an experiment a patient associates "threads" to the stimulus word, "heart," because "two hearts are linked as by a thread." A hebephrenic [a type of schizophrenic patient] defines "hay" as a "means of maintenance of the cow." (Bleuler 1911, 1950:13–20)

Observations like these led Bleuler to believe that patients who display this kind of associative thinking suffer from a particular type of mental illness. In his 1911 book on this form of illness, he referred to these patients as *schizophrenic* and named their disorder *schizophrenia.* Thus

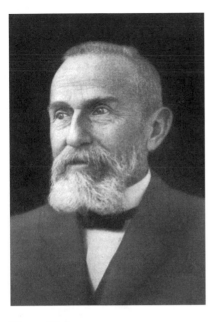

Figure 11.1
Eugen Bleuler (1857 1933), director of the famous Burghölzli Hospital near
Zürich. His research on word associations in normal and mentally disordered
people led him to form the concept of schizophrenia that we still use today.

the arguably most devastating of all mental disorders was for the first
time defined and clearly distinguished by a given set of symptoms.

About one in a hundred human beings develops an episode of schizophrenia over his or her lifetime. The disorder strikes men and women to
the same degree, although men, on average, become sick about five years
earlier (men in their early twenties, women in their late twenties). The
disorder may have a chronic progressive or an episodic course, or it may
even be limited to a single episode with no permanent further dysfunction. Because schizophrenic patients often suffer from somatic disorders,
which are either not diagnosed or not treated, these patients run a higher
than normal risk of mortality from such illnesses. About half of schizophrenic patients attempt suicide at some point, and between 10 and 15
percent of them are successful (Häfner 1993, M. Bleuler 1983, Kaplan
et al. 1994).

In dizygotic twins, the relative frequency of the disorder in one twin
when the other suffers from it (the *concordance rate*) is 12 percent, which

is the same as in nontwin siblings. In monozygotic twins, however, the concordance rate is about 50 percent. These numbers can be, and have been, interpreted quite differently—depending upon whether you see the glass as half full or half empty. Some take the 50-percent concordance rate in monozygotic twins as a sure sign of a genetic and, hence, biological causation of the disorder, whereas others point out that as monozygotic twins, who have the same genetic makeup, have only a 50-percent concordance rate, environmental and psychosocial factors must surely be important. Findings that schizophrenic patients from intensely emotional families (the technical term is *high expressed emotions*) and those living in the dense population areas of big cities are comparatively more likely to suffer relapses further suggest the importance of psychosocial factors (Gottesman 1991, Kaplan et al. 1994).

Madness and Craziness

When people talk about *madness,* they are usually referring to the symptoms of schizophrenia. Psychiatrists, of course, do not use words like *crazy* and *mad,* but rather refer to disturbances in the form and content of thought. In particular, their diagnoses mention schizophrenic *formal thought disorder* and schizophrenic *delusions.* They still, like Bleuler, define the former in terms of disturbed associative processes, as in the official definition of formal thought disorder in the fourth edition of the *Diagnostic and Statistical Manual of Mental Disorders* (*DSM-IV*):

Because of the difficulty inherent in developing an objective definition of "thought disorder," and because in a clinical setting inferences about thought are based primarily on the individual's speech, the concept of *disorganized speech* has been emphasized in the definition for Schizophrenia used in this manual. The speech of individuals with Schizophrenia may be disorganized in a variety of ways. The person may "slip off the track" from one topic to another ("derailment" or "*loose associations*"); answers to questions may be *obliquely related* or completely unrelated ("tangentiality"); and, rarely, speech may be so severely disorganized that it is nearly incomprehensible and resembles receptive aphasia in its linguistic disorganization ("incoherence" or "word salad"). Because mildly disorganized speech is common and nonspecific, the symptom must be severe enough to substantially impair effective communication. (American Psychiatric Association 1994:276, italics added)

Bleuler assumed that the normal psychological laws of association remain valid in schizophrenic patients; that is, that their associations are guided by the same principles as normal people's. What these patients lack, he believed, is the ability to concentrate on what they want to say; in other words, they cannot focus their thoughts on the intended subject, the content at issue. The overt speech of these patients, therefore, is guided to a decreased extent by intentional thinking and the contextual constraints of the immediate actions and interactions, and to an increased extent by the idling apparatus of language production itself. We have already encountered one example of the language-production mechanism taking over functions usually performed by intentional thought: In normal people, rhyming words are actively inhibited from disturbing the flow of thought-directed speech. When this inhibition is no longer present, however, as in some schizophrenic patients, utterances are determined by clang and rhyme (i.e., by purely linguistic features) instead of by thoughts.

A second look at figure 10.1 helps to clarify what happens: If higher cortical areas no longer function properly, lower areas become comparatively more influential, even for high-level information processing.

Connections with accidentally aroused ideas, condensations, clang associations, intermediate associations. . . . All these thought-connections are not foreign to the normal psyche either. But they occur only exceptionally and incidentally, whereas in schizophrenia they are exaggerated to the point of caricature and often actually dominate the thought-processes. (Bleuler 1911/1950:23)

This view of schizophrenic formal thought disorder has not changed much up to the present time, and recent research findings are in clear support of this view. For example, in order to investigate the language capabilities and proficiencies of schizophrenic patients in relation to those of normal subjects, Allen and coworkers (1993) had subjects produce words of a given category ("name as many animals as come to mind now for one minute"). Schizophrenic patients performing this task produce fewer words than normal subjects. However, if they do the task five times on different days, and if the answers are lumped together, the differences in the number of names produced by schizophrenic patients and normal subjects disappear. This supports Bleuler's view that the associations are all there in schizophrenic patients but cannot be put to use. In other words, it is not the store of words that is missing but goal-directed *access* to the store.

Dysfunctional Lexical Access

In the mid-1980s, several studies of formal thought disorder in schizo-phrenic patients were performed at Harvard University, guided by the hypothesis that these patients suffer from dysfunctional access to stored words and meanings. Researchers used, in particular, *lexical-decision tasks* to investigate semantic priming effects in schizophrenic patients (figure 11.2).

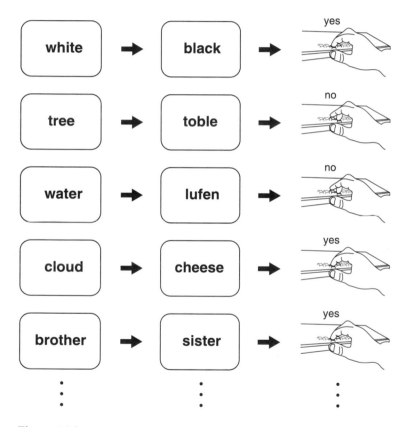

Figure 11.2
Experimental procedure for a study of semantic-priming effects using a lexical-decision task. Each row of the drawing represents the crucial aspects of a lexical-decision task. Only the first word (*prime*) is read by the subject. Then the subject has to decide whether the subsequent string of characters (*target*) is a word or not. The decision is made by pressing one of two buttons on the

If thought-disordered schizophrenic patients produce fewer normal associations than healthy subjects, we would expect them to show a decreased semantic priming effect when we experimentally probe their responses to normal associations by using lexical-decision tasks. After all, what is being measured in semantic priming is the presence of the normal associations that guide a simple behavioral response; accordingly, people with *decreased* normal associations should show a *decreased* semantic priming effect. It therefore came as a big surprise to find just the opposite: Thought-disordered schizophrenic patients show an *increased* semantic priming effect.

The reader will recall that the semantic priming effect tells us how much faster (either in milliseconds or in percentage) a word is recognized when it is preceded by a meaningfully related word. The effect, therefore, must be caused by normal associations. How, then, can the effect be larger in patients suffering from a *deficit* of normal associations?

The field of schizophrenia research is littered with strange, nonreplicated results that are due to chance, the high variability of anything measured in schizophrenic patients, and the thousands of studies carried out by diligent psychiatrists and psychologists vexed by this most enigmatic disorder. Hence, if a strange result is found, one should not think much about it but, instead, try to replicate it.

The first study in semantic priming in schizophrenic patients was carried out in the United States with eighteen patients—twelve with and six without formal thought disorder—and eleven control subjects. A similar study conducted in Heidelberg, Germany, with seventy patients—thirty-six with and thirty-four without formal thought disorder—produced the very same result (figure 11.3): an increased semantic priming effect in the thought-disordered schizophrenic patients (Spitzer et al. 1994b). How can we explain this result?

computer's keyboard. Only correct positive responses are subjected to further analysis. The mean of the reaction times for both conditions (related words, unrelated words) and the difference between the mean times for the two conditions (the *semantic priming effect*) are calculated. This difference tells how much faster subjects recognize target words associated with the primes than those not associated with them.

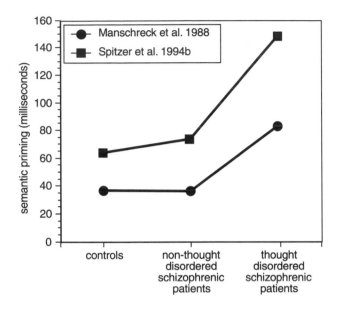

Figure 11.3
Semantic-priming effect in normal subjects, non–thought-disordered (NTD) schizophrenic patients, and thought-disordered (TD) schizophrenic patients. Results from two studies are shown. Although the absolute numbers are somewhat different (possibly due to a number of methodical details), the results published by Manschreck, Maher, and their coworkers in 1988 are strikingly similar to a replication study performed in Germany (Spitzer et al. 1994b). The main thrust of the findings is identical: thought-disordered schizophrenic patients display comparatively larger semantic-priming effects. In other words, patients who, by definition, suffer from disordered associative processes show a larger gain in their behavioral responses in a lexical-decision task than normal subject when they are provided with normally associated words. The effect is specific to thought disorder, since schizophrenic patients who do not suffer from thought disorder show the same priming effects as normal subjects.

As already suggested by Eugen Bleuler, thought-disordered schizophrenic patients may suffer from *dysfunctional access* to stored information about the meaning (the semantics) of words. This dysfunctional access may also be characterized as *less focused*.

The degree of focus of the access to a certain node in a semantic network may be described by a bell-shaped probability function (see figure 11.4). This bell-shaped curve indicates, for a specific node in the semantic network, the probability of the represented information being

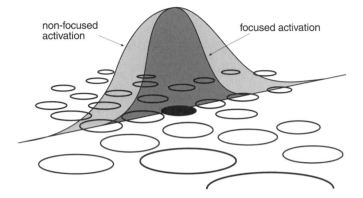

non-focused activation

focused activation

Figure 11.4

Semantic network (cf. figure 10.6, top), showing the degree of activation resulting from the intention to access the black node drawn in the vertical axis. The curves have to be mentally rotated around their highest point in the vertical axis in order to represent the activation properly. Because this effect cannot be drawn well in two dimensions, the figure shows only a cross section of this three-dimensional activation function. The entire process of activation should also be visualized as a dynamic process (cf. figure 10.6, bottom), of which we see only a snapshot at some point after lexical access has started. In normal subjects, this curve is usually quite steep and the activation spreads only slightly to immediately adjacent nodes (dark gray). In contrast, when the activation is less focused (light gray), it spreads farther and adjacent—and even more remote nodes—become activated. The wider focus, then, decreases the differences in activation of the intended node and other nodes; it therefore, increases the chances that other nodes will become active and influence actual speech production. Further activity at other locations in the net—wobbling around in the net, for example—may activate an entirely different node than the intended node and result in a formally disordered utterance.

accessed as intended. In other words, it tells us how accurately you "shoot," in your mind's lexicon, at a certain word. You may be very sharp and miss only rarely (and by a small margin), or your shooting may be less focused; that is, you may hit other nodes around the intended one rather often. If the curve is flat, the latter is the case, and on average, there will be little difference in the activation of the intended node and adjacent nodes. In this case, however, two things happen. (1) If the plan of your utterance requires use of a certain semantic content, the language-production system will call up a node but may incorrectly activate one at a higher level in the same neighborhood; your speech will therefore be full of associative intrusions, that is, unusual, oblique, and indirect associations. In short, your utterances will be formally thought disordered. (2) Within the (admittedly quite arbitrary) framework of a lexical-decision task, however, this dysfunction will become a virtue, in that the appearance of the prime will activate adjacent nodes and, hence, facilitate your performance of the task. This is why semantic priming occurs. Notice that this explanation accounts for both clinically abnormal associations and improved performance in a task involving the processing of normal associations.

Indirect Associations

The theory of semantic networks, spreading activation, and a larger activation focus in thought-disordered patients can explain the clinical phenomena and the counterintuitive experimental results quite well. However, a theory is only as good as its ability to generate *new* predictions (sometimes referred to as its *heuristic value*) and its ability to integrate a wide range of otherwise inexplicable or at least unrelated findings (referred to as its *integrative potential*). In the following section, we discuss an experiment (motivated by the careful observation of numerous patients) that exemplifies the heuristic value of the theory. Examples of its integrative potential are described in subsequent sections.

Bleuler described the relatively high frequency of indirect, oblique, or remote, associations in schizophrenic patients. This type of association, observed either in spontaneous speech or in the word-association test, goes from one word to another word via a not overtly spoken intermediate word. One of Bleuler's examples is *wood–dead cousin*. At first glance, this association appears to be a complete word salad. However, if you know that a cousin of the patient had died recently and was buried in a wooden coffin, it becomes obvious that this was in fact an indirect association, from *wood* to *wooden coffin* to *dead cousin*. One of my own patients who was severely formally thought disordered once had the association "*computer–no city*," another apparently complete word salad. I was curious enough to ask the patient what he meant, and he said: "It is obvious: Computer–Nixdorf–no city." Nixdorf is a German computer maker, *Dorf* is the German word for village, and *nix* is internationally understood. So the patient had gone from a concept (*computer*) to a related concept (the computer maker, *Nixdorf*) to an association of a part of the name of the computer maker (*village–city*).

In the word-association task, thought-disordered schizophrenic patients produce more indirect associations than non–thought-disordered schizophrenic patients and normal control subjects (Spitzer 1997). Bleuler commented on this phenomenon as follows: "In experimental investigations of association, we find a notable frequency of 'mediate associations.' I suspect that only the lack of sufficient observation has been responsible for our inability to demonstrate them more frequently in the thought-processes of our patients" (Bleuler 1911/1950:26).

With reference to figure 11.4, the theory of unfocused activation of semantic networks allows us to make the following prediction: If the priming effect for indirectly related words is measured, it should be smaller than the effect for related words, whereas the difference between thought-disordered schizophrenic patients and normal controls should be particularly marked. Figure 11.5 depicts this prediction in more detail.

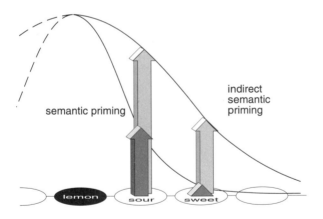

Figure 11.5
Activation characteristics soon after access to the *lemon* node in the semantic network. When the activation is tightly focused, it spreads to *sour* to some extent, but goes no farther than that (i.e., it does not spread to *sweet*). When the activation is unfocused, it should go not only to *sour* but also to *sweet*. Notice that the indirect associations should always be smaller than direct ones but should distinguish better between thought-disordered and non–thought-disordered subjects. These ideas guided the experiment on indirect semantic priming discussed below.

At the Psychiatric Clinic of the University of Heidelberg, we conducted a study of fifty schizophrenic patients and fifty normal subjects matched for age, gender, and education. (The latter is especially important when conducting research on language and related subjects.) We determined the direct semantic priming effect (see above) as well as the indirect semantic priming produced by introducing an indirectly related condition—in which the prime is related to the target via an intermediate association. The indirect pairs were produced by making a direct association to a direct association of the prime; for example, *lemon–sweet, lion–stripes, flower–thorn,* and *summer–snow* (cf. Spitzer 1993a,b,c). The results were in line with the predictions. Normal control subjects did not show a significant indirect semantic priming effect, and non–thought-disordered patients showed only a small, nonsignificant effect. In marked contrast, thought-disordered schizophrenic patients showed a marked and highly significant indirect semantic priming effect. The activation in their semantic network spreads through the network farther and faster (see below) than in the networks of people without thought disorder (see figure 11.6).

The increased indirect semantic priming effect in thought-disordered schizophrenic patients was replicated in subsequent studies. We further demonstrated that normal subjects will display indirect semantic priming if there is a pause of half a second between the prime and the target. This priming effect is still smaller than the effect in thought-disordered schizophrenic patients; however, if there is enough time, there appears to be some activation of indirectly related words in normal subjects. This finding suggests that the activation within semantic networks of schizophrenic patients not only spreads comparatively farther, but also faster.

What Pauses during Speech Reveal about Thoughts

There are many possible reasons for silence within speech. The speaker may be anxious or may not know exactly what to say, or may know what to say but have to search for the right sentence structure or the appropriate word. He or she may want to emphasize something and pause to capture the listener's attention, or may have articulation difficulties, or may simply want to take a breath.

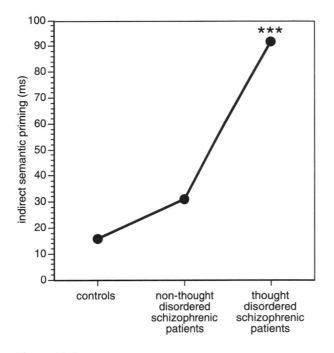

Figure 11.6
Indirect semantic priming in 50 normal control subjects, 21 non–thought-disordered patients, and 29 thought-disordered schizophrenic patients. The indirect semantic-priming effect in the thought-disordered patients as well as the differences in indirect semantic priming between this group and the control subjects are highly significant (as indicated by ***). The indirect semantic-priming effects of the other two groups are small and not significant. The difference between the two patient groups is significant (p 0.019; two-tailed t-test; data from Spitzer et al. 1993b).

The measurement of pauses in spontaneous speech can reveal dynamic aspects of the access to the mental lexicon. Psycholinguists know that the distribution of pauses in the spontaneous speech of normal subjects follows certain rules. Pauses are made between sentences and before content words within sentences, especially if the content is new and unexpected and the word is infrequently used in the language (Goldman-Eisler 1958, Butterworth 1973, 1975). Pauses between sentences are therefore the result of strategic planning processes, whereas pauses within sentences tell us something about how at ease the speaker is with subsequent words (Beattie & Butterworth 1979).

If the clinically observed disordered thinking of schizophrenic patients is the result of unreliable access to the stored semantic aspects of words, this should show up in the length of the pauses in their spontaneous speech. In particular, we should expect pauses before words that are clinically "strange" to be comparatively brief, because these words, according to the proposed model, are associative intrusions. (They are not, for example, the result of willful acts of the patients.) A study of the length of pauses in the spontaneous speech of schizophrenic patients and normal subjects demonstrated that this was in fact the case.

In order to obtain comparable speech samples, all participants in the experiment were asked to describe the same image rich in detail, Breughel's *Wedding Feast* (figure 11.7). Hence, subjects had to choose from the same set of many words denoting the things, people, or events illustrated in the picture. Their descriptions of the picture were audiotaped and transcribed as well as digitized for further sound analysis on a computerized sound system. The latter procedure permitted the measurement of the length of a pause with an accuracy of a few milliseconds. Only words within sentences were studied. From the verbatim tran-

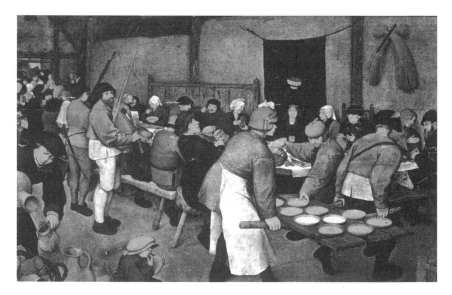

Figure 11.7
Picture used in the experiment: Breughel's *Wedding Feast.*

scripts, the words were divided into those suggested by the context of the picture and those that were not. The context words occurred in most descriptions and clearly referred to items in the picture. Each noncontext content word occurred only once in all the descriptions and did not refer to the picture in any simple way. (To give an example: If someone said, "I do not see a submarine in the picture," and if no one else has used the word *submarine* in any of the descriptions, then *submarine* was counted as a noncontext content word.)

In normal control subjects, there was a clear difference between the length of pauses before context versus noncontext words, in that people paused longer before noncontext words. This difference was also present in non–thought-disordered schizophrenic patients, who talked more slowly and made longer pauses altogether. In contrast, this difference in the length of pauses before context and noncontext words was not present at all in thought-disordered schizophrenic patients (figure 11.8).

In other words, whereas for healthy subjects the words denoting items on the picture were faster "at hand" to the speech-production system than words not suggested by the context—because subjects had to search in their minds for them, which presumably takes time—this was not the case in patients with formal thought disorder. The language-production system of these patients clearly does not differentiate between words denoting what is there and at issue (i.e., context words) and what is not (i.e., noncontext words). Words denoting strange and farfetched items pop into the mind without much control; hence, pauses before these words are no longer than the pauses before words that are appropriate.

Remote Ideas

Before you continue reading, please answer the following question: What is it that a table and a married couple have in common?

Maybe you thought that this is a silly question; maybe you have stopped pondering it after a few attempts. However, maybe briefly after the question the answer "four legs" struck through your brain like lightning. In this case you are either highly creative or better see your psychiatrist soon.

In the 1960s, the Russian psychologist Poljakov (1973) conducted experiments involving such strange questions with normal subjects and

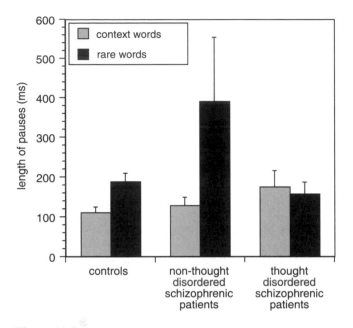

Figure 11.8
Contextually determined length of pauses in spontaneous speech (in milliseconds) in 36 control subjects and in 8 non–thought-disordered and 22 thought-disordered schizophrenic patients. The absolute heights of the columns are not important, but the *differences* in their heights are. The difference in the mean pause before context and noncontext words is clearly visible in normal subjects and non–thought-disordered patients. No such difference was found in the group of patients diagnosed with formal thought disorder (cf. Spitzer et al. 1994c).

schizophrenic patients. Asking for common features of far-apart concepts, he learned that schizophrenic patients were sometimes comparatively better at the task. This finding can be directly related to the hypothesis of a less tightly focused activation in semantic networks in some (viz., thought-disordered) schizophrenic patients. If the focus is tight, then each concept becomes activated for itself, and we have to use willful attention to plow through the associative connections of each of the concepts in order to solve the task. In contrast, if the focus of semantic network activation is spread out, there may be some spontaneous overlap of activation in the network (see figure 11.9). This should automatically produce activation of an association to both concepts, and the solution should pop into the mind without any conscious effort.

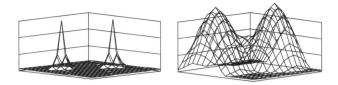

Figure 11.9
Schematic rendering of the focused and unfocused activation of a semantic network. If two concepts are presented to the subject, unfocused activation can lead to the spontaneous overlap of spreading activation.

How do different activation functions come about? What determines the width of the focus in our semantic networks?

Dopamine, Neuromodulation, Signal, and Noise

In 1952 it was discovered that chlorpromazine, a substance used to treat allergies, also alleviated the symptoms of schizophrenia. In the early 1960s, the Swedish pharmacologist Arvid Carlson related this discovery to biochemical findings about the effects of chlorpromazine and other substances that were by then being used to treat schizophrenia. Research in animals showed that these substances blocked receptors of neurons for the substance *dopamine,* which is released by special neurons in the brain. Carlson found a correlation between the clinical effect of a substance and its blocking effect on a specific subgroup of dopamine receptors. From this finding, he developed the *dopamine hypothesis* of schizophrenia. According to this hypothesis, schizophrenia is caused by too much dopamine in the brain (i.e., overactivity of the dopamine system). Agents that block the dopamine system (called *dopamine antagonists*), therefore, can be used to treat the disorder. These agents became widely known as *neuroleptic agents* or *neuroleptics.*

At the present time, this hypothesis is widely known, simple, compelling, and elegant. However, it suffers from one drawback: It is wrong.

In the brain, dopamine plays a role in three different functional systems: the system involved in motor control (the *nigro-striatal system*); the system governing release of the hormone prolactine, which activates milk production in the mammary glands (the *tubero-infundibular system*); and the system that influences the cortex and, hence, the higher cognitive functions (the *mesolimbic-mesocortical system*). The therapeutic actions of the neuroleptic agents obviously are brought about by their effects on the third dopaminergic system.

When dopamine antagonists are given to a schizophrenic patient, the effects on the motor control system are immediately visible: The patient may develop a tremor, muscle rigidity, and a highly unpleasant restlessness. These side effects of neuroleptics are highly stigmatizing and severely limit their therapeutic use. The desirable therapeutic effects, in contrast, come about days or even weeks after neuroleptic therapy has begun. This indicates that whereas blockade of the dopamine system happens immediately (as the side effects indicate), the therapeutic actions occur later and may be only indirectly related to the dopamine blockade.

Current discussion of the role of dopamine in the genesis of schizophrenia is conducted at a highly sophisticated level; a simple idea has become a highly complex model whose complex ramifications arouse considerable controversy. In brief, the following are the important points to keep in mind. First, it is generally assumed that schizophrenia involves, at different times, both increased and decreased activity of the dopaminergic system (Davis et al. 1991, Grace 1991, Heritch 1990). Second, the acute effect of neuroleptics is to block the dopamine system; but during chronic administration, something else may happen, perhaps even an increase in dopaminergic activity. Third, schizophrenia may not be a disorder of the dopamine system at all. Instead, it may result from some primary microanatomical deficit: a slightly faulty wiring of certain neurons, a loss of neurons in the frontal or temporal cortex, or a migration of neurons to the wrong location or wrong cortical layer. In any of these cases, the dopamine system would play only a secondary role within a compensatory process. In acute psychosis (not rarely triggered by stressful life events), this compensatory system would break down and lead to manifestation of the disorder. All of these possibilities are currently subjects of intense research.

Neuromodulation

Whatever the findings of research on the primary cause of schizophrenia, there is no doubt that dopamine plays some role in the disorder. This being so, the question arises how a small molecule relates to such signs and symptoms of schizophrenia as formal thought disorder and delusions.

Until a few years ago, this question was beyond the reach of scientific inquiry. Of course, we knew something about biochemical processes in the brain and were familiar with how the many symptoms of schizophrenia changed under neuroleptic (i.e., biochemical) treatment. The gap between biochemistry on the one hand and psychopathology on the other hand, however, appeared unbridgeable. Network models have changed all that.

To obtain a better understanding of the processes involved and to clarify the problem, let us start with the basic distinction between *neurotransmission* and *neuromodulation*. So far in this book, we have discussed only the first term (cf. chapters 2 and 3, figures 2.1 and 3.3). In this process, a neuron releases a substance (e.g., glutamate) at a synapse, which causes the opening of an ion channel at the other side of the synaptic cleft and, thereby, changes the membrane potential. This happens at a highly exact location (a single synapse) and within a few milliseconds.

There are, in addition to such rapid and spatially exact information processing carried out by glutamatergic and GABAergic neurons, other processes in which less than 1 percent of the brain's neurons are involved. These neurons do not, in a strict sense, carry out information processing but, rather, release substances such as norepinephrine, dopamine, serotonin, and acetylcholine diffusely across large areas of the cortex (figure 11.10). The effects of these substances are not mediated by receptors coupled to fast ion channels, but by receptors coupled to biochemical reactions inside the cell (*G-protein-coupled receptors*). These reactions take time and need several hundred milliseconds to complete.

In short, these neurons are, first, small in number, second, connected in a nonspecific, nontopological way, and, third, slow. Hence, they cannot do the job of fast and specific information processing. However, they do influence the functioning of the fast glutamatergic (and quite likely, the GABAergic) neurons—that is, the very neurons that do carry out information processing in the brain.

This influence over information processing by these few slow, diffusely wired neurons is called *neuromodulation*. Kaczmarek and Levitan define

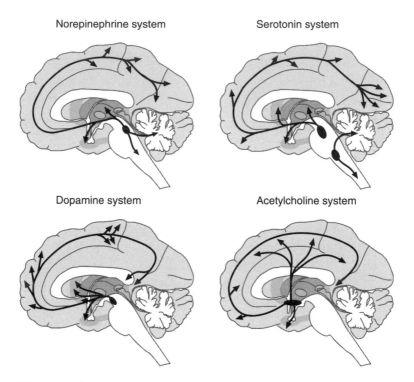

Figure 11.10
Schematic rendering of four neuromodulatory systems. Arrows indicate the cortical areas into which each neuromodulator is predominantly released.

neuromodulation as "the ability of neurons to alter their electrical properties in response to intracellular biochemical changes resulting from synaptic or hormonal stimulation" (1987:3). Neuromodulators do not directly carry out information processing, but they do affect it." How?

An analogy to a television set may provide an intuitive hint to how neuromodulators function. Fast information processing based upon neurotransmission corresponds to the signals coming in through the antenna or cable. Every picture element (pixel) of the screen is refreshed about every thirty milliseconds, and the detail displayed on the screen entirely depends on this signal. However, there is another, rather crude way to influence the image on a television screen: One can change brightness, contrast, or color by turning hand knobs. This change is slow and influences the entire display. The changes of brightness or contrast on the television screen correspond to the effects of neuromodulators in the brain. Just as we adapt the television screen image to the environment by changing contrast or brightness, neuromodulators fine-tune the general parameters of information processing to adapt to the particular demand characteristics of the organism's environment.

With respect to which aspects of information processing are changed by neuromodulatory processes, we can recognize from a purely subjective point of view the general changes that occur in our mental processes (i.e., thinking, perceiving, sensing, etc.): We know when we are more or less awake, can concentrate more or less well, and find ourselves in different mood states; and, depending on the particular state, we experience different sensations, perceptions, and thoughts.

Let's take an example. When we daydream and are free from anxiety, we may experience an endless stream of loosely associated ideas and internal images. Under such conditions we may come across unusual ideas and may actually be more than usually creative. The history of science is full of anecdotes describing how unexpected solutions to long-standing problems just sprang to mind without conscious effort—as it were, out of the blue. Some companies make use of this phenomenon when creative solutions are needed by holding brainstorming sessions in which anyone can say anything, free of the fear of criticism. In contrast, when there is imminent danger, or when anxiety is high, such "lateral," creative thinking no longer takes place. This makes sense, since lengthy streams of more or less well-connected associations are not adaptive in circumstances that call for rapid action. Any action performed in such conditions should be well trained and familiar, so that it can be carried out without much thought in an automatic sequence of actions. Conditions of anxiety and stress, therefore, exclude creativity. This makes sense from an evolutionary point of view, but it can be detrimental for a modern man or woman facing, for example, an oral examination. In sum, just as changes in brightness and contrast adapt the television image to the environmental conditions, changes in the general characteristics of information processing in the brain can be adaptive. Neuromodulation sets the general processing parameters and adjusts them to the demands of the environment.

We are used to thinking of neural transmission in terms of *activation* and *inhibition* and have frequently used these terms to describe what happens at the interface of nerves and muscles (the neuromuscular coupling). The terms are highly useful in this context, because they allow us to express relations between incoming impulses and muscular force. However, these concepts are not sufficient to capture complex neuromodulatory processes. Take, for example, the effects of norepinephrine and dopamine. Single-cell studies have shown that small concentrations of these agents have neither a directly activating nor an inhibitory effect. Instead, norepinephrine and dopamine *amplify strong signals and dampen weak signals*. To continue the analogy to visual images, these substances do not make the image brighter or darker but rather increase its contrast (figure 11.11). In neurocomputational terms, the amplification of a strong signal and the dampening of a weak signal result in an increase in the ratio between the signal and the system's background activity (which includes any small, spontaneous, and irrelevant activity). In short, norepinephrine and dopamine increase the *signal-to-noise ratio* in neuronal systems (cf. Cohen & Servan-Schreiber 1992).

Noise: Not a Bug, but a Feature

At first glance, a large signal-to-noise ratio may appear beneficial under all circumstances. After all, the music system in your living room doesn't have a knob you can turn to *increase* the background noise. However, we have already discussed cases in which noise may have positive effects under certain circumstances. For example, highly sharpened thoughts— that is, maximal signal and very little noise—may be detrimental if you want to come up with creative solutions to long-standing problems. Conversely, a lower signal-to-noise ratio with some "intrusions" of "far-fetched" thoughts may help. In chapter 7 we demonstrated by way of simulations that noise can facilitate the reorganization of networks of the self-organizing feature-map type (cf. figures 7.7 to 7.11). Similar processes in the nervous system are quite likely to help an organism adapt to new experiences. In fact, we may assume that the noise level is crucial to optimizing learning in neural systems.

From an evolutionary point of view, it is important to note that, compared to the silicon chips used in present-day computers, neurons are

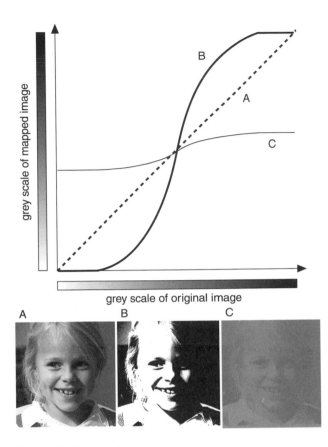

Figure 11.11

A source image mapped onto a target image by three different functions. These functions determine the contrast of the target image. Each gray value of the source image (A) is mapped onto a new gray value, as determined by the mapping function. If the function is steep, contrast is increased, since many dark pixels of the source image are mapped onto black pixels and light pixels are mapped onto white ones. The resulting image (B) has high contrast. If the function is almost flat, any gray levels from black to white are mapped onto a small band of gray values and the resulting image (C) is flat. The identical mapping (A) produces a target image that is like the source image. Similar mappings can be performed on any signal. The contrast of pictures roughly corresponds to the signal-to-noise ratio in general signal processing.

lousy pieces of hardware. As discussed in chapter 1, a neuron is about a billion times more prone to errors than a silicon chip. In the terminology of this chapter, the noise in neuronal systems is several orders of magnitude larger than the noise in silicon-based computers. If this is so, it is likely that systems built out of millions or even billions of such noisy devices—brains—have evolved in a way that puts this noise to some use rather than permanently fighting it off. If noise is a feature of systems (and not a bug), then the amount of noise in systems must be a crucial parameter, since noise can be either beneficial or detrimental, possibly depending on the computational task at hand. If so, then a mechanism to regulate the amount of noise in a computational system must itself have developed in response to evolutionary pressures. For example, if an organism needs a somewhat lower signal-to-noise ratio for learning and creativity than for responding rapidly to danger, then natural selection will ensure that the organism develops a way to modulate signal to noise. As a corollary, we can state that a generally too high or too low signal-to-noise ratio is maladaptive.

In semantic networks, a high signal-to-noise ratio leads to a tight focus of activation of nodes representing meaningful content. Under conditions of danger (e.g., approach of a large predatory animal), a high signal-to-noise ratio will make sure that the organism's well-learned response (perhaps to run away or climb a tree) will be carried out with high reliability. This is evolutionarily adaptive. Like all higher animals, human beings have evolved so that under conditions of incipient danger they don't fool around thinking laterally but respond quickly and efficiently with sequences of well-learned actions It would be highly dangerous and, hence, maladaptive to develop and try out new responses under such circumstances (although human children do so during play, as we saw in chapter 3). Researchers have used the old-fashioned word-association task to demonstrate that lateral thinking and creativity are blocked under conditions of perceived danger. In normal subjects, stress and anxiety lead to increased production of standard associations (such as *black–white, mother–father,* etc.) and, therefore, to a decrease in unusual associations (Mintz 1969). While this pattern of responses to danger worked well for early humans living on the savanna, it may produce maladaptive behavior in civilized society. We know, for example, that the anxious student or employee is unlikely to produce creative solutions under the very circumstances that call for such solutions. Anxious people, generally speaking, only reproduce what they already know. Moreover, we know that learning—whether in school or in a psychotherapeutic session—is facilitated by an open and unintimidating environment.

Formal Thought Disorder as the Result of Decreased Signal-to-Noise

In 1990, Jonathan Cohen and David Servan-Schreiber, two young psychiatrists from Pittsburgh, proposed on the basis of network simulations that formal thought disorder in schizophrenic patients is caused by a decreased signal-to-noise ratio, which in turn is caused by a decreased level of the dopamine needed to modulate the signal-to-noise ratio. This hypothesis, for the first time, integrated neurobiological and psychological facts, allowing us to relate psychopathological symptoms directly to brain functions. Mind and brain pathology could finally be viewed within a single common framework.

The Pittsburgh psychiatrists were able to demonstrate that a number of inexplicable, or at least unrelated, results could be easily explained within the framework they proposed. They described a series of network simulations in which an increase of noise resulted in dysfunctional network behavior analogous to the symptomatic dysfunctions of thought-disordered schizophrenic patients (Cohen et al. 1992, 1993). In short, under specific circumstances the researchers were able to simulate schizophrenic symptoms in neural network models. Their research fueled the tradition of network simulations of psychopathology begun by Yale psychiatrist Ralph Hoffman (cf. chapter 8) and provided new ideas to inspire further work in this field.

If their theory is correct and we extend it to the issue at hand, then dopamine should have an effect on human semantic networks. Such an effect should be demonstrable if both the spreading-activation theory and the focus hypothesis are correct. This line of reasoning led to another experiment using the lexical-decision method. If dopamine determines the signal-to-noise ratio in semantic networks, and if the width of focus in semantic networks is nothing but a larger or smaller amount of noise in such networks, then the focus should become tighter when subjects are under the influence of dopamine. As the size of the focus can be measured through semantic and indirect semantic priming effects (which decrease with a smaller, tighter focus), dopamine should decrease these effects. This was directly tested in a placebo-controlled, double-blind study in which normal subjects received either an oral placebo or L-dopa, a molecule that is transformed into dopamine in the brain (Kischka et al. 1996). (L-dopa is a precursor of dopamine.) As predicted, priming effects decreased under L-dopa; especially the indirect semantic priming effect, the more sensitive measure of the width of the activation focus, decreased significantly (see figure 11.12).

In the brain, L-dopa is transformed into dopamine as well as into norepinephrine. As both these agents are supposed to increase the signal-to-noise ratio, it might be argued that norepinephrine causes the obtained results. However, as norepinephrine is released into cortical areas that process sensations of touch and control motor behavior (the

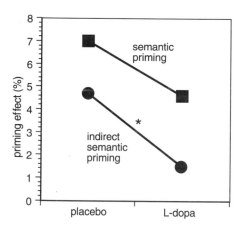

Figure 11.12
Direct (squares) and indirect (circles) semantic-priming effect in normal control subjects receiving either L-dopa (a precursor of dopamine) or placebo. Experimental procedures were identical to those described in figure 11.2, with the indirect condition added (as described in the text). To induce indirect priming in the normal control subjects under the placebo condition, researchers introduced a pause of half a second between prime and target. (This procedure had produced indirect priming in normal subjects in earlier studies.) As can be seen, the priming effects decreased under L-dopa, as predicted. This decrease was significant for the indirect priming effect, as indicated by * (data from Kischka et al. 1996).

primary sensorimotor areas), and as dopamine is released into regions involved in language processing, we may assume that the changes in the priming effects were in fact caused by dopamine.

Intermediate Result

We can summarize the facts, experimental results, and hypotheses regarding formal thought disorder in schizophrenic patients as follows:

1. Semantic networks have a maplike structure.

2. The access to such maps can be described by the spreading-activation model.

3. The width of the spread of activation corresponds to the accuracy of the activation. It is controlled by the neuromodulator dopamine.

4. If dopamine is decreased, the focus becomes wider and lexical access is less reliable and sharp. This can be captured by saying that the signal-to-noise ratio of the system is low. If dopamine is increased, then the signal-to-noise ratio is raised and the focus tightens (see figure 11.13).

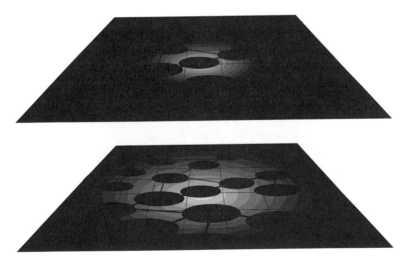

Figure 11.13
Focusing in a semantic network (cf. figures 10.5, 10.6, 11.4, and 11.9). In a network activation with a tight focus (i.e., a clear signal), above, a particular node should become most active (high dopaminergic tone; high signal-to-noise ratio). By contrast (below), in a loosely activated network (wide focus, low dopaminergic tone, and low signal-to-noise ratio) the signal determining which node is activated is relatively weak.

5. If the dopaminergic tone is comparatively low, signal-to-noise ratio is low and lexical access is unreliable. Clinically, this results in loose associations and an increase in indirect, remote associations.

6. The signal-to-noise ratio in semantic networks can be measured experimentally by obtaining priming effects. In formal thought-disordered schizophrenic patients, direct and indirect semantic priming effects are higher than in other populations. This implies that dopaminergic activation of language-related areas in these patients is comparatively low.

Meaning Electrified: EEG and Semantics

Whenever reaction times are measured, all the many processes that compose a given response are lumped together and are represented by a single number. For example, when a subject is shown a stimulus and has to make a decision to respond, perceptual, cognitive, and motor processes are all involved. A single process can only be investigated by measuring reaction times when several conditions are compared to each other. For example, in the lexical-decision experiments described above, the perceptual input and the motor output components of the task were assumed to be equal across all trials. Therefore, any differences in reaction times when different relations between the prime and target words are implemented must be due to semantic differences. This method has a long history, and its logic is widely used in the field of experimental psychology (cf. Posner 1986, Posner & Raichle 1994).

When carried over to experimental psychopathology, the method can still be used, but with caution. Schizophrenic patients may suffer from perceptual deficits (cf. Braff 1993), and we know that they have difficulties with decision making (Mundt 1984, Saß 1989) as well as with motor behavior. For these reasons, results from measuring reaction times in schizophrenic patients have great variability. When priming effects are measured, the variability caused by the above-mentioned factors will be combined with the differences in reaction times caused by semantic processing. In other words, the patient with formal thought disorder can carry out a lexical-decision task, but his or her performance will be affected by perceptual, decision-making, and motor deficits. This implies that differences in lexical access between normal subjects and thought-disordered schizophrenic patients will not be as easily detectable as they would be if we were able to measure lexical access directly.

Wouldn't it be nice if we could tap into semantic processing directly, bypassing (supposedly unreliable) overt behavioral (button press) responses? Given some technical sophistication, this is exactly what is possible.

For decades we have known that the small electrical currents produced by active neurons pass through the skull and can be recorded at the surface (figure 11.14). Such electroencephalographic (EEG) recording can be done while the person is performing, for example, a lexical-decision task, thereby giving us a direct view of semantic information processing. Since the early 1980s, researchers have known that semantic incongruencies produce a negative electrical potential, which is strongest in the middle of the scalp (Kutas & Hillyard 1980, cf. review by Kutas & van Petten 1994). For example, when you read the sentence "This morning, we had bread, butter, and socks," your brain produces a negative potential about four hundred milliseconds after you read "socks." Because of its polarity and timing, this potential is called the *N400*. In order to calculate the N400, we take the mean of many potentials generated under similar conditions—just as in reaction-time measurements we always use the mean to get rid of variations in the results. (See Regan 1989 for further methodological details.)

As figure 11.15 demonstrates, the N400 potential is clearly visible after the presentation of unrelated word pairs, whereas after related word pairs it is practically absent.

Obviously, we regard *black–white* as a fit, but don't see *cloud–cheese* the same way. In figure 11.15 the potential curves differ markedly at about 400 milliseconds post–stimulus onset, suggesting that we are looking specifically at semantic information processing. With respect to method, it is important to note once more that differences in the potentials caused by different experimental conditions are the most revealing.

Electrical recordings from many locations on the scalp allow for inferences regarding the location as well as the exact timing of computational processes. Using this method of high-resolution, event-related potentials (ERP), researchers can clearly map differences in access to semantic networks of thought-disordered schizophrenic patients and control subjects (Spitzer et al. 1997, Spitzer and Kammer 1997). When indirectly related words are presented, the potential curve of normal control subjects resembles the potential curve when unrelated words are presented.

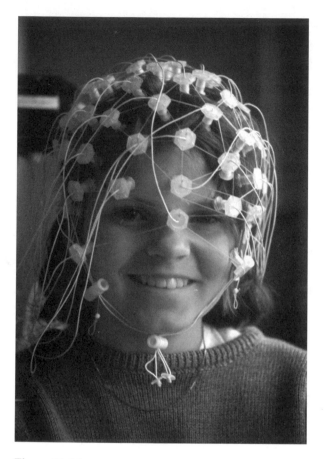

Figure 11.14
Sixty-four-channel geodesic electrode net for recording high-resolution event-related potentials. Electrode nets of this type were developed by Don Tucker at the University of Oregon (cf. Curran et al. 1993, Tucker 1994). They allow the comparatively quick application of many electrodes and have been used, for example, in the study of small children's language development mentioned in chapter 9 (Dehaene-Lambertz & Dehaene 1994).

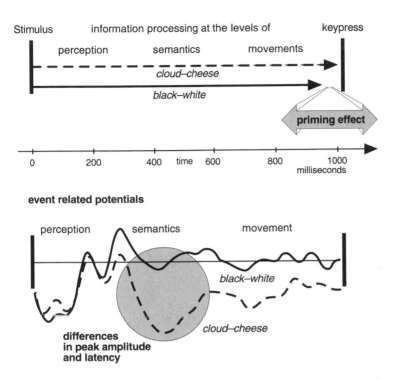

Figure 11.15
Reaction-time studies reveal preliminary, approximate, and comparatively rough estimates of differences in central nervous information processing. The example demonstrates that lexical decisions involve perceptual, cognitive, and motor processes. As all of these processes may be disturbed in a schizophrenic patient; differences specifically related to lexical access may not show up in experimental reaction-time studies, because the error variance in a patient's data may be so high that the semantic effect cannot be distinguished from it. Event-related potentials, by contrast, provide a window on the entire time span from stimulus perception to motor output and thus permit the direct (on-line) investigation of language-system components situated between perceptual input and motor output.

In other words, electrophysiologically speaking, normal subjects process indirectly related word pairs just as they do unrelated word pairs. Schizophrenic patients, however, do not. They process indirectly related words as if they were related words; their ERP-potential curve for indirectly related words looks like the curve produced for directly related word pairs. Accordingly, the curves produced by indirectly related word pairs and unrelated word pairs are significantly different. In sum, N400 potentials nicely reflect the results from the reaction-time studies and lend further support to that work.

Associative and Working Memory

Whenever we utter a thought, a very small fraction of our large repertoire of stored meanings is actualized. When I say something, I use a few of my thousands of words to convey just a few semantic items. These few words are "at hand" for a few hundred milliseconds, then disappear from my conscious stream of thought and speech. The mental function that holds on line the content relevant to any given short period of time is called working memory (see chapter 8). Working memory is clearly distinct from long-term memory, which stores the memory of episodes (specific events) as well as of the generalizations extracted from experience—most notably, semantic associative memory. Working memory stores what we currently need for action (including verbal action). For example, to understand a sentence, an action, or a story (Mazoyer et al. 1993), we have to keep in mind the appropriate contexts of single words or behaviors and string them together into a meaningful gestalt.

Several clinical observations suggest that schizophrenic patients have difficulty using relevant contextual information to guide thought- and decision-making processes. As we explained in chapter 8, these functions are carried out in the frontal lobes, which are known to be involved in the organization and planning of goal-directed behavior. According to a large number of neuroimaging studies (Andreasen 1994), schizophrenic patients suffer from *hypofrontality,* that is, failure to activate the frontal lobes for tasks that require them to be activated in order to be carried out properly. In other words, schizophrenic patients suffer from a dysfunction of working memory, which severely impairs goal-directed thinking (Park & Holzman 1992, Spitzer 1993).

As shown in figure 11.10, dopamine is released in the frontal lobes. It has been demonstrated that dopamine increases the capacity of working memory, and it may be assumed that the lack of dopamine impairs the function of the frontal lobes. These assumptions allow us to relate the clinical symptoms of schizophrenia to the general model of language comprehension and production discussed in chapter 10 (cf. figure 10.1). According to this model, we not only have to look for neuromodulatory changes in a *single* area or network but also to pay attention to whether interactions occur between areas. Within the framework of the model, it follows that a frontal lobe in which dopamine release is decreased will no longer provide the top-down input needed by other language areas. This top-down input encompasses contextual information, gestalt formation, and analytic and focusing processes bearing on the proper functioning of lower-level areas. This decreased influence from "above" causes lower-level areas to process information solely according to their own immanent structures and computational capabilities. Hence, language becomes less goal- and thought-directed, less influenced by the internal structure of the long-term store in which words and their meanings are kept. In short, a dysfunctional frontal lobe will lead to utterances driven more by associative chains, or even by clang relations (presumably one more level down from the semantic network), than by goal-directed thinking (figure 11.16).

This view is corroborated by a British study (Dolan et al. 1995), during which twelve healthy subjects and twelve schizophrenic patients had to either repeat words or produce words of a given category. The activation of the brain produced by performing these tasks was measured using positron emission tomography (PET). The first phase of the experiment uncovered the well-known (and above-described) decreased activation of the frontal lobes in the schizophrenic patients. When normal subjects spoke new words ("name as many animals as possible as quickly as possible"), their frontal lobes became active, whereas the frontal lobes of schizophrenic patients did not. In the second phase of the experiment, the task was repeated after giving all twenty-four subjects apomorphine, a substance that stimulates dopamine receptors and, hence, mimics the effects of dopamine release. In this phase, only the patients had increased frontal activity, and only when they had to produce new words. In other words, strengthening the dopaminergic system had an effect only on the

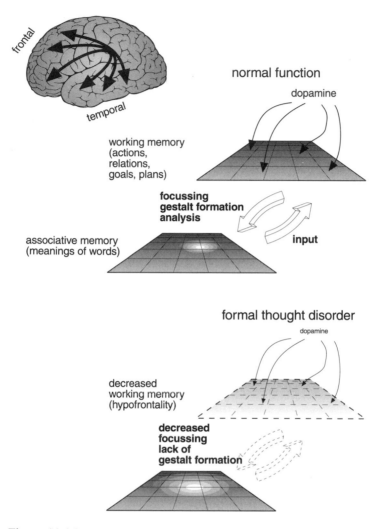

normal function

formal thought disorder

Figure 11.16
The frontal lobe is connected to semantic associative maps that—at least in part—are located in the temporal lobe (top left). When the frontal lobes are sufficiently "irrigated" by dopamine, they function normally and provide enough focus for lower-level semantic (and phonological) maps. If dopamine irrigation dries up, the frontal lobes no longer do their job properly, and utterances are guided to a lesser degree by frontal functioning. They become less planned and less goal and thought directed. Instead, the internal structures of long-term memory take over, producing speech governed by associations and phonological similarities.

group in which it was initially decreased and only on the task for which it was needed. Furthermore, the frontal activation was found in a specific frontal region, the *cingulate gyrus,* which we know to be involved in directing attention.

It is known that the frontal cortex has intricate connections to the temporal cortex, which traditionally has been regarded as the seat of associative memory. The anterior cingulate cortex is likely to mediate, through these connections, the integration and structure-formation processes. Studies in primates have demonstrated the direct influence of the cingulate cortex on the temporal cortex (Müller-Preuss & Ploog 1981), and studies in humans suggest that a similar influence is also present in our species (Fletcher et al. 1995).

Finally, it should be noted that recent studies suggest that long-term neuroleptic treatment increases the dopaminergic tone of the frontal lobes and, accordingly, decreases the heightened priming effects of thought-disordered schizophrenic patients to normal levels (Spitzer et al. 1994, Spitzer 1997, Young et al. 1995).These studies demonstrate that dopamine may improve language and thought processes in schizophrenic patients and indirectly corroborate the idea that disordered thought is the result of a decreased dopaminergic tone in the frontal lobes.

In the following section, I apply the model of the interaction of associative and working memory to resolve a long-standing dispute in psychiatry.

Metaphors and Concretism

Our common language is full of metaphoric phrases, which often go unnoticed in everyday speech and understanding. We do not really hurt ourselves; nor do we engage in grasping motions when we hit the hay to catch some Zs; people biting bullets or the dust or even chewing the fat don't really move their jaws; and you need not work on a farm to get the cream of the crop, spill the beans, hold your horses, take the bull by the horns, put all your eggs in one basket, or look for a needle in a haystack.

In order to comprehend a metaphor, we need to put the words of a sentence into context; only then can the metaphoric meaning be constructed. When I say, "Hans is skating on thin ice," neither winter sports nor snow are at issue. Instead, I am saying that Hans is taking a *risk*. None of the words in the sentence is associatively linked with risk, however, and only the interaction of the words within the sentence conveys the metaphoric meaning.

The term *concretism* denotes the inability of patients—mostly schizophrenics—to generalize, which shows up in their thought, speech, and behavior. Such patients tend to comprehend only the concrete meaning of words or sentences, rather than their general or metaphoric meaning. For example, if schizophrenic patients have to interpret proverbs that express a general idea by mentioning a concrete object (e.g., "My love is like a red, red rose"), they are able to identify the latter, but not the former (cf. Holm-Hadulla & Haug 1984).

Schizophrenic thinking has been described not only as overly concrete but also as overly abstract (cf. American Psychiatric Association 1994:278). The fact that schizophrenic patients often produce remote associations to a given content has often been taken as evidence for their ability to "transgress" concept boundaries and think in a highly abstract manner. Thus, there appears to be an unresolved puzzle about the way schizophrenic thinking differs from normal thinking. Since abstractness and concreteness are the two ends of a continuum in which normal thinking takes up the middle ground, the question remains: Is schizophrenic thinking overly abstract or overly concrete?

To answer the question of when and to what extent the concrete and abstract meanings of a sentence are present during the process of understanding, we employed, again, the lexical-decision method. Instead of words, we used phrases as primes, while words denoting or associated with, respectively, the concrete and the abstract meaning of the phrases were the targets. For example, we used *He is skating on thin ice* as a prime, and *winter* as well as *risk* were the related targets. Hearing this prime should activate, within a few hundred milliseconds, its sound pattern, the semantic codes for the words making up the phrase, and, finally, the code for the meaning of the entire phrase. During this process, as the nodes in the semantic network become activated, the activation may spread to adjacent nodes—for example, from *ice* to *winter* and *snow*. If the statement has an additional metaphoric meaning, then this meaning (in our example, *risk*) should also be activated during the time it takes the individual to comprehend the phrase. This process may take some time, as sometimes happens when we do not immediately "get the picture." The time it takes to understand the metaphoric meaning is not only subjectively noticeable but can also be objectively measured in psychological experiments (Alonso-Quercy & Vega 1991, Cacciari & Tabossi 1988, Clark & Lucy 1975, Janus & Bever 1985; for a review, see Spitzer et al. 1994a).

Such a study in normal subjects and schizophrenic patients (figure 11.17) demonstrated that four hundred milliseconds after the prime sentence was presented only the concrete meaning was active. At this point, normal subjects presented with *He is skating on thin ice* showed a priming effect for *snow* but not for *risk*. A little later, twelve hundred milliseconds after presentation of the prime, normal subjects showed a priming effect for both *snow* and for *risk;* that is, both the concrete and the metaphoric meanings were mentally present. In marked contrast, at this point schizophrenic patients showed a large concrete priming effect but none for the metaphoric target (i e , *snow* was highly active, but *risk* was not active at all).

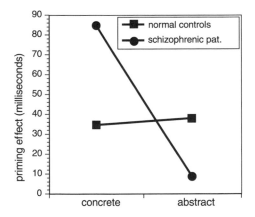

Figure 11.17
Concrete and metaphoric priming effects in 43 normal control subjects and 35 schizophrenic patients (data from Spitzer et al. 1994a). The interaction between group (patients versus normal subjects) and condition (concrete versus metaphoric) was significant.

Automatic priming effects for word pairs such as *ice* and *snow* were, obviously, more pronounced in the patients than in the control subjects. The active process of constructing the metaphoric meaning from the components of the phrase, on the other hand, was either severely impaired or unusually slow in the patients. The results again suggest that activation of semantic associative memory in schizophrenic patients is less focused than it is in normal subjects (as indicated by a larger concrete priming effect). Moreover, the data point to a dysfunctional working memory, since this cognitive function is essential to the process of constructing metaphoric meaning. Recognition of the metaphoric meaning cannot result from automatic processing of the spreading-activation type. Instead, the words of the phrase have to be held on line as the new, metaphoric meaning is actively constructed.

In sum, the above-mentioned psychopathological puzzle—that schizophrenic patients appear to be overly concrete as well as overly abstract (metaphoric)—can be resolved as follows. Schizophrenic patients *seem* to be overly abstract, because they access meanings unreliably, thereby producing remote associations and easily transgressing concept boundaries. In fact, however, these features are not indicative of abstract thinking but of unreliable lexical access. The true hallmarks of abstract thinking— planning, the production of new ideas by keeping several items on line, and using them creatively to form new gestalts (thereby thinking *beyond* the associative halos of single words)—all are impaired in schizophrenic patients.

Delusions

Delusions, a frequent symptom of schizophrenia, are by definition ideas with an unlikely, impossible, or false content, or with a metaphysical or religious content beyond empirical truth value. To the person experiencing a delusion, its reality is beyond doubt, denial, or refutation by others. The contents of a patient's statements about a delusion, as well as the way they are put forward, is important to the diagnosis. A person with delusions will cling to them even in the face of clear negative evidence.

Acute delusions are often accompanied by strong emotions and increased vigilance. The state of mind that facilitates the occurrence of delusions is called the *delusional mood*. Anxiety, suspiciousness, and increased vigilance lead to the overinterpretation of unimportant and trivial events; these events are given a special meaning, and relationships between events are fabricated without reason. Once delusional statements enter the mind, coupled with intense emotion and determined by the person's motivational state, they are woven tightly into the stream of the patient's subjective experience, where they become completely and inextricably entrenched and no longer subject to doubt.

Acute delusions tend to become chronic. The patient works his or her delusions—often together with the content of auditory hallucinations and real experiences—into a *delusional system* that encompasses pathology as well as true life history. Hence, chronic delusions are not so much a mental state as a part of a person's thoughts, values, attitudes, hopes, and aims. In some cases, chronic delusions are the result of a long developmental process that does not begin with some initial acute delusion. Unusual experiences coupled with suspiciousness and a certain readiness to jump to unfounded conclusions may, in the absence of social contacts and corrections, lead to development of systematic ideas that eventually become indistinguishable from a delusional system. For example, if a single person prone to suspiciousness and anxiety is alone in a foreign country and without social interaction and feedback or mastery of the local language, he or she may develop delusions (Allers 1920, Herschmann 1921). By the same token, people with partial deafness are also more than usually prone to develop delusions (Kraepelin 1909, cf. Fuchs 1993).

Acute delusions can often be effectively treated with neuroleptic drugs, whereas chronic delusions often do not respond to pharmacotherapy, or only respond to some degree or after a long time.

Acute Delusions and Neuromodulation

Several researchers have linked acute delusions and hallucinations to a hyperactive dopaminergic system (Davis et al. 1991, Grace 1991). Such a relationship is suggested by the fact that amphetamine—an indirect dopamine agonist—can cause psychotic states characterized by delusions and hallucinations (Angrist 1983, Bell 1965, Sano 1956). In contrast to hallucinogens like LSD, psilocybin, and mescaline, which cause visual hallucinations, amphetamine causes acute delusions, increased vigilance, irritability, high levels of activity, and suspiciousness. It acts by increasing the activity of dopamine and norepinephrine.

According to the model of the action of dopamine and norepinephrine discussed above, these two neuromodulators then increase the signal-to-noise ratio, making it possible to access stored semantic information with a high degree of reliability, but also decreasing the likelihood that representations in the network will change. Under such circumstances, it is conceivable that small environmental signals (i.e., perceptions to which we would normally pay little or no attention at all) may become amplified and result in experiences of "significant events" when merely ordinary events are in fact occurring. Once such spurious meanings are activated and become subject to further thought processing, they are less likely than normal to be forgotten (passively, through some decay mechanism) or actively discarded. Competing concepts, ideas, and "hypotheses" about reality are then less likely to become activated, so that there is less interference with the delusional meaning. Thus, an increased signal-to-noise ratio leads, in several ways, to an increased likelihood that ordinary things or events will gain unusual significance and to a decreased likelihood that such spurious significances—once generated—will either passively decay or be actively erased. The reduced width of the focus of the "mental spotlight" is experimentally suggested by the finding that patients with delusions show reduced semantic priming (Henik et al. 1992).

Chronic Delusions and Neuroplasticity

Delusions become part of the sufferer's experience. Hence, delusions are not just experienced but are also processed further. In this view, acute delusions can be seen as the *input,* which reaches progressively higher cortical maps and is laid down there, together with other experiences of acute psychosis. As the degree of any input-driven change of cortical representations depends on their relevance and frequency of occurrence, we can deduce that the longer the state of psychosis, the larger will be the long-term impact of the psychotic state on the patient's mental functioning.

Chronic delusions can therefore be regarded as distortions of the high-level cortical semantic-representation maps. Historically, a similar view was proposed in the 1960s by the Heidelberg psychiatrist Werner Janzarik (1988), who derived the concept of *structural deformation* from his clinical observations and interpretation. The term was later used by neurobiologists to denote similar changes that result from the neuroplasticity of maps (cf. Merzenich et al. 1988). This concept implies that cortical representations change their size (and, hence, that maps of these representations change their structure) and enlarge or shrink, depending on the input over time.

Once such deformations exist, you cannot get rid of them easily. They are stored representations, just as other representations are stored; and, because of their emotional salience, they may even be more tightly associated with other emotional content. From research in normal psychology, we know that even normal people do not readily change their views, even when faced with contradictory evidence. Changes, if they happen, are usually gradual. Moreover, we know—not least from psychotherapeutic experience—that marked changes in our views of things are often accompanied by anxious feelings. This is particularly the case for patients with delusions, as they are already predisposed to tension and anxiety. As a consequence, even if the neuromodulatory changes that led to acute delusions are no longer present, the deformations brought about by this state of mind are hard to correct. Any such attempt is likely to cause anxiety, which, in turn, will decrease the likelihood of change.

It should be noted that chronic delusions, namely, deformations of high-level representations (as simulated in artificial neural networks), may be caused by highly restricted input. Our model does not, therefore, contradict psychological models of the development of delusions postulated by clinicians (cf. Kretschmer 1927/1974). Rather, it provides the neurobiological and neurocomputational underpinnings of a process of delusional development caused by a restricted environment.

To summarize, clinical, pharmacological, and psychological evidence all suggest that increased activity of the neuromodulator dopamine plays a role in acute delusion. The acute delusional state is characterized not only by increased suspicion, anxiety, and vigilance but also, in neural networks carrying out higher cognitive functions, by an increased signal-to-noise ratio. Such an increased signal-to-noise ratio impairs neuroplasticity, that is, the likelihood of change.

This view is of immediate relevance for the treatment of patients with delusions. It is known that acute delusions respond rather well to neuroleptic treatment, whereas chronic delusions do not. This follows from the fact that neuroleptics can affect neuromodulatory states but cannot change the deformed semantic maps that store long-term, high-level representations. In order to change these representations, new input—that is, new experience—is needed. Accordingly, a low-key, monotonous psychosocial environment is not helpful in the treatment of chronically delusional patients. Thus one of the most important therapeutic consequences of the proposed neurobiological and neurocomputational model of delusions is the recommendation not simply to dispense drugs but, instead, to provide an environment that facilitates new experiences within a milieu that does not evoke anxiety. In some chronically deluded patients who also suffer from chronic neuromodulatory dysregulations, the use of drugs is indicated to stop the acute delusions from occurring repeatedly. However, even in these patients, this is only the first step. *All* patients must have new experiences. This corresponds well to the clinical impression that under circumstances of increased pressure of reality created by, for example, a somatic illness, death of a close relative, or a move to a different hospital, delusional symptoms temporarily decrease.

Recap

Schizophrenia, a severe mental disorder, afflicts approximately 1 percent of people, influencing their perceptions, volitions, emotion, thought, and behavior. In this chapter we have focused on the disorders of thought characteristic of schizophrenia. We saw that early in this century, using an experimental approach to study word associations, the Swiss psychiatrist Eugen Bleuler and his resident Carl-Gustav Jung were able to provide detailed descriptions of schizophrenic formal thought disorder. Bleuler also suggested that patients with formal thought disorder suffered from dysfunctional access to stored high-level representations, a hypothesis that was experimentally confirmed a decade ago. Clinically, schizophrenic patients with formal thought disorder display highly unusual associative connections between ideas, because activation in their semantic networks is extremely unreliable. The concepts of signal and noise introduced in chapter 7 usefully capture this unreliability, as schizophrenic patients with formal thought disorder suffer from a low signal-to-noise ratio, compared to normal subjects and patients without formal thought disorder.

The neuromodulator dopamine controls the signal-to-noise ratio in the cortex. Especially in the frontal cortex—the brain area that carries out the functions of working memory and selective attention—there has to be enough dopamine for access to associative memory to occur within a tight focus. If there is a lack of dopamine in the frontal lobe, it can no longer provide the structure, ability to form gestalts, processing power, and on-line context needed for clear, goal-directed thinking. Instead, thoughts and utterances are influenced to a larger degree by the internal structure of the associative store, that is, by associative chains determined by the structure of semantic networks, or even by sound similarities stored in (even lower-level) sound maps.

Acute delusions are caused by dysfunctional neuromodulation, whereas chronic delusions are a product of the neuroplasticity of cortical representations.

There have always been mentally ill people everywhere on earth. One of the major cultural advances of our time has been the recognition that they are ill. Only this view allows us to understand, as well as help, these patients. Together with neurobiological advances, neural network simulations provide a deeper understanding of mental illness and a framework within which biological as well as psychological knowledge and therapeutic strategies can be integrated. Such a framework is dearly needed by present-day psychiatry. We can now abandon dogmatic fights between brain- and mind-based schools of thought, which did nothing but harm to our patients.

12

Thoughts and Impressions

What are the consequences of our understanding of neural networks for understanding ourselves? Can computer models, vector transformations, and the algebra of matrices really help us grasp the essence of human beings?

The variety of models discussed in the chapters of this book leaves many questions open. Which model best fits our own brain? Should we built a large computer and simulate all the known neurons and connections of the brain in order to really learn about ourselves? I take up such critical issues, among others, in this final chapter. However, I also demonstrate that such questions rest upon misconceptions about the nature of science in general and of models in particular.

Once we have looked at these misleading arguments, it will be time to consider what neural network models offer us: namely, a new perspective on human mental functions—not only perception and thought, but also mood, affect, and emotions. The new neuroscientific framework may even allow us to develop previously unfeasible research and ideas about temperament and personality.

Understanding neural networks, therefore, implies nothing less than an enhanced understanding of ourselves. Such an improved self-understanding is the ultimate goal of this book. Moreover, if this understanding is in fact really new and better than the one we had before, it should have immediately practical consequences for the ways we deal with ourselves and with others.

Back to the Basics: What Are Models?

As explained in chapter 1, models are a simplification of reality. If models did not simplify matters, they would not be models but, instead, reality itself. Models, as it were, have a right to exist only insofar as they are simple. The small toy network for pattern recognition described in chapter 2 may serve as an example: There is no real brain that is built like it (nor is the model by any means intended to represent a real brain). Because of its simplicity, however, it permits us to develop insights that would be impossible to derive from examination of a real brain. The degree of simplification varies from model to model, depending on the phenomenon under study and the question being investigated. In all cases, the goal is to find a model of maximal simplicity that nonetheless captures all the features to be studied (Rall 1995).

Principles

Because of their marked simplification, the network models currently discussed in psychology are likely to be wrong. They are insufficient to represent the complex reality of the brain, just as (to return to the metaphor introduced in chapter 1) the law of gravity does not sufficiently describe the swirling leaves in an autumn forest. Like any model, a neural network model seeks to reduce the aspect of the real world it represents to its essential components. As mentioned earlier, model building, an integral part of doing science, necessarily involves *generalization* (i.e., disregarding details) and simplification of the complex phenomena under study. A good model represents only those aspects of a complex data set that are essential from a certain perspective. This explanation may sound vague—and it is! Model building is just as much an art as it is a part of science. The art lies in finding the essential features of the phenomena under study and separating them from the contingent ones. Models are therefore neither true nor false. Instead, they are useful or not; they either explain many phenomena or only a few; and they fit either well or poorly. With good models we can identify general principles that would be difficult to detect if we were not disregarding peculiarities.

In the course of our discussion we encountered several such general principles. We learned, for example that modules—that is, networks of networks—work better than a single large network. We found that neural networks are capable of generalizing and forming prototypes and that they self-organize and build meaningful structures that change when the input changes. Networks also detect structures in time and, therefore, can make predictions. We have learned that networks under development are able to extract more complexity from their environments than static networks.

Within the past ten or fifteen years, researchers have developed many different network structures for modeling various biological or psychological processes and solving vexing problems in these fields. The differences among the models reflect differences in the fields' levels of knowledge, research strategies and questions, and scientific cultures. Needless to say, a number of different principles have been discovered. James McClelland, a leading figure in neural network research in psychology, summarizes very clearly the leading idea of network modeling: "All my models may be wrong, but some of the principles we have discovered using them may be right" (personal communication).

It is plainly wrong to ask for a "biologically correct" network. This demand is not suited to the general nature of models and how they work. Moreover, the question implies a level of uniformity of the subject under study that does not exist. It has to be assumed that, in the course of evolution, different types of biological neural networks have developed within central nervous systems to meet different computational demands (Eichenbaum 1993). For example, the function of the cortex can be modeled with self-organizing feature maps (as in a Kohonen network), whereas the hippocampus appears to more closely resemble an auto-associative (Hopfield) network. The interaction of different cortical areas that are still under development may be simulated with Elman networks. In sum, the search for a "correct" network model of the brain would be naive from the point of view of the philosophy of science and inappropriate to the subject of investigation.

Realistic and Abstract Models

Neural network models differ greatly with respect to their biological plausibility. At present there are highly realistic models of the information processing that occurs at the dendrites of single neurons (Segev 1995), of clusters of cells in simple ganglia (Hooper 1995), and of the brain functions of insects and amphibians (Engelhaaf & Borst 1993). There are also models of cell membranes and receptors that, by means of differential equations, allow researchers to simulate molecules docking at receptors. Such models are quite close to biological reality. However, this fact alone does not render them "better" than other models. They merely have a different purpose than the more abstract models discussed in this book. Most of the psychologically and psychiatrically relevant neural network models are of this kind; they are abstract in nature because they are analogous to biological structures only in a certain respect.

Learning algorithms also differ with respect to their biological plausibility, that is, whether or not they could be implemented in biological nervous systems. For example, Francis Crick has used the following arguments to criticize the widely used backpropagation algorithm (in which the errors made by the network are fed back into it) (1988, 1989). First, he points out that in biological systems the optimal output is not known a priori (i.e., there is no "trainer" to teach the network a certain function). Second, there is no known biological mechanism by means of which the necessary feedback of errors could be implemented. However, functional reciprocity (as described in chapters 6 and 8) *has* been established for almost all anatomically interconnected cortical areas (Fellemann & van Essen 1991, Mumford 1992). In the visual system, for example, information does not flow in one direction—namely, from simple to complex areas. On the contrary, anatomical connections exist in both directions, which is why the perception of nonexistent contours in visual illusions (see figure 6.7) is paralleled by activation of contour neurons in the primary and secondary visual cortex. This activation cannot be driven by the stimulus, since the stimulus does not actually consist of the perceived contours. Rather, the contour is the result of an interpretive process by higher cortical centers, which feed the result of their activity back to the lower level. Since they—as it were—"figured out" that there *should* be contours, they send back a pattern of activation that corresponds to the contours, which is why the pattern exists in the lower areas. Thus the contours of such a well-ordered gestalt are seen (cf. figure 6.7), even though there is no input corresponding to it (Metzger 1975).

With respect to the first point of Crick's critique, we have already noted that biologically more plausible learning algorithms that produce results similar to those of the backpropagation algorithm have been developed.

In other words, not only is there a lot of feedback in the brain, but there are also theoretical ways of network learning that correspond rather nicely to known brain properties. Finally, we could point to several of the striking similarities between computer simulations and human behavior that we described in earlier chapters.

Models in Medicine

Brain disorders can be investigated in various ways. Psychologists describe pathological phenomena from the realms of subjective experience and objective behavior and use them to construct *psychological models* of pathology. Research data from animal studies and deceased humans allow other researchers to fashion *biological models* of pathology. More recently, *computational models* have been added to the psychological and biological ways of modeling brain disorders. Neural network models are not special, they are simply a new way of constructing models in the enterprise called science.

The medical and psychiatric research discussed in this book have demonstrated that neural network models allow us to investigate categorically different phenomena within a single unifying model. The factors that influence human subjective experience and objective behavior— whether the effects of environmental stress (psychological level) or the effects of dying neurons, pruned connections, or neuromodulatory agents (biological level)—cannot be studied in isolation but must be viewed within an interactive framework. The network perspective provides new and unexpected insights in several areas of research: from the need for modularity in brain architecture, to the necessary role of connectivity in the production of abstract representations, to the causes of critical periods in language acquisition. In psychiatry, neural network research has been conducted for a mere ten years, but it has already created network models for almost every major mental dysfunction.

Neural network research by no means leads to an inadequate view of human beings, or even reduces the human organism to a mere machine, a computer. The phantom sensations described in chapter 7 and the discussion of schizophrenia in chapter 11 should provide enough material to demonstrate that these models of neurological and psychiatric disorders are quite compatible with detailed descriptions of subjective experiences. The argument that computer models would eliminate the subjective viewpoint in the fields of psychiatry and neurology is, therefore, not only short-sighted, but plainly wrong. For one thing, computer simulations are likely to contribute to an unprejudiced and unbiased description of experience. Second, computer simulations often open, or at least sharpen, the eyes of observers to phenomena and experiences they would otherwise not notice. For example, patients' assertions that a teardrop running down the cheek caused the sensation of a second drop running down the phantom limb lacked any validity for generations of neurologists adhering to the peripheral model of phantom causation (cf. chapter 7). Third, findings from research into neuroplasticity emphasize the primary importance of experience (including motivation and attention) for brain functioning. Statements like, "Humans are nothing but a complicated piece of chemical machinery" clearly do not capture the computational aspect in all its ramifications and therefore fall short of comprehensively describing human existence. In other words, there is hardly a branch of science that emphasizes the importance of subjective psychological experience for brain function *more* strongly than the current computational models in neurobiology!

Computational Models of Emotions?

Even if we take for granted that computational models in neurobiology enhance our understanding of such higher cognitive functions as perception, thinking, and decision making, we might question their use in the study of affect and emotion. In fact, computer models of emotions at first glance appear to be a contradiction in terms, as expressed by LeDoux and Fellous:

Using computers to understand emotions has always been a challenge. Popular beliefs define computing devices as inherently incapable of exhibiting and experiencing any emotions and, at present, no definite claims have been made that computers are (or may be) suitable for such a task. Nevertheless . . . computers can be and have begun to be used as tools for modeling certain aspects of emotional processing. (1995:358)

One of the major hurdles to research on affect and emotions lies in the fact that there is no generally accepted theory of emotion or affect. It is generally agreed, however, that the concepts of emotion and affect encompass a wide range of mental and physical phenomena: mental representations, states and responses of the autonomic nervous system, and behaviors, as well as subjective experiential qualities.

Emotions and affective states can be implemented within neural network models in two completely different ways. First, affect may be conceived of as a node in a semantic network (Segal et al. 1996). Such a node could represent an affective valence (e.g., *good/pleasant* versus *bad/unpleasant*) or an object of knowledge that is tightly connected with affective valences (such as *mother, spider, weapon, death,* etc.). Second, in contrast, affect may be viewed as a general parameter of network function, such as the signal-to-noise ratio. Looked at in this way, affect would not denote a particular part of the network but, rather, a state of the entire network.

In biological reality, affect is both these things and more. The meaning of a pattern of dots on the retina is recognized (semantic network) and judged with respect to its value for the organism (*pleasant/dangerous*). In fact, this judgment is based upon a crude black-and-white image of the perceived object that is sent to the amygdala in about two hundred milliseconds (Aggleton 1992). Thus, the value of the object is judged very quickly, long before (in the psychological sense of "long") a complete, detailed, full-color percept of the object has been worked out by the respective cortical areas. For example, your amygdala and related emotional brain structures have figured out that you are in imminent danger from the crude black-and-white image they received several hundred milliseconds before you consciously perceive the nearby lion in full color. Once these structures signal danger, they send the message down to neuromodulatory centers that release neuromodulators such as norepinephrine across large areas of the cortex, thereby setting the stage for adaptive information processing. In the case of danger, the networks may be "pulled tightly"; that is, the signal-to-noise ratio may be set to "high," so that you do very quickly what you have learned to do best, without much lateral, creative, time-consuming thinking. The neuromodulators, in this instance, represent the connection between knowledge and modulatory mechanisms. These neuromodulators affect your predispositions to behavioral responses, including such overt behavior as facial expressions and gestures. The neuromodulatory centers are also related to the hormone system and, by releasing molecules like epinephrine into the blood stream, prepare your entire body to respond to the evaluative quality (e.g., the danger) of the perceived object. You experience this state, in turn (cf. Damasio 1994), along with the percept and its semantic and emotional meaning and, possibly, changes in the mode of thinking caused by the neuromodulators. All this is called *affect*.

This sketch of emotional processes should clarify how neural network models can be used to better understand affects and emotions. Such an understanding will go beyond qualities subjectively experienced and beyond semantic analyses. We would expect that what are currently called *affect* and *emotion* in a very broad sense will be disentangled into different subcomponents (Davidson & Sutton 1995). We could then study these subcomponents by themselves and in detail, developing and empirically testing specific hypotheses. To see how we might do this, let us look at the an example from psychopathology: depression.

The Depression Spiral

Semantic networks are crucial to the operation of certain network models of depression. The *cognitive theories of depression* assert that negative affects are overrepresented in the semantic networks of depressed patients, causing a negative bias in the evaluation of new experiences as well as in the evaluation of remembered past experiences. Such mood-congruent recall facilitates the conscious experience of, for example, depressing memories (cf. Blaney 1986). If we assume that semantic networks contain nodes for emotional content (cf. Bower 1981), and further assume the spreading-activation model of semantic access described in chapter 10, we can easily explain the phenomena of negative bias and mood-congruent recall. In depressed patients, there is a downward spiral of negative evaluations of new experiences, which facilitates negative thoughts and negative associations. This, in turn leads to the increased negative evaluation of future experiences and their association with negatively "charged" nodes, even before there is a chance for neutral or even positive associative connotations to form (Ackermann-Engel 1993, Teasdale 1988).

This spiral of negative evaluation can be simulated with network models that contain nodes for affective valence within their semantic networks. When these networks are trained selectively with affectively negative content, they develop predominantly negative representations. Once these representations are in place, they bias the training of neutral material toward a negative evaluation (Siegle et al. 1995). In sum, these models capture the effect of experience on depression and, vice versa, the effect of depression on further experience. This explains the specifically depressed responses of depressive patients in everyday life as well as in experimental test situations. It also opens the door for new therapeutic strategies that can be developed and tested with the model and then clinically applied.

Temperament, Character, and Personality

The foregoing ideas about the influence of experience on depression, however, appear to contradict other models of depression, which see a disturbance of the neuromodulator serotonin (5-hydroxytryptamine, 5-HT) as the primary culprit. This view is supported by the genetic component of depression—after all, we are born with subtle differences in our neuromodulatory systems—as well as by findings of decreased 5-HT levels in the cerebrospinal fluid of some depressed patients and of successful treatment of depressive patients with 5-HT-enhancing drugs. But how is the 5-HT system related to subjective experiences and behavior?

Several lines of research are of interest. Most important are findings that the 5-HT system is involved in even very subtle forms of social behavior. This has been demonstrated in certain mammals, especially primates living in hierarchically organized groups (Raleigh & McGuire 1984). The highest 5-HT levels are found in the blood of the alpha male in each group. As an animal moves down the social-dominance scale, its 5-HT blood levels decline; if it climbs upward on the social ladder, its 5-HT blood levels increase. To investigate the direction of causality, the researchers manipulated 5-HT levels experimentally. The results were clear-cut. When an animal had more 5-HT, it moved up the social scale; when 5-HT levels were decreased, it declined socially (Raleigh et al. 1991). Similar changes in the personality of human patients with changes in the availability of 5-HT are nicely described in Peter Kramer's best-selling book, *Listening to Prozac* (1993).

All of this appears to suggest that depression, as well as certain aspects of temperament (see below), are "nothing but chemistry"; that is, that they are causally dependent on certain neurochemical processes. This is not so! For one thing, we know that self-confidence in children is affected by their family experiences; warmth, respect, and clear limits set by parents facilitate self-confidence (Coopersmith 1967, quoting Kramer 1993). Second, the above-mentioned cognitive models of depression suggest that chronic frustration can bring about depressiogenic neuromodulatory effects. Third, animal studies provide direct evidence that the effects of neuromodulators depend on experience, as the following example demonstrates.

Male crayfish display a marked territorial defense behavior. They defend their river-bottom living quarters against competitors by engaging in a fight. Such a fight ordinarily lasts for about half an hour and decides which crayfish will be master of the territory. Most interestingly, the outcome of the fight also markedly affects the animals' social behavior. Yeh and coworkers (1996) demonstrated that a certain neuron governing the upright posture of the animal's tail, a sign of dominance, is controlled by 5-HT. Moreover, they showed that this neuron responds differentially to exogenous (injected) 5-HT, depending on the outcome of the fight. The neuron of the winning animal given 5-HT increased its firing rate, whereas the very same amount of 5-HT had the opposite effect on the firing rate of the loser's neuron: its activity decreased. (The mechanism of this difference most likely involves expression of different subtypes of 5-HT-receptors.) This experiment shows for the first time that social behavior—in fact, a single social interaction—can have a marked influence on the effect of a neuromodulator.

It might be argued that crayfish differ genetically and that whether they are "strong" or "weak" affects some of their neurons' response to 5-HT. This possibility was ruled out by further experiments in which two previous losers were put into an experimental territory (an aquarium), fought each other, and established a new winner. Within about two weeks after the fight, this winner developed the winner's response to 5-HT. When two winners were placed in the same aquarium, the new loser had a hard time adapting to its nondominant social status. It tended to repeatedly intrude into the territory of the new winner, provoking the very animal it had just lost to. More than 70 percent of these new losers did not survive the first five days after the fight! Those who did adapted to their newly gained lower status slowly and within about four weeks were showing the loser's response to exogenous 5-HT.

Think of the ramifications of these results! For the first time research had demonstrated that, down to the level of single neurons, the effects of a neuromodulatory agent depend on the organism's experience—in this case, a single social interaction. Of course, during the course of evolution, more complex social interactive behaviors evolved, and higher organisms developed the ability to adapt to the complex situations brought about by these behaviors. The importance of neuromodulatory systems, which implemented the long-term changes in behaviors and response tendencies, increased. Temperament and character thus became variables that were shaped by the environment.

We can assume that every human being is born equipped with a certain neuromodulatory makeup. This makeup determines—in a way, *is*—his or her temperament. According to Cloninger (1986), the neuromodulators 5-HT, norepinephrine, and dopamine determine the general parameters of human behavior. Individual differences in the amounts of these agents are the basis of differences in response biases and dispositions to behave in certain ways. However, we are not completely genetically determined, as the crayfish-model illustrates. Rather, the amounts of neuromodulators present in someone's brain, as well as the effects of those neuromodulators, are the product of individual experience.

It remains largely unknown how a person's genetic makeup and experience interact, but it appears highly plausible that what may be good for one child may not be beneficial to another. Unfortunately, it is extremely difficult to conduct studies to increase our knowledge in this field. Hundreds of children would have to be studied for years, if not for decades. Given the politics of current science, the pursuit of such a line of inquiry does not lend itself to quick results and long publication lists. Hence, we have very few hard facts from long-term developmental research on temperament and personality, and the little knowledge we have corresponds to a plethora of unfounded speculation about influences on child development. Nonetheless, the neuroscientific and neurocomputational approaches now present opportunities to ask the right questions and plan the right studies.

What Is Good for Children

What do children need? What conditions are beneficial to their development? What can we reasonably say in answer to these questions?

First of all, children need structure. Without structured experiences, children cannot form stable internal structures. It is well known that children themselves demand structure: The fairy tale must be told exactly the same way each time; nursery rhymes are repeated over and over again, always in the same way, just as the same games are played over and over again. Such rituals enable the child to build up stable representations of its world, that is, its immediate physical and social environment. Most important are the caregivers and immediate peers: mother, father, brothers and sisters.

Since the groundbreaking monkey studies carried out in the 1950s by H. F. Harlow, we have known that young monkeys most dearly need a soft cozy place to be, even more than they need adequate food (Harlow & Zimmerman 1959). Further studies conducted by a student of Harlow's demonstrate that monkeys reared separately from their parents display behavioral deficits, behaving more aggressively toward members of their group and, later in life, tending to neglect their children (Suomi 1991a,b,c).

The interactions between experience and development are often quite complex. Monkeys reared by either their mothers or their peers do not differ upon superficial observation. Later in life, however, animals reared by their mothers can tolerate a several-days' separation from their social group much better than peer-raised animals can. Under such circumstances, the animals reared by animals other than their mothers tended to display depressed behaviors and release more stress hormones into their bloodstream (Suomi 1991a,b,c). Most notably, the differences between the differently reared monkeys tended to increase with age. The theory of depression discussed above would predict this outcome, as each new experience of separation becomes associated with anxiety and depression and, therefore, increases the likelihood of similar reactions in the future. Once certain behaviors are set in motion, as it were, they are reinforced and become the main cause of further similar behaviors.

Such spirals are at the heart of many pathological personality traits. A person disappointed by others several times will expect further frustrations and be unlikely to behave in an outgoing manner and welcome new contacts with others. Accordingly, his or her social contacts will be governed by distrust and shyness—that is, by factors that may trigger in others the very responses (lack of interest or even aversion) that are anticipated. The self-confident, open person is likely to experience just the opposite. It is important to realize that these social-response biases are to some extent present at birth and develop further during childhood. Finally, we need to remember that developmentally the human nervous system deals with biochemistry and neuromodulators (temperament) early in life; then, somewhat later, with modifications to neuromodulatory systems brought about by experience; and, lastly, with the generation of internal meaningful structures from experience through production of semantic and emotional maps (character, personality) to guide the behavior of the adult.

The most comprehensive studies of these long-term developmental issues were carried out over the last few decades by Jerome Kagan (1992, 1994) at Harvard University. He first studied three hundred children at the age of twenty-one months with respect to inhibition and shyness. At later points—for example at seven and a half years—he carried out detailed behavioral observations of various group situations. These studies demonstrated that shyness is a stable personality trait that may wane when the child has warm and supportive parents. As adults, only a fraction of the original 15 percent of shy children were still shy. However, shyness can also result from certain childhood and adolescent experiences.

Stability and Teddy Bear

The small child needs stability and a soft place to cuddle. It is no wonder, therefore, that one of the few well-established facts about the long-term dysfunctional effects of early childhood experience is that loss of the mother in early childhood leads to an increased incidence of anxiety disorders later in life (Kendler et al. 1992). <u>That lack of stability and ever-changing new experiences are harmful to the child is demonstrated by the finding that the repeated loss of a parent is more harmful than a single but definitive loss.</u> For example, a pilot or a truck driver who leaves the child every week is more detrimental to the child's mental health than a parent who dies early. In other words, a father who leaves the child about a thousand times during the first eighteen years of its life is more harmful than a nonexistent, dead father. <u>The most likely explanation is that the father who leaves and returns repeatedly produces instability and a lack of structure that is hard on a child striving to form stable representations, especially in the interpersonal realm.</u> Another finding, similarly counterintuitive at first glance, points to the importance of structure: The loss of a family member is more harmful in a large family than in a small one. We might expect that loss of a member of a large family would count for relatively less than a similar loss in a small family; but it's just the opposite. Like the comparison of the father who leaves repeatedly with the father who dies, structure is important in the second case and the percentage of people lost is not. In a small family, after a family member dies or leaves, the distribution of roles among the remaining members can be worked out fairly quickly. In a large family, by contrast, this process may take a long time and lead to an extended period of insecurity and instability. <u>This instability, this lack of a clear social structure, has a demonstrable pathogenic effect upon the future life of the children in the family</u> (Sklar & Harris 1985).

Children not only need stable structure but also the *right* experiences. In this respect, the possibilities of modern society are wider than ever before—for better or for worse. In chapter 7, we discussed the therapeutic possibilities presented by neural network models for children with language and reading difficulties. Knowledge of the underlying cause—the dysfunctional decoding of rapid sounds—as well as the research findings on neuroplasticity, have made it possible to develop therapeutic strategies specifically tailored to the primary dysfunction. And the therapy seems to work!

We have reason to believe that, because of their marked postnatal development, the brains of children themselves take care, at least in part, to provide the child with experiences suitable to its developmental state (cf. chapter 8). However, the simulations reported by Elman also show that the right input—that is, experience that fits the developmental stage—leads to more rapid learning than the wrong input. A good teacher knows this and will teach whatever the child of a given age can learn and wants to learn.

Modern society, however, has a stockpile of traps for children. The child who daily experiences horror and violence, either in real life or on television, will learn violence as a behavioral strategy; horror and violence will become widely represented on the brain's maps of the meaningful experiences. Since semantic and emotional maps exist to guide future behavior, they will henceforth bias the child's actions toward thrills and violence. Moreover, such maps do not change easily, as we saw in the discussions of schizophrenia and depression. Rather, they tend to be self-perpetuating, in that they either directly lead to experiences that reinforce them or to the interpretation of ordinary experiences within their framework. No wonder, given the situation in many United States inner cities, that about one in eight male African Americans between fifteen and thirty-five spends his life in prison—an environment hardly likely to introduce helpful changes in the semantic maps of the inmates! In Germany, ill-informed caretakers of small children and teachers (often supported by some half-baked pop-psychology idea) tend not to intervene when children treat each other with violence, arguing that children should settle their own disputes. These caregivers do not see that this practice leads children to accept violence as a good means of solving conflicts. In the 1960s and 1970s, it was standard (antiauthoritarian) theory and practice in education to let children do as they liked. No strategy could be worse for children.

It is worth repeating that children need structure to attain the ability to develop their own structured representations. Therefore, what we most urgently need are people who can serve as models for children; responsible people who treat children according to their needs; and people who will speak and act in a way that helps the child learn how to behave. Children need warmth, structure, and the right experiences, especially in their interactions with other children. They do not get any of this from television. Nor do they get it from computer games or badly run kindergartens and schools. In our institutions, we need well-paid, bright, and responsible people to guide our children, mainly by consistently representing the right model. Our children are our future. It is disturbing to realize how carelessly we treat them.

Psychotherapy

Psychotherapists are people who can endure, or have learned to endure, people who are difficult to deal with because of their genetic makeup, or because of an unfortunate life history, or because of both. Psychotherapists do not have an easy task, which is why, the American psychotherapist Harry S. Sullivan asserted, they do not live to an old age.

At first glance, psychotherapy and computational neurobiology seem unrelated. But only at first glance! Neurocomputational models may in fact be helpful to understanding the therapeutic mechanisms of psychotherapy, because they make it clear how learning—and every psychotherapy involves some form of learning—works. Every good psychiatrist, for example, knows about the importance for the outcome of the therapy of a warm, anxiety-free, and empathic atmosphere. As we saw in chapter 11, anxiety has a negative impact on learning. Furthermore, we know that insight, as well as repetitive training, may have therapeutic effects.

This comes as no surprise to the neurobiologist working in neuroplasticity research. The studies conducted by Merzenich and coworkers of cochlea-implant patients, for example, should open our eyes to the principles of psychotherapeutic change. The reader will recall that in these patients the completely new input from the implant is fed into the nerve, which formerly received its signals from the inner ear and conducted them directly to the brain. There the new input drives reorganization of sound maps that analyze the input patterns and make it possible for the majority of the patients, eventually, to understand spoken language again. For this to happen, however, training with repetitive input must take place. Moreover, reorganization of the auditory and phonetic maps have to take place in a way that allows the newly formed representations to be well connected to higher-level maps representing semantic and contextual structures. In sum, the change is input-driven but, at the same time, not independent of preexisting meaningful structures; it is, rather, guided by these high-level structures.

There are analogies in this process to what happens during psychotherapy. The *insight-oriented psychotherapist* works by talking to the patient. Such "talking cures" operate by accessing remote associations, thinking through problems, seeing them within new and tentative frameworks, and forming new connections between formerly separate facts and understandings. In order to be successful, the talking cure has to be put to work; that is, it has to be translated into appropriate behavior. *Behavioral therapists* too emphasize this step as well as the repetitive training aspect of therapy. But training, by itself, does not effect change; the patient must be motivated and emotionally disposed toward change. Thus any good behavioral therapist will work to motivate and educate the patient.

It is time for the field of psychotherapy we get rid of irrationality and dogmatism and replace these habits of thinking with openness, new knowledge, and rational decision making. We now have the needed new framework. Neurobiology and neurocomputational models have provided this new, clear, and open framework—not merely for psychotherapy, but for psychiatry as a whole. Therapists and their mentally ill patients can only benefit from it.

The results from neurobiology make it clear that the distinction between organic disorders and psychological disorders, which is currently still in use, will become, and must become, obsolete. "Can this disorder be treated by talking or by pills?" turns out to be the wrong question! Most patients need both appropriate medication and the right word at the right time, in the right combination and timing. As we have seen above, a "problem"—from the heartless mother to a lost fight—may lead to clearly demonstrable biological changes in the brain. In turn, a purely "organic" disorder, as, for example a slowly growing brain tumor, may lead to changes in the behavior and life of a patient, who may need psychotherapy after surgery in order to sort out his past and plan for the future.

Problem or disease—this distinction formed the basis of psychiatric diagnosis and therapy for more than a century. It will have to be replaced by a more detailed and at the same time more holistic view of human beings. Only then will truly integrative therapeutic strategies become possible. As the psychiatrist and neuroscientist Eric Kandel has put it,

The boundary between behavioral studies and biology is arbitrary and changing. It has been imposed not by the natural contours of the disciplines, but by the lack of knowledge. As our knowledge expands, the biological and behavioral disciplines will merge at certain points, and it is at these points that our understanding of mentation will rest on secure ground. (1991:1030)

User's Manual for Your Brain

Just as detailed knowledge of how the heart works enables cardiologists to give rational and well-grounded advice for a way of life that is good for your heart, insights into the workings of the brain have immediate practical consequences. These are especially important with respect to child development, but they can also be applied to our entire lives. Understanding the function of neural networks changes the way we see ourselves. Here are some essential points we should all keep in mind.

• *Provide examples, not rules.* During the developmental stage, the brain needs not rules but good examples. If you teach your children rules by the use of force and repression, don't be surprised when they generalize over the many examples of repression and violent force and act in a similar way. Teaching children this way fosters aggressive behavior and creates experiences of anxiety in human interactions. Remember, children do not learn rules by rote; they produce them from the examples they see and hear. If rules are taught the wrong way, children will learn the bad ways in which they are taught.

• *Children need structure.* Such structure can only be extracted from examples if these examples are not completely random. They need to reflect some underlying order or internal structure. In other words, unconnected or even contradictory experiences make it hard or impossible for the child to extract clear-cut rules. It bears repeating: Children need structure.

• *First things first.* Learning proceeds faster and more smoothly when simple, basic things are learned first. Once these are learned, more complex concepts and behaviors can be more easily digested. For example, we sing children's songs with our children first—simple songs that go up and down a few notes. In doing this, we provide the input from which the child can generate the major scale (which, by the way, consists of mathematically complex ratios between the basic harmonic frequencies of the tones). Once "twinkle, twinkle, little star" and other such songs are mastered, we can turn to more complex melodies and harmony.

- *There are natural stages in development.* The brain develops as learning occurs. Because these two things happen at the same time (and we need not assume anything else!), there are phases or stages of development. To return to the musical example, we can point out that the father who thinks he will facilitate his child's musical development by beginning with a John Cage composition and complex modern jazz is just as ill-advised as the mother who tries to teach higher mathematics at the earliest possible time in the life of her child. The child will learn that complex mixtures of tones (or numbers) are hard to disentangle (or may not learn anything), and could well decide that learning is hard and no fun. Both lessons are contradictory to the natural tendencies of a child to be curious, to like music and numbers, and to enjoy learning.

- *Watch your mental diet!* The brain is plastic throughout our lifetime, and this neuroplasticity calls for responsibility, for, in effect, "psychohygiene." We should take care that the experiences we arrange for ourselves and for others are appropriate to their (and our) development and potential for growth. To put it bluntly, he who watches movies rife with horror and violence for two hours a day (or, even worse, lets his children watch them) should be aware that such experiences produce brain changes that facilitate similar behavior and, ultimately, lead to a more horrific and violent society. While we are accustomed to watching carefully the "input" of our stomachs, the very idea of taking comparable care with the dietary input to our most important organ, the brain, sounds strange. But this is all the more important since, unlike the stomach, the brain remains as malleable as a wax tablet throughout life. In the future, let's take better care of the impressions!

Glossary

accommodation Adaptation of an organism to its environment. The term was used specifically by the developmental psychologist Jean Piaget to denote changes in an organism caused by the acquisition of knowledge.

acetylcholine Substance liberated at the terminals of certain nerve fibers. Neurons that use acetylcholine are called *cholinergic neurons*. A group of such neurons resides in the **nucleus basalis Meynert,** which is located deep in the brain. These neurons have connections that can distribute acetylcholine across wide areas of the cortex.

action potential Brief change of the difference in charge between the inner and the outer part of a neuron's cell membrane. An action potential travels along the main output fiber of the neuron, the *axon*, at speeds of up to 100 meters per second.

afferent A nerve fiber providing input to the brain.

agonist A substance that causes a receptor to become activated.

algorithm A systematic logical procedure that leads to solution of a mathematical problem by carrying out a finite number of steps. For example, we learned in school how to divide a large number by a smaller number by using an algorithm that reduces the problem to a succession of statements about the relationships of small numbers.

amnesia Loss of memory. The terms *anterograde* and *retrograde* specify the temporal relation of the memory loss to its cause. Memory loss for events that occurred after the cause (i.e., brain damage) is called anterograde amnesia, whereas memory loss for events that took place before the brain was damaged is called retrograde amnesia.

amygdala Structure located deep in the temporal lobes that, when electrically stimulated, produces strong emotional and responses such as anxiety and anger, as well as vegetative responses such as relaxation and calmness.

antagonist A substance that blocks the activation of a receptor.

aphasia A disorder of speech in which the patient has relatively intact speech-production mechanisms and thought processes but experiences difficulty in speaking or in understanding what others say. In *motor aphasia*, the patient's ability to speak is mainly affected, whereas in *sensory aphasia* understanding is principally disturbed.

assimilation   Making the world more similar to the organism. The concept was used by Jean Piaget to denote changes introduced to the world as perceived by the organism. The concepts of **assimilation** and **accommodation** are related terms denoting changes in the world and the organism that occur during learning.

association norm   Most-frequent word association spontaneously produced by a representative sample of people when presented with a word. Researchers have presented hundreds, or even thousands, of subjects with lists of words, one by one, asking them to say aloud the word that immediately comes to mind. The word that is produced most often is the association norm, that is, the statistically normal association to a given word. For example, the norm for *table* is *chair*, the norms for *sun* and *hot* are, respectively, *moon* and *cold*.

attractor   The stable state of a system. The concept is derived from physics, where it is used to describe dynamic systems. An attractor may be a single point (as in a pendulum system, where the pendulum swings until it reaches a stable point, its stable resting state).

autism   Inability to make and sustain social contact. In psychiatry, autism denotes a severe disorder that affects one in every thousand children. It is characterized by a qualitative impairment of social relations (autistic isolation), an impairment of communication and fantasy (failure to generalize), and by a highly decreased repertoire of activities and interests (monotonous thoughts and actions). Some autistic people have "islands" of intact functions, most often in skills related to rote memory.

backpropagation algorithm   A learning rule for training certain types of simulated neural networks; it feeds back the errors produced by the network in order to adjust the weights of the connections to a small degree. The backpropagation algorithm is an extension and generalization of the delta rule.

deafferentation   Disconnection of input fibers to the brain.

decade of the brain   In 1989 the president of the United States declared the 1990s the decade of the brain and predicted that the workings of the brain would be a major subject of research in the decade ahead (cf. Goldstein 1990).

delta rule   The learning rule for training two-layered neural networks; it feeds back the errors produced by the network in order to adjust the weights of the connections to a small degree.

delusions   Disorders of thought content. A patient with delusions maintains some—in most cases rather strange—thought content in spite of evidence to the contrary. In many cases, delusions are easy to recognize, because of their strangeness ("I am Jesus," "the CIA is after me"), but in other cases the only way to diagnose them is to observe how the person maintains them in conversation.

dementia   Loss of mental functions during later life, most frequently caused by Alzheimer's disease or multiple vascular strokes.

disambiguation Process during which an ambiguous pattern is resolved and thereby supplied with a clear meaning.

dopamine A substance released at the synapses of dopaminergic neurons in the brain. There are several centers containing such dopaminergic neurons; one of them sends fibers diffusely to the cortex, thereby providing dopaminergic activation.

dual-task method Procedure in experimental psychology in which a subject has to perform two tasks at the same time. This allows researchers to draw inferences about the influence of one mental function upon a second function.

EEG (electroencephalogram) A recording of the electric potentials from the scalp by means of electrodes. Amplifying the small currents measured allows researchers to detect changes in frequency and amplitude.

efference Nerve fibers traveling away from the brain.

Elman network A simulated neural network with an architecture that allows it to represent temporal context.

entorhinal cortex Phylogenetically the oldest part of the cortex, it resides at the bottom of both hemispheres.

event-related potential (ERP) Stimulus (event)-induced change of the electrical potential recorded from the scalp. The potential is very weak, with amplitudes of only a few (or even fractions of a) millionth of a volt. Researchers detect such small changes against the background of higher-amplitude EEG activity by presenting many similar stimuli and averaging the electrical signals that occur within a given interval after the stimulus. The amplitude and the latency of the peaks occurring after the stimulus are the major focus of interest.

fMRI *See* **Magnetic resonance imaging.**

forebrain In the human brain, both hemispheres of the forebrain lie on top of all the other brain structures. The surface of the forebrain is characterized by *sulci* (shallow furrows) and *gyri* (convolutions). The neurons are located in the cortex, the 3- to 5-millimeter-thick folded surface that contains about 100,000 neurons per cubic millimeter. The size of the cortex is about 2,500 square centimeters.

formal thought disorder Disturbance of thinking that is manifested as disordered language. Formal thought disorder is a common symptom of schizophrenic patients, whose utterances may slip off the track, contain newly formed words (neologisms), or may simply be incomprehensible.

G-proteins A class of intracellular proteins, which are coupled to certain types of receptors in the cell membrane and which cause intracellular changes when the receptor is stimulated by a neuromodulatory agent. The name *G-protein* is derived from the fact that these proteins are bound to guanine nucleotides.

ganglion Aggregation of neurons.

Gestalt (usually lower case) shape, form, figure. Within psychology, the term (upper case) denotes a school of thought (*Gestalt psychology*) that seeks to account for perception, thought, and behavior in terms of an organism's unified response to configurational wholes. This school is opposed to atomistic or elemental analyses of perception and behavior.

glutamate A substance released at synapses of glutamatergic neurons that has an excitatory effect on the connected neuron. Such neurons have point-to-point connections and carry out the bulk of information processing in the brain.

glutamate receptors Structures to which glutamate binds and that, thereby, affect the connected neuron. There are two basic types of glutamate receptors: The *Q/K-receptors* carry the signal forward, whereas the *NMDA-receptors* are involved in changes of synaptic strength—that is, in learning and memory.

graceful degradation Gradual loss of function resulting from the buildup of faults in a system. This feature of simulated and biological neural networks is in marked contrast to conventional digital computers, which often respond to small defects by crashing.

hallucinations Experiences similar to perceptions. They may occur in any perceptual modality; for example, patients may see objects or persons or hear voices. In most cases, hallucinations are not exactly like perceptions but merely somewhat similar.

Hebb's learning rule This rule states that the connection between two neurons increases if both of them are active at the same time.

hippocampus A phylogenetically old part of the brain situated in the medial temporal lobe. The hippocampus integrates information from many cortical areas and is essential for learning and memory.

Hopfield network A neural network with a special architecture in which each neuron is connected to every other neuron in the network.

interference Superimposition of signals that may result in an increase in the signals but can also result in their mutual cancellation. Interference may occur in neural networks during learning if learning of a new content is detrimental to storage of content learned earlier.

interleaved learning A process of learning in which presentation of new material is integrated into re-presentation of material that has already been learned.

introspection Literally, watching within. This method in psychology attempts to understand mental functions by directly observing one's own thoughts and feelings.

invasive techniques Procedures that may be harmful to the subject in some way and, therefore, either cannot be used at all or can be used in only a limited way in research using healthy volunteers. In patients, however, such procedures are permissible if the potential benefit outweighs the risks of potential harm. For example, a neurosurgeon trying to remove all traces of a brain tumor located dangerously close to the language areas of the brain has to be sure not to cut into those areas, which might leave the patient aphasic. In such cases, the skull is removed under local anesthesia, exposing the brain (which has no pain receptors); the brain is then stimulated directly with tiny wires carrying electrical current while the patient is awake. This procedure allows the surgical team to map the areas of the patient's brain that are crucial to such functions as language.

logic The aspect of philosophy that deals with correct reasoning, its forms, structure, and laws. **Propositional logic** deals with the logical relationships between propositions. The basic operations of this area of logic are *and*, *or*, and negation.

magnetic resonance imaging (MRI) Imaging technique using the magnetic property of hydrogen atomic nuclei that aligns them in the presence of a strong magnetic field. When these aligned nuclei are then given a brief pulse from a second magnetic field, they emit electromagnetic waves (i.e., something like radio waves). These radio signals can then be recorded and used to create an image whose features correspond to the presence or absence of hydrogen nuclei (i.e., water). In **functional MRI (fMRI)**, the different magnetic properties of oxygenated and deoxygenated blood are used to generate a contrast and, hence, to image brain function.

matrix calculation (computation/operation) Part of linear algebra, a branch of mathematics. In a matrix, the elements are ordered by rows and columns. Matrices may be added or multiplied or manipulated by other computations.

membrane potential Voltage difference between the outside and the inside of a cell membrane.

meninges The protective and nutritive layers of hard and soft tissues (or membranes) that cover the brain and spinal cord.

mesocortical system Dopaminergic pathway leading from the midbrain to the frontal cortex; it is important for higher cognitive functions.

migration, neuronal During brain development, the movement of brain cells to the site of their final destination in the brain. Neuronal migration is an important process for understanding normal as well as abnormal brain development.

modularity Principle of organization for a system made up of functional subsystems (modules). According to the definition of J. Fodor, who proposed the principle of *strong modularity* for mental information processing, information is processed in separate modules and what is processed in one module is not available to other modules. Throughout this book, the principle of modularity is used in a *weak* form. In this view, modules are characterized by the way they work closely together.

motor neuron Neuron that sends a fiber to the muscles and causes them to contract.

neuroleptic drugs A subclass of psychoactive agents used to treat schizophrenic patients. When neuroleptic agents are given infrequently, they block dopamine receptors (i.e., they act as dopamine **antagonists**). When used chronically in a moderate dose, they may act as dopamine **agonists**.

neuromodulation Relatively global and nonspecific regulation of neurotransmission.

neuron   A nerve cell that differs from other cells by being specialized for the rapid reception, processing, and transmission of information.

neuroplasticity   Adaptation to changing information-processing needs caused by environmental and experiential changes. It is based upon synaptic plasticity; that is, the ability of synapses to change their connecting strength.

neurotransmission   Specific and rapid point-to-point information transmission at synapses.

neurotransmitter   *See* **Transmitter**.

nigro-striatal system   A dopaminergic pathway leading from the *substantia nigra* (an assembly of neurons deep in the brain) to the *corpus striatum* (a rather large body of neurons beneath the cortex). This system is involved in the control of movement.

noise   Concept from information theory denoting randomness in a (transmitted) signal. If this randomness is distributed equally across all the frequencies of the signal, it is called **white noise**.

noninvasive techniques   Procedures for investigating the specific functions of the normal brain in normal subjects that do not harm subjects in any way. Such techniques did not exist until a few years ago. The advent of such harmless noninvasive techniques as high-resolution event-related potentials, functional magnetic resonance imaging, and magnetoencephalography has dramatically changed brain research.

nucleus basalis Meynert   An assembly of neurons deep in the brain that produces acetylcholine and spreads it widely over parts of the cortex.

paraplegia   Loss of sensory-motor control of the legs resulting from injury to the spinal cord. A patient suffering from paraplegia is called a *paraplegic*.

phantom   Sensation of a body part that is not present. In most cases, the respective body part, such as an arm or a leg, has been removed by amputation.

phoneme   The smallest unit of the sound system of a language.

phrenology   Doctrine originated by Viennese physician Franz-Joseph Gall (1758–1828); it proposes that the form of the skull provides clues to the functions of the underlying brain.

population vector   Sum of vectors. Neurophysiologists assume that each vector summed up by the population vector codes the same variable, but from the "point of view" of a single neuron. When the activities of the neurons representing a common variable are summed up, the result represents the "sum of the votes" on that variable—that is, the population vector.

positron emission tomography (PET)   Imaging technique that employs radioactive material (isotopes) to investigate body functions (including brain function). When the isotopes decay, positrons (positively charged particles) are released and are transformed into gamma rays when they collide with electrons. The PET machine detects these gamma rays and uses their signals to form an image of the brain. If the isotope is coupled to a substance that binds to specific receptors, the image will capture their respective distribution in the brain. However, PET can also be used for imaging brain function. In this case, researchers use radioactive sugar or oxygen, because both substances are distributed according to the energy needs of functioning neurons and, hence, indicate brain function.

psycholinguistics A branch of linguistics that investigates the psychological aspects of language development and understanding and the production of speech in children.

pyramidal cell Type of neuron located in the brain. These cells are relatively large and have—if you allow for some fantasizing—a somewhat pyramidal shape. Pyramidal cells release the transmitter glutamate (among others) and thereby excite other neurons.

receptor A structure within the cell membrane sensitive to a specific chemical. More specifically, a chemoreceptor that senses a certain chemical substance, such as a neurotransmitter or neuromodulator, and thereby transduces a signal.

regression A "going back"; psychoanalytic term denoting either the movement of psychic energy, the course of a disorder, the course of the development of a person, or features of a proposed intrapsychic entity, such as the ego or superego. In statistics, the term **regression** denotes a procedure that determines the correlation of a variable, or a set of variables, with another variable.

schizophrenia A severe mental disorder. At any time, one in three to five hundred people suffer from it. Schizophrenia most often starts in early adulthood, hits women and men equally, and is characterized by disordered thought, affect, volition, and behavior.

semantic priming The facilitatory effect of a meaningfully related word on recognition of a second word.

silent connection A pathway between neurons that does not transmit signals. Silent connections may be reactivated under some circumstances.

somatosensory area Part of the brain that deals with the sensations coming in from the body.

synapse Connecting structure between neurons. The functional connection is mediated by the release of a neurotransmitter at the synapse.

syncytium A cellular structure without real boundaries between the cells. The brain was once conceived of as a syncytium.

transmitter A substance liberated at a synapse that carries a signal to the postsynaptic site of the next neuron.

tubero-infundibular system Dopaminergic system involved in the regulation and release of certain hormones.

two-point discrimination The smallest distance between two points of touch that is discernible to a subject. When two pointed pencils touch the back of a human body simultaneously, they may be as far as three inches apart but may still be felt as one pencil touching one point, whereas at the fingertips or the tongue, two touches that are very close together may still be sensed as separate.

vegetative nervous system The parts of the nervous system that deals with basic body functions—such as breathing, digestion, circulation, hormonal secretion, and so on—that are regulated with little or no conscious activity.

References

Ackermann-Engel, R., and DeRubeis, R. J. 1993. The role of cognition in depresssion. In Dobson K. S., and Kendall, P. C., eds. *Psychopathology and Cognition*, pp. 83–119. San Diego: Academic Press.

Aggleton, J. P., ed. 1992. *The Amygdala: Neurobiological Aspects of Emotion, Memory, and Mental Dysfunction*. New York: Wiley.

Ahissar, E., Vaadia, E., Ahissar, M., Bergman, H., Arieli, A., and Abeles, M. 1992. Dependence of cortical plasticity on correlated activity of single neurons and on behavioral context. *Science* 257: 1412–1415.

Aitchison, J. 1994. *Words In the Mind*. Oxford: Blackwell.

Allard, T., Clarc, S. A., Jenkins, W. M., and Merzenich, M. M. 1991. Reorganization of somato-sensory area 3b representations in adult owl monkeys after digital syndactyly. *Journal of Neurophysiology* 66: 1048–1058.

Allen, H. A., Liddle, P. F., and Frith, C. D. 1993. Negative features, retrieval processes and verbal fluency in schizophrenia. *British Journal of Psychiatry* 163: 769–775.

Allers, R. 1920. Über psychogene Störungen in sprachfremder Umgebung. *Zeitschrift für die gesamte Neurologie und Psychiatrie* 60: 281–289.

Allgaier, C., Stangl A., Warnke, P., and Feuerstein,T. J. 1995. Effects of 5-HT receptor agonists on depolarization-induced [^{3}H]-noradrenaline release in rabbit hippocampus and human neocortex. *British Journal of Pharmacology* 116: 1769–1774.

Alonso-Quecuty, M. L., and de Vega, M. 1991. Contextual effects in a metaphor verification task. *European Journal of Cognitive Psychology* 3: 315–341.

American Psychiatric Association. 1994. *Diagnostic and Statistical Manual of Mental Disorders*, 4th ed. Washington, D.C.: American Psychiatric Press.

Amit, D. J. 1989. *Modeling Brain Function*. Cambridge: Cambridge University Press.

Anderson, J. A. 1995. *An Introduction to Neural Networks*. Cambridge: MIT Press.

Anderson J. A., and Rosenfeld, E., eds. 1988. *Neurocomputing: Foundations of Research*. Cambridge: MIT Press.

Anderson, J. A., Pellionisz, A., and Rosenfeld, E., eds. 1990. *Neurocomputing 2: Directions for Research*. Cambridge: MIT Press.

Andreasen, N. C. 1994. *Schizophrenia: From Mind to Molecule*. Washington, D.C.: American Psychiatric Press.

Andreasen, N. C., Rezai, K. R., Alliger, R., Swayze, V. W., Flaum, M., Kirchner, P., Cohen, G., and O'Leary, D. S. 1992. Hypofrontality in neuroleptic-naive patients and in patients with chronic schizophrenia: Assessment with Xenon 133 single-photon emission computed tomography and the Tower of London. *Archives of General Psychiatry* 49: 943–948.

Angrist, B. 1983. Psychosis induced by central nervous system stimulants and related drugs. In Creese, I, ed., *Stimulants: Neurochemical Behavioral and Clinical Perspectives*. New York: Raven Press.

Anonymus. 1994. Smart microwave is a touch easier. *New Scientist* (22 October): 24.

Antonini, A., and Stryker, M. P. 1993. Rapid remodeling of axonal arbors in the visual cortex. *Science* 260: 1819–1821.

Arbib, M. A. 1995. *Handbook of Brain Theory and Neural Networks*. Cambridge: MIT Press.

Aristotle. 1975. On memory and recollection. In *Aristotle*, vol. 8, *On the Soul, Parva Naturalia, on Breath*, W. S. Hett, transl. Loeb Classical Library. Cambridge: Harvard University Press.

Aroniadou-Anderjaska, V., and Keller, A. 1995. LTP in the barrel cortex of adult rats. *Neuroreport* 6: 2297–2300.

Arthur, C. 1994. IBM enters the field in Pentium battle. *New Scientist* 24 (31 December): 18.

Aschaffenburg, G. 1896. Experimentelle Studien über Assoziationen I. In Kraepelin, E., ed., *Psychologische Arbeiten* 1: 209–299. Leipzig: Engelmann.

Aschaffenburg, G. 1899. Experimentelle Studien über Assoziationen II. In Kraepelin, E., ed., *Psychologische Arbeiten* 2: 1–83. Leipzig: Engelmann.

Aschaffenburg, G. 1904. Experimentelle Studien über Assoziationen III. In Kraepelin, E., ed., *Psychologische Arbeiten* 4: 235–373. Leipzig: Engelmann.

Bach y Rita, P. 1990. Brain plasticity as a basis for recovery of function in humans. *Neuropsychologia* 28: 547–554.

Baddeley, A. 1986. *Working Memory*. Oxford: Oxford University Press.

Baddeley, A. 1992. Working memory. *Science* 255: 556–559.

Baddeley, A. 1995. Working memory. In Gazzaniga, M. S., ed., *The Cognitive Neurosciences*, pp. 755–764. Cambridge: MIT Press.

Barinaga, M. 1996. Giving language skills a boost. *Science* 271: 27–28.

Barnden, J. A. 1995. Semantic networks. In Arbib M., ed., *Handbook of Brain Theory and Neural Networks*, pp. 854–857. Cambridge: MIT Press.

Barondes, pp. H. 1995. *Moleküle und Psychosen*. Heidelberg: Spektrum Verlag.

Basso, A., Capitani, E., and Laiacona, M. 1988. Progressive language impairment without dementia: A case with isolated category-specific semantic defect. *Journal of Neurology, Neurosurgery and Psychiatry* 51: 1201–1207.

Bates, E. A., and Elman, J. L. 1993. Connectionism and the study of change. In Johnson, M. H., ed., *Brain Development and Cognition*, pp. 623–642. Oxford: Blackwell.

Baudry, M., and Davis, J. L., eds. 1991. *Long-Term Potentiation: A Debate of Current Issues*. Cambridge: MIT Press.

Baudry, M., and Davis J. L., eds. 1994. *Long-Term Potentiation*, vol. 2. Cambridge: MIT Press.

Baudry, M., Thompson, R., and Davis, J., eds. 1993. *Synaptic Plasticity: Molecular, Cellular, and Functional Aspects*. Cambridge: MIT Press.

Baxt, W. G. 1994. A neural network trained to identify the presence of myocardial infarction bases some decisions on clinical associations that differ from accepted clinical teaching. *Medical Decision Making* 14: 217–222.

Bear, M., and Kirkwood, A. 1993. Neocortical long-term potentiation. *Current Opinion in Neurobiology* 3: 197–202.

Bear, M. F., and Cooper, L. N. 1987. A physiological basis for a theory of synapse modification. *Science* 237: 42–48.

Beattie, W. G., and Butterworth, B. L. 1979. Contextual probability and word frequency as determinants of pauses and errors in spontaneous speech. *Language and Speech* 22: 201–211.

Bechtel, W., and Abrahamsen, A. 1991. *Connectionism and the Mind: An Introduction to Parallel Processing in Networks*. Oxford: Blackwell.

Bell, D. S. 1965. Comparison of amphetamine psychosis and schizophrenia. *British Journal of Psychiatry* 111: 701–707.

Bellemann, M., Spitzer, M., Brix, G., Kammer, T., Loose, R., Schwartz, A., and Gückel, F. 1995. Neurofunktionelle MR-Bildgebung höherer kognitiver Leistungen des menschlichen Gehirns. *Der Radiologie* 35: 272–283.

Belliveau, J. W., Kennedy, D. N., McKinstry, R. C., Buchbinder, B. R., Weisskoff, R. M., Cohen, M. S., Vevea, J. M., Brady, T. J., and Rosen, B. R. 1991. Functional mapping of the human visual cortex by magnetic resonance imaging. *Science* 254: 716–719.

Bickerton, D. 1996. *Language and Human Behavior*. London: UCL Press.

Blaney, P. 1986. Affect and memory: A review. *Psychological Bulletin* 99: 229–246.

Bleuler, E. 1911. *Dementia praecox oder die Gruppe der Schizophrenien*. Leipzig: Franz Deutecke.

Bleuler, M. 1983. *Lehrbuch der Psychiatrie*. Berlin: Springer.

Bliss, T. V. P., and Lømo, T., 1973. Long-lasting potentiation of synaptic transmission in the dentate area of the anaesthesized rabbit following stimulation of the perforant path. *Journal of Physiology* 232: 331–356.

Bliss, T. V. P., and Collingridge, G. L. 1993. A synaptic model of memory: Long-term potentiation in the hippocampus. *Nature* 361: 31–39.

Bloom, F. E., and Lazerson, A., eds. 1988. *Brain, Mind, and Behavior*, 2nd. ed. New York: Freeman.

Bloom, P. 1994. Controversies in language acquisition. In Bloom P., ed., *Language Acquisition: Core Readings*, pp. 5–48. Cambridge, MIT Press.

Boon, M. E., and Kok, L. P. 1993. Neural network processing can provide means to catch errors that slip through human screening of pap smears. *Diagnostic Cytopathology* 9: 411–416.

Boone, J. M., Seshagiri, S., and Steiner, R. M. 1992. Recognition of chest radiograph orientation for picture archiving and communication systems display using neural networks. *Journal of Digital Imaging* 5: 190–193.

Bors, E. 1951. Phantom limbs of patients with spinal cord injury. *Archives of Neurology and Psychiatry* 66: 610–631.

Borst, A., and Egelhaaf, M. 1994. Dendritic processing of synaptic information by sensory interneurons. *Trends in Neuroscience* 17: 257–263.

Bower, G. 1981. Mood and memory. *American Psychologist* 36: 129–148.

Braff D. L., Heaton, R., Kuck, J., Cullum, M., Moranville, J., Grant, I., and Zisook, S. 1991. The generalized pattern of neuropsychological deficits in outpatients with chronic schizophrenia with heterogeneous Wisconsin card sorting test results. *Archives of General Psychiatry* 48, 891–898.

Braff, D. L. 1993. Information processing and attention dysfunctions in schizophrenia. *Schizophrenia Bulletin* 19: 233–259.

Braitenberg, V., and Schüz, A. 1989. Cortex: Hohe Ordnung oder größtmögliches Durcheinander. *Spektrum der Wissenschaft* (May): 74–86.

Bregman, A. S. 1994. *Auditory Scene Analysis: The Perceptual Organization of Sound*. Cambridge: MIT Press.

Breidbach, O. 1993. Nervenzellen oder Nervennetze? Zur Entstehung des Neuronenkonzepts. In Florey, E., and Breidbach, O., eds., *Das Gehirn—Organ der Seele? Zur Ideengeschichte der Neurobiologie*, pp. 81–126. Berlin: Akademie-Verlag.

Brix, G., Gückel, F., Bellemann, M., Röther, J., Schwartz, A., Ostertag, H., and Lorenz, W. 1994. Functional MR mapping of activated cortical areas. *Nuclear Medicine* 33: 200–205.

Brown, T. H., and Chattarji, S. 1995. Hebbian synaptic plasticity. In Arbib, M., ed., *Handbook of Brain Theory and Neural Networks*, pp. 454–459. Cambridge: MIT Press.

Bumke, O., ed. 1935. *Handbuch der Geisteskrankheiten*, vols. 1 and 9. Berlin: Springer.

Bunsey, M., and Eichenbaum, H. 1996. Conservation of hippocampal memory function in rats and humans. *Nature* 379: 255–257.

Butterworth, B. 1973. The science of silence. *New Society* 26: 771–773.

Butterworth, B. 1975. Hesitation and semantic planning in speech. *Journal of Psycholinguistic Research* 4: 75–87.

Cacciari, C., and Tabossi, P. 1988. The comprehension of idioms. *Journal of Memory and Language* 27: 668–683.

Cacioppo, J. T., and Tassinary, L. G., eds. 1990. *Principles of Psychophysiology: Physical, Social, and Inferential Elements*. Cambridge: Cambridge University Press.

Campenhausen, C. v. 1993. *Die Sinne des Menschen*, 2nd. ed. Stuttgart: Thieme.

Caramazza, A., Hillis, A., Leek, E. C., and Miozzo, M. 1994. The organization of lexical knowledge in the brain: Evidence from category- and modality-specific deficits. In Hirschfeld, L. A., and Gelman, S. A., eds. *Mapping the Mind*, pp. 68–84. Cambridge: Cambridge University Press.

Carlen, P. L., Wall, P. D., Nadvorna, H., and Steinbach, T. 1978. Phantom limbs and related phenomena in recent traumatic amputations. *Neurology* 28: 211–217.

Carlsson, A. 1988. The current status of the dopamine hypothesis of schizophrenia. *Neuropsychopharmacology* 1: 179–203.

Caudill, M., and Butler, C. 1990. *Naturally Intelligent Systems*. Cambridge: MIT Press.

Caudill, M., and Butler, C. 1992. *Understanding Neural Networks*, 2 vols. Cambridge: MIT Press.

Cherniak, C. 1990. The bounded brain: Toward quantitative neuroanatomy. *Journal of Cognitive Neuroscience* 2: 58–68.

Chomsky, N. 1972. *Language and Mind*. New York: Harcourt Brace Jovanovich.

Chomsky, N. 1978. *Rules and Representations*. New York: Columbia University Press.

Chomsky, N. 1988. *Language and Problems of Knowledge*. Cambridge: MIT Press.

Churchland, P. M. 1995. *The Engine of Reason, the Seat of the Soul*. Cambridge: MIT Press.

Churchland, P. S., and Sejnowski, T. J. 1988. Perspectives in cognitive neuroscience. *Science* 242: 741–745.

Churchland, P. S., and Sejnowski, T. J. 1992. *The Computational Brain*. Cambridge: MIT Press.

Cipra, B. 1995. How number theory got the best of the Pentium chip. *Science* 267: 175.

Clark, A. 1993. *Associative Engines*. Cambridge: MIT Press.

Clark, H. H., and Lucy, P. 1975. Understanding what is meant from what is said: A study in conversationally conveyed requests. *Journal of Verbal Learning and Verbal Behavior* 14: 56–72.

Clark, S. A., Allard, T., Jenkins, W. M., and Merzenich, M. M. 1988. Receptive fields in the body-surface map in adult cortex defined by temporally correlated inputs. *Nature* 332: 444–445.

Cloninger, C. R. 1986. A systematic method for clinical description and classification of personality variants. *Archives of General Psychiatry* 44: 573–588.

Cohen, I. 1994. An artificial neural network model of autism. *Biological Psychiatry* 36: 5–20.

Cohen, J. D., and Servan-Schreiber, D. 1992. Context, cortex, and dopamine: A connectionist approach to behavior and biology in schizophrenia. *Psychological Review* 99(1): 45–77.

Cohen, J. D., and Servan-Schreiber, D. 1993. A theory of dopamine function and its role in cognitive deficits in schizophrenia. *Schizophrenia Bulletin* 19: 85–104.

Cohen, J. D., Servan-Schreiber, D., and McClelland, J. L. 1992. A parallel distributed processing approach to automaticity. *American Journal of Psychology* 105(2): 239–269.

Cohen, J. D., Forman, S. D., Braver, T. S., Casey, B. J., Servan-Schreiber, D. and Noll, D. C. 1994. Activation of the prefrontal cortex in a nonspatial working memory task with functional MRI. *Human Brain Mapping* 1: 293–304.

Collins, A. M., and Loftus, E. F. 1975. A spreading activation theory of semantic processing. *Psychological Review* 82: 407–428.

Comrie, B. 1990. *The World's Major Languages*. Oxford: Oxford University Press.

Corbetta, M., Miezin, F. M., Dobmeyer, S., Shulman, G. L., and Petersen, S. E. 1991. Selective and divided attention during visual discriminations of shape, color, and speed: Functional anatomy by positron emission tomography. *Journal of Neuroscience* 11: 2383–2402.

Corbetta, M. 1993. Positron emission tomography as a tool to study human vision and attention. *Proceedings of the National Academy of Science* 90: 10901–10903.

Corkin, S. 1984. Lasting consequences of bilateral medial temporal lobectomy: Clinical course and experimental findings in H.M. *Seminars in Neurology* 4: 249–259.

Costin, D. 1988. MacLab: A Macintosh system for psychology labs. *Behav Res Meth Instr Comp* 20: 197–200.

Creutzfeld, D. O. 1995. *Cortex Cerebri: Performance, Structural and Functional Organization of the Cortex*. Oxford: Oxford University Press.

Crick, F. 1988. *What Mad Pursuit*. Basic Books, New York.

Crick, F. 1989. The recent excitement about neural networks. *Nature* 337: 129–132.

Cronholm, B. 1951. *Phantom Limbs in Amputees.* Stockholm:

Cross, S. S., Harrison, R. F., and Kennedy, R. L. 1995. Introduction to neural networks. *Lancet* 346 (21 October): 1075–1079.

Cummings, J. L. 1993. Amnesia and memory disturbances in neurologic disorders. In Oldham, J. M., Riba, M. B., and Tasman, A., eds. *Review of Psychiatry,* vol. 12. Washington, D.C.: American Psychiatric Press.

Curran, T., Tucker, D. M., Kutas, M., and Posner, M. I. 1993. Topography of the N400: Brain electrical activity reflecting semantic expectancy. *Electroencephalography and Clinical Neurophysiology* 88: 188–209.

Damasio, A. 1994. *Descartes' Error: Emotion, Reason and the Human Brain.* New York: Putnam.

Damasio, A., and Geschwind, N. 1984. The neural basis of language. *Annual Review of Neurocience* 7: 127–147.

Daugherty, K., and Seidenberg, M. S. 1992. Rules or connections? The past tense revisited. In *Proceedings of the 14th Annual Meeting of the Cognitive Science Society,* pp. 259–264. Hillsdale, N.J.: Erlbaum.

Davidson, R. J., and Sutton, S. K. 1995. Affective neuroscience: The emergence of a discipline. *Current Opinion in Neurobiology* 5: 217–224.

Davis, K. L., Kahn, R. S., Ko, G., and Davidson, M. 1991. Dopamine in schizophrenia: A review and reconceptualization. *American Journal of Psychiatry* 148: 1474–1486.

Decety, J., Perani, D., Jeannerod, M., Bettinardi, V., Tadary, B., Woods, R., Mazziotta, J. C., and Fazio, F. 1994. Mapping motor representations with positron emission tomography. *Nature* 371: 600–602.

DeFelipe, J., and Jones, E. G. 1988. *Cajal on the Cerebral Cortex: An Annotated Translation of the Complete Writings.* Oxford: Oxford University Press.

Dehaene, S. 1995. Electrophysiological evidence for category-specific word processing in the normal human brain. *Neuroreport* 6: 2153–2157.

Dehaene-Lambertz, G., and Dehaene, S. 1994. Speed and cerebral correlates of syllable discrimination in infants. *Nature* 370: 292–295.

Dennis, M. 1976. Dissociated naming and locating of body parts after left anterior temporal lobe resection: An experimental case study. *Brain and Language* 3: 147–163.

De Renzi, E., and Lucchelli, F. 1994. Are semantic systems separately represented in the brain? The case of living category impairment. *Cortex* 30: 3–25.

Devor, M. 1984. The pathophysiology and anatomy of damaged nerve. In Wall, P. D., Melzack, R., eds., *Textbook of Pain,* 2nd. ed. Edinburgh: Livingstone Churchill.

Dolan, R. J., Fletcher, P., Frith, C. D., Friston, K. J., Frackowiak, R. S. J., and Grasby, P. M. 1995. Dopaminergic modulation of impaired cognitive activation in the anterior cingulate cortex in schizophrenia. *Nature* 378: 180–182.

Douglass, J. K., Wilkens, L., Pantazelou, E., and Moss, F. 1993. Noise enhancement of information transfer in crayfish mechanoreceptors by stochastic resonance. *Nature* 365: 337–340.

Dudai, Y. 1994. *The Neurobiology of Memory: Concepts, Findings, Trends.* New York: Oxford University Press.

Ebell, M. H. 1993. Artificial neural networks for predicting failure to survive following in-hospital cardiopulmonary resuscitation. *Journal of Family Practice* 36: 297–303.

Eichenbaum, H. 1993. Thinking about brain cell assemblies. *Science* 261: 993–994.

Eichenbaum, H., and Otto, T. 1993. LTP and memory: Can we enhance the connection? *Trends in Neuroscience* 16: 163–164.

Elbert, T., Flohr, H., Birbaumer, N., Knecht, S., Hampson, S., Larbig, W., and Taub, E. 1994. Extensive reorganization of the somatosensory cortex in adult humans after nervous system injury. *Neuroreport* 5: 2593–2597.

Elbert, T., Pantev, C., Wienbruch, C., Rockstroh, B., and Taub, E. 1995. Increased cortical representation of the fingers of the left hand in string players. *Science* 270: 305–307.

Elman, J. L. 1990. Finding structure in time. *Cognitive Science* 14: 179–211.

Elman, J. L. 1991. Incremental learning, or The importance of starting small. In *Proceedings of the Thirteenth Annual Conference of the Cognitive Science Society*, pp. 443–448. Hillsdale, N.J.: Erlbaum.

Elman, J. L. 1994. Implicit learning in neural networks: The importance of starting small. In Umilta, C., and Moscovitch, M., eds., *Attention and Performance,*vol. 6: *Conscious and Nonconscious Information Processing*, pp. 861–888. Cambridge: MIT Press.

Elman, J. L. 1995. Language processing. In Arbib, M., ed., *Handbook of Brain Theory and Neural Networks*, pp. 508–513. Cambridge: MIT Press.

Engelhaaf, M., and Borst, A. 1993. A look into the cockpit of the fly: Visual orientation, algorithms and identified neurons. *Journal of Neuroscience* 13: 4563–4574.

Farah, M. J., and Wallace, M. A. 1992. Semantically-bounded anomia: Implications for the neural implementation of naming. *Neuropsychologia* 30: 609—621.

Felleman, D. J., and van Essen, D. C. 1991. Distributed hierarchical processing in primate cerebral cortex. *Cerebral Cortex* 1: 1–47.

Feuerstein, T. J., Lehmann, J., Sauermann, W., v. Velthoven, V., and Jackisch, R. 1992. The autoinhibitory feedback control of acetylcholine release from human neo tissue. *Brain Research* 572: 64–71.

Finger, S. 1994. *Origins of Neuroscience*. Oxford: Oxford University Press.

Flechsig P. 1929. *Anatomie des menschlichen Gehirns und Rückenmarks auf myelogenetischer Grundlage*. Leipzig: Thieme.

Fletcher, P. C., Frith, C. D., Grasby, P. M., Shallice, T., Frackowiak, R. S. J., and Dolan, R. J. 1995. Brain systems for encoding and retrieval of auditory-verbal memory: An in vivo study in humans. *Brain* 118: 401–416.

Flohr, H., Elbert, T., Knecht, S., Wienbruch, C., Pantev, C., Birbaumer, N., Larbig, W., and Taub, E. 1995. Phantom-limb pain as a perceptual correlate of cortical reorganization following arm amputation. *Nature* 375: 482–484.

Florio, T., Einfeld, S., and Levy, F. 1994. Neural networks and psychiatry: Candidate applications in clinical decision making. *Australian and New Zealand Journal of Psychiatry* 28: 651–666.

Fodor, J. A. 1983. *The Modularity of Mind*. Cambridge: MIT Press.

Frackowiak, R. S. J. 1994. Functional mapping of verbal memory and language. *Trends in Neuroscience* 17: 109–115.

Frege, G. 1879/1977. *Begriffsschrift, eine der arithmetischen nachgebildete Formelsprache des reinen Denkens*. Halle: Nebert.

Frégnac, Y. 1995. Hebbian synaptic plasticity: Comparative and developmental aspects. In Arbib, M., ed., *Handbook of Brain Theory and Neural Networks*, pp. 459–464. Cambridge: MIT Press.

Frégnac, Y., Shulz, D., Thorpe, S., and Bienenstock, E. 1992. Cellular analogs of visual cortical epigenesis. I. Plasticity of orientation selectivity. *Journal of Neuroscience* 12: 1280–1300.

Freud, S. 1895/1966 Project for a scientific psychology. In Strachey, J., ed., *The Standard Edition of the Complete Works of Sigmund Freud*, vol. 1, pp. 295–397. London: Hogarth Press.

Frith, U. 1992. *Autismus*. Heidelberg: Spektrum Verlag.

Fuchs, T. 1993. Wahnsyndrome bei sensorischer Beeinträchtigung—Überblick und Modellvorstellungen. *Fortschritte der Neurologie und Psychiatrie* 61: 257–266.

Funahashi, S., Bruce, C. J., and Goldman-Rakic, P. S. 1989. Mnemonic coding of visual space in the monkey's dorsolateral prefrontal cortex. *Journal of Neurophysiology* 61: 331–349.

Fuster, J. M. 1991. The prefrontal cortex and its relation to behavior. *Progress in Brain Research* 87: 201–211.

Fuster, J. M. 1993. Frontal lobes. *Current Opinion in Neurobiology* 3: 160–165.

Fuster, J. M. 1995. *Memory in the Cerebral Cortex*. Cambridge: MIT Press.

Gabor, A. J., and Seyal, M. 1992. Automated interictal EEG spike detection using artificial neural networks. *Electroencephalography and Clinical Neurophysiology* 83: 271–280.

Galton, F. 1879. Psychometric experiments. *Brain* 2: 149–162.

Galton, F. 1883. *Inquiries into Human Faculty and Its Development.* London: MacMillan.

Galton, F. 1910. *Genie und Vererbung,* Neurath, O., and Schapire-Neurath, A., transl. *Philosophisch-soziologische Bücherei,* vol. 19. Leipzig: Verlag Dr. Klinkhardt.

Gardner, D., ed. 1993. *The Neurobiology of Neural Networks.* Cambridge: MIT Press.

Gehlen, A. 1978. *Der Mensch: Seine Natur und seine Stellung in der Welt,* 12th. ed. Wiesbaden: Akademische Verlagsgesellschaft Athenaion.

Georgopoulos, A. P., Kettner, R. E., and Schwartz, A. B. 1988. Primate motor cortex and free arm movements to visual targets in three-dimensional space. II. Coding of the direction of movement by a neuronal population. *Journal of Neuroscience* 8: 2928–2937.

Georgopoulos, A. P., Schwartz, A. B., and Kettner, R. E. 1986. Neuronal population coding of movement direction. *Science* 233: 1416–1419.

Georgopoulos, A. P., Taira, M., and Lukashin, A. 1993. Cognitive neurophysiology of the motor cortex. *Science* 260: 47–52.

Gilbert, C. D. 1993. Rapid dynamic changes in adult cerebral cortex. *Current Opinion in Neurobiology* 3: 100–103.

Globus, G. G., and Arpia, J. P. 1994. Psychiatry and the new dynamics. *Biological Psychiatry* 35: 352–364.

Gluck, M, A., and Rumelhart, D. E., eds. 1990. *Neuroscience and Connectionist Theory.* Hillsdale, N.J.: Erlbaum.

Goldman-Eisler, F.1958. The predictability of words in context and length of pauses in speech. *Language and Speech* 1: 226–231.

Goldman-Rakic, P. S. 1990. Cellular and circuit basis of working memory in prefrontal cortex of nonhuman primates. In Uylings, H. B. M., Van Eden, C. G., De Bruin, J. P. C., Corner. M. A., and Feenstra, M. G. P., eds. *Progress in Brain Research 85,* pp. 325–236. New York: Elsevier.

Goldman-Rakic, P. S. 1991. Cortical dysfunction in schizophrenia: The relevance of working memory. In Carroll, B. J., and Barrett, J. E., eds., *Psychopathology and the Brain.* New York: Raven Press.

Goldman-Rakic, P. S. 1994. Working memory dysfunction in schizophrenia. *Journal of Neuropsychiatry and Clinical Neuroscience* 6: 348–357.

Goldman-Rakic, P. S. 1995. Cellular basis of working memory. *Neuron* 14: 477–485.

Goldman-Rakic, P. S., and Friedman, H. R. 1991. The circuitry of working memory revealed by anatomy and metabolic imaging. In Levin, H. S., Eisenberg, H. M., and Benton, A. L., eds., *Frontal Lobe Function and Dysfunction,* pp. 72–91. Oxford: Oxford University Press.

Goldman-Rakic, P. S., Funahashi, S., and Bruce, C. J. 1990. *Neocortical Memory Circuits.* Cold Spring Harbor Symposia on Qualitative Biology, vol.55, pp. 1025–1038. Cold Spring Harbor, N.Y.: Cold Spring Harbor Laboratory Press.

Goldstein, M. 1990. The decade of the brain. *Neurology* 40: 321.

Goodglass, H., Klein, B., Carey, P., and James, K. J. 1966. Specific semantic word categories in aphasia. *Cortex* 2: 74–89.

Gottesman, I. I. 1991. *Schizophrenia Genesis: Theories of Madness.* New York: Freeman.

Grace, A. A. 1991. Phasic versus tonic dopamine release and the modulation of dopamine system responsivity: A hypothesis for the etiology of schizophrenia. *Neuroscience* 41: 1–24.

Greenwald, A. G. 1992. New look 3: Unconscious cognition reclaimed. *American Psychologist* 47: 766–779.

Gregory, R. L., and Gombrich, E. H., eds. 1973. *Illusion in Nature and Art.* London: Duckworth.

Gregory, R. L. 1986. *Odd Perceptions.* New York: Routledge.

Grossberg, S., Schmajuk, N., and Levine, D. S. 1992. Associative learning and selective forgetting in a neural network regulated by reinforcement and attentive feedback. In Levine, D. S., and Leven, S. J., eds. *Motivation, Emotion, and Goal Direction in Neural Networks,* pp. 37–62. Hillsdale, N.J.: Erlbaum.

Guyton, A. 1992. *Basic Neuroscience.* Philadelphia: Saunders.

Häfner, H. 1993./94. *Weshalb erkranken Frauen später an Schizophrenie?* Proceedings of the Heidelberg Academy of Science: Mathematics and Natural History section.

Handel, S. 1989. *Listening.* Cambridge: MIT Press.

Harlow, H. F., and Zimmerman, R. R. 1959 Affectional responses in the infant monkey. *Science* 130: 421–432.

Hart, J. J., and Gordon, B. 1992. Neural subsystems for object knowledge. *Nature* 359: 60–64.

Hart, J. J., Sloan Berndt, R., and Carramazza, A. 1985 Category-specific naming deficit following cerebral infarction. *Nature* 316: 439–440.

Hasselmo, M. E. 1994. Runaway synaptic modification in models of cortex: Implications for Alzheimer's disease. *Neural Networks* 7(1): 13–40.

Hebb, D. O. 1949 *The Organization of Behavior.* Wiley, New York.

Hecht-Nielsen, R. 1990. *Neurocomputing.* Reading, Mass.: Addison-Wesley.

Heden, B., Edenbrandt, L., Haisty, W. K., Jr., and Pahlm, O. 1994. Artificial neural networks for the electrocardiographic diagnosis of healed myocardial infarction. *American Journal of Cardiology* 74: 5–8.

Henik, A., Priel, B., and Umansky, R. 1992. Attention and automaticity in semantic processing of schizophrenic patients. *Neuropsychiatry, Neuropsychology, and Behavioral Neurology* 5: 161–169.

Herder, J. G. 1772/1960. *Abhandlung über den Ursprung der Sprache*. Hamburg: Meiner.

Heritch, A. J. 1990. Evidence for reduced and dysregulated turnover of dopamine in schizophrenia. *Schizophrenia Bulletin* 16: 605–615.

Herschmann, H. 1921. Bemerkungen zu der Arbeit von Rudolf Allers: "Über psychogene Störungen in sprachfremder Umgebung". Der Verfolgungswahn der sprachlich Isolierten. *Zeitschrift für Neurologie* 66: 346.

Hillis, A. E., and Caramazza, A. 1991. Category-specific naming and comprehension impairment: A double dissociation. *Brain* 114: 2081–2094.

Hilts, P. J. 1995. *Memory's Ghost: The Strange Tale of Mr. M and the Nature of Memory*. New York: Simon & Schuster.

Hinton, G. E., and Shallice, T. 1991. Lesioning an attractor network: Investigations of acquired dyslexia. *Psychological Review* 98: 74–95.

Hoeffner, J. 1992. Are rules a thing of the past? The acquisition of verbal morphology by an attractor network. *Proceedings of the Fourteenth Annual Conference of the Cognitive Science Society*, pp. 861–866. Hillsdale, N.J.: Erlbaum.

Hoffman, R. E. 1987. Computer simulations of neural information processing and the schizophrenia-mania dichotomy. *Archives of General Psychiatry* 44: 178–185.

Hoffman, R. E. 1992. Attractor neural networks and psychotic disorders. *Psychiatric Annals* 22: 119–124.

Hoffman, R. E. 1996. Exploring psychopathology with simulated neural networks. In Spitzer, M., and Maher, B. A., eds., *Experimental Psychopathology*. Cambridge University Press.

Hoffman, R. E., and Dobscha, S. 1989. Cortical pruning and the development of schizophrenia: A computer model. *Schizophrenia Bulletin* 15: 477–493.

Hoffman, R. E, and McGlashan, T 1993. Parallel distributed processing and the emergence of schizophrenic symptoms. *Schizophrenia Bulletin* 19: 119–140.

Hoffman, R. E, Rapaport, J., Ameli, R., McGlashan, T. H., Harcherik, D., and Servan-Schreiber, D. 1995. The pathophysiology of hallucinated "voices" and associated speech perception impairments in psychotic patients. *Journal of Cognitive Neuroscience* 7: 479–496.

Hoffmann, N. 1993. *Neuronale Netze*. Braunschweig: Vieweg.

Holm-Hadulla, R., and Haug, F. 1984. Die Interpretation von Sprichwörtern als klinische Methode zur Erfassung schizophrener Denk-, Sprach- und Symbolisations-störungen. *Nervenarzt* 55: 496–503.

Holmes, B. 1996. The creativity machine. *New Scientist* (20 January): 22–26.

Hooper, S. L. 1995. Crustacean stomatogastric system. In Arbib, M., ed., *Handbook of Brain Theory and Neural Networks*, pp. 275–278. Cambridge: MIT Press.

Hopfield, J. J. 1982. Neural networks and physical systems with emergent collective computational abilities. *Proceedings of the National Academy of Science* 79: 2554–2558.

Hopfield, J. J. 1984. Neurons with graded response have collective computational properties like those of of two state neurons. *Proceedings of the National Academy of Science* 81: 3088–3092.

Hubel, D. H. 1989. *Auge und Gehirn: Neurobiologie des Sehens*. Heidelberg: Spektrum Verlag.

Hubel, D. H., and Wiese, T. N. 1962. Receptive fields, binocular interaction and functional architecture in the cat's visual cortex. *Journal of Physiology* 160: 106–154.

Inhelder, B., and Piaget, J. 195?

Iriki, A., Pavlides, C., Keller, A., and Asanuma, H. 1991. Long-term potentiation of thalamic input to the motor cortex induced by coactivatoin of thalamocortical and cortico-cortical afferents. *Journal of Neurophysiology* 65: 1435–1441.

James, W. 1892/1984. *Psychology: Briefer Course*. Cambridge: Harvard University Press.

Janus, R. A., and Bever, T. G. 1985. Processing of metaphoric language: An investigation of the three-stage model of metaphor comprehension. *Journal of Psycholinguistic Research* 14: 473–487.

Janzarik, W. 1988. *Strukturdynamische Grundlagen der Psychiatrie*. Stuttgart: Enke.

Jenkins, W. M., Merzenich, M. M., and Recanzone, G. 1990. Neocortical representational dynamics in adult primates: Implications for neuropsychology. *Neuropsychologia* 28: 573–584.

Jensen, T. S., Krebs, B., Nielsen, J., and Rasmussen, P. 1984. Non-painful phantom limb phenomena in amputees: Incidence, clinical characteristics and temporal course. *Acta Neurologica Scandinavica* 70/6: 407–414.

Jensen, T. S., and Rasmussen, P. 1989. Phantom pain and related phenomena after amputation. In Wall, P. D., and Melzack, R., eds., *Textbook of Pain*, 2nd. ed. Edinburgh: Livingstone Churchill.

Johnson, J. S., and Newport, E. L. 1993. Critical period effects in second language learning: The influence of maturational state in the acquisition of English as a second language. In Johnson, M. H., ed., *Brain Development and Cognition*, pp. 248–282. Oxford: Blackwell.

Jones, W. P., and Hoskins, J. 1987. Back-propagation. A generalized delta learning rule. *BYTE* (October): 155–162.

Jonides, J., Smith, E. E., Koeppe, R. A., Awh, E., Minoshima, S., and Mintun, M. A. 1993. Spatial working memory in humans as revealed by PET. *Nature* 363: 623–625.

Jung, C. G., and Riklin, F. 1906/1979. Experimentelle Untersuchungen über Assoziationen Gesunder. *Gesammelte Werke*, vol. 2, pp. 13–213. Freiburg: Walter.

Just, M. A., Miyake, A., and Carpenter, P. A. 1994. Working memory constraints in comprehension: Evidence from individual differences, aphasia, and aging. In M. A. Gernsbacher, ed., *Handbook of Psycholinguistics*, pp. 1075–1122. New York: Academic Press.

Just, M. A., and Carpenter, P. A. 1992. A capacity theory of comprehension: Individual differences in working memory. *Psychological Review* 99: 122–149.

Kaczmarek, L. K., and Levitan, I. B. 1987. *Neuromodulation: The Biochemical Control of Neuronal Excitability*. New York: Oxford University Press.

Kagan, J. 1992. The nature of shyness. *Harvard Magazine* 94: 40–45.

Kagan, J. 1994. *Galen's Prophecy: Temperament in Human Nature*. New York: Basic Books.

Kandel, E. R., Schwartz, J. H., and Jessell, T. M. 1991. *Principles of Neural Science*. New York: Elsevier.

Kaplan, H. I., Sadock, B. J., and Grebb, J. A. 1994. *Synopsis of Psychiatry*, 7th ed. Baltimore: Williams & Wilkins.

Karmiloff-Smith, A. 1995. Developmental disorders. In Arbib, M., ed., *Handbook of Brain Theory and Neural Networks*, pp. 292–294. Cambridge: MIT Press.

Katz, J. 1992. Psychophysiological contributions to phantom limbs. *Canadian Journal of Psychiatry* 37: 282–298.

Katz, L. C. 1993. Cortical space race. *Nature* 364: 578–579.

Katzner, K. 1995. *The Languages of the World*, new ed. London: Routledge.

Kelso, S. R., Ganong, A. H., and Brown, T. H. 1986. Hebbian synapses in hippocampus. *Proceedings of theNational Academy of Science* 83: 5326–5330.

Kendler, K. S., and Neale, M. C. 1992. Childhood parental loss and adult psychopathology in women: A twin study perspective. *Archives of General Psychiatry* 49: 109–116.

Kent & Rosanoff 1910?

Kiernan, V. 1994. Pentagon sets sights on breast cancer. *New Scientist* (29 October): 10.

Kilgard, M. P., and Merzenich, M. M. 1995. Anticipated stimuli across skin. *Science* 373: 663.

Killackey, H. P., [W RR, Name left out here?], and Bennett-Clarke , C. A. 1995. The formation of a cortical somatotopic map. *Trends in Neuroscience* 18: 402–407.

Kischka, U., Kammer, T., Weisbrod, M., Maier, S., Thimm, M., and Spitzer, M. 1996. Dopaminergic modulation of semantic network activation. *Neuropsychologia* 34: 1107–1113.

Kleiner, K. 1995. Language deaths: Bad for us all? *New Scientist* (4 March): 15.

Kneale, W., and Kneale, M. 1984. *The Development of Logic.* Oxford: Clarendon Press.

Kohonen, T. 1982. Self-organized formation of topologically correct feature maps. *Biological Cybernetics* 43: 59–69.

Kohonen, T. 1989. *Self-Organization and Associative Memory.* New York: Springer.

Komuro, H., and Rakic, P. 1993. Modulation of neuronal migration by NMDA receptors. *Science* 260: 95–97.

Kosslyn, S. M., and Koenig, O. 1992. *Wet Mind: The New Cognitive Neuroscience.* New York: Free Press.

Kraepelin, E. 1892. Über die Beeinflussung einfacher psychischer Vorgänge durch einige Arzneimittel. Jena: G. Fischer.

Kraepelin, E. 1896. Der psychologische Versuch in der Psychiatrie. In Kraepelin, E., ed., *Psychologische Arbeiten*, vol. 1, pp. 1–91. Leipzig: Engelmann.

Kraepelin, E. 1909. *Psychiatrie*, vol. 1, Leipzig: Barth.

Kramwer, P. D. 1993. *Listening to Prozac.* New York: Viking Penguin Press.

Kretschmer, E. 1927/1974. *Der sensitive Beziehungswahn*, 4th ed. Berlin: Springer.

Kutas, M., and Hillyard, S. A. 1980. Reading senseless sentences: Brain potentials reflect semantic incongruity. *Science* 207: 203–205.

Kutas, M., and van Petten, C. K. 1994. Psycholinguistics electrified. In Gernsbacher, M. A., ed., *Handbook of Psycholinguistics*, pp. 83–143. San Diego: Academic Press.

Kwong, K. K., Belliveau, J. W., Chesler, D. A., Goldberg, I. E., Weiskoff, R. M., Poncelet, B. P., Kennedy, D. N., Hoppelt, B. E., Cohen, M. S., Turner, R., Cheng, H. M., Brady, T. J., and Rosen, B. R. 1992. Dynamic magnetic resonance imaging of human brain activity during primary sensory stimulation. *Proceedings of the National Academy of Science* 89: 5675–5679.

Lahav, O., Naim, A., Buta, R. J., Corwin, H. G., de Vaucouleurs, G., Dressler, A., Huchra, J. P., van den Bergh, S., Raychaudhury, S., Sodré Jr., L., and Storrie-Lombardi, M. C. 1995. Galaxies, human eyes, and artificial neural networks. *Science* 267: 859–862.

Lapuerta, P., Azen. S. P., and LaBree, L. 1995. Use of neural networks in predicting the risk of coronary artery disease. *Computers in Biomedical Research* 28: 38–52.

LeDoux, J. E., and Fellous, J-M. 1995. Emotion and computational neuroscience. In Arbib, M., ed., *Handbook of Brain Theory and Neural Networks*, pp. 356–359. Cambridge: MIT Press.

Lehky, S. R., and Sejnowski, T. J. 1988. Network model of shape-from-shading: neural function arises from both receptive and projective fields. *Nature* 333: 452–454.

Lehky, S. R., and Sejnowski, T. J. 1990 Neural network model of visual cortex for determining surface curvature from images of shaded surfaces. *Proceedings of the Royal Society* 240: 251–278.

Lenneberg, E. H. 1967. *Biological Foundations of Language.* New York: John Wiley.

Levelt, W. J. M. 1989. *Speaking: From Intention to Articulation.* Cambridge: MIT Press.

Leven, S. J. 1992. Learned helplessness, memory, and the dynamics of hope. In Livine, D. S., and Leven, S. J., eds., *Motivation, Emotion, and Goal Direction in Neural Networks,* pp. 259–299. Hillsdale, N.J.: Erlbaum.

Llinás, R. R. 1988. *The Biology of the Brain: From Neurons to Networks.* New York: Freeman.

Lovinger, D. M., White, G., and Weight, F. F. 1989. Ethanol inhibits NMDA-activated ion current in hippocampal neurons. *Science* 243: 1721–1724.

Lowell, W. E., and Davis, G. E. 1994. Predicting length of stay for psychiatric diagnosis-related groups using neural networks. *Journal of the American Medical Association* 1: 459–466.

Lurito, J. T., Georgopoulos, T., and Georgopoulos, A. P. 1991. Cognitive spatial-motor processes: 7. The making of movements at an angle from a stimulus direction: Studies of motor cortical activity at the single cell and population levels. *Experimental Brain Research* 87: 562–580.

Maclin, P. S., Dempsey, J., Brooks, J., and Rand, J. 1991. Using neural networks to diagnose cancer. *Journal of Medical Systems* 15: 11–19.

Maddox, J. 1994. Bringing order out of noisiness. *Nature* 369: 271.

Maher, B. A., Manschreck, T. C., Hoover, T. M., and Weisstein, C. C. 1987. Thought disorder and measured features of language production in schizophrenia. In Harvey, P., and Walker, E., eds., *Positive and Negative Symptoms in Psychosis: Description, Research and Future Directions.* Hillsdale, N.J.: Erlbaum.

Maher, B. A., and Spitzer, M. 1993. Thought disorder and language behavior in schizophrenia. In Blanken, G., Dittmann, J., Grimm, H., Marshal, J. C., and Wallesch, C. W., eds., *Linguistic Disorders and Pathologies: Handbücher der Sprach- und Kommunikationswissen-schaf* 9: 522–533. Berlin: De Gruyter.

Mainen, Z. F., and Sejnowski, T. J. 1995. Reliability of spike timing in neokortikal neurons. *Science* 268: 1503–1506.

Mamelak, A., Quattrocchi, J., and Hobson, J. 1991. Automated staging of sleep in cats using neural networks. *Electroencephalography and Clinical Neurophysiology* 79(1): 52–61.

Manschreck, T. C. 1992. Clinical and experimental analysis of motor phenomena in schizophrenia. In Spitzer, M., Uehlein, F. A., Schwartz, M. A., and Mundt, C., eds. *Phenomenology, Language, and Schizophrenia,* pp. 258–273. New York: Springer.

Manschreck, T. C., Maher, B. A., Milavetz, J. J., Ames, D., Weisstein, C. C., and Schneyer, M. L. 1988. Semantic priming in thought-disordered schizophrenic patients. *Schizophrenia Research* 1: 61–66.

Marcus, G. F. 1995. The acquisition of the English past tense in children and multilayered connectionist networks. *Cognition* 56: 271–279.

Marlsburg, C. v. D 1995. Self-organization and the brain. In Arbib, M., ed., *Handbook of Brain Theory and Neural Networks*, pp. 840–843. Cambridge: MIT Press.

Martin, J. H., and Ghez, C. 1985. Task-related coding of stimulus and response in cat motor cortex. *Experimental Brain Research* 57: 427–442.

Martin, A., Haxby, J. V., Wiggs, C. L., and Ungerleider, L. G. 1996. Discrete cortical regions associated with knowledge of color and knowledge of action. *Science* 270: 102–105.

Martin, A., Wiggs, C. L., Ungerleider, L. G., and Haxby, J. V. 1996. Neural correlates of category-specific knowledge. *Nature* 379: 649–652.

Massing, W. 1989. Schizophrenie und die Theorie neuronaler Netzwerke. *Fortschritte der Neurologie und Psychiatrie* 57: 70–73.

Mazoyer, B. M., Tzouria, N., Frak, V., Syrota, A., Murayama, N., Leurier, O., Salomon, G., DeLaene, S., Cohen, L., and Mehler, J. 1993. The cortical representation of speech. *Journal of Cognitive Neuroscience* 5: 467–479.

McCarthy, G., Blamire, A. M., Puce, A., Nobre, A. C., Bloch, G., Hyder, F., Goldman-Rakic, P., and Shulman, R. G. 1994. Functional magnetic resonance imaging of human prefrontal cortex activation during a spatial working memory task. *Proceedings of the National Academy of Science* 91: 8690–8694.

McClelland, J. L. 1989. Parallel distributed processing: Implications for cognition and development. In Morris. R. G. M., ed., *Parallel Distributed Processing: Implications for Psychology and Neurobiology*, pp. 9–45. Oxford: Clarendon Press.

McClelland, J. L. 1994. The interaction of nature and nurture in development: A parallel distributed perspective. In Bertelson, P., Eelen, P., and d'Ydevalle, G., eds., *International Perspectives on Psychological Science*, vol.1, pp. 57–88. Hillsdale, N.J.: Erlbaum.

McClelland, J. L., and Plunkett, K. 1995. Cognitive development. In Arbib, M., ed., *Handbook of Brain Theory and Neural Networks*, pp. 193–197. Cambridge: MIT Press.

McClelland, J. L., McNaughton B. L., and O'Reilly, R. C. 1995. Why there are complementary learning systems in the hippocampus and neocortex: Insights from the success and failures of connectionist models of learning and memory. *Psychological Review* 102: 419–457.

√ McCulloch, W. S., and Pitts, W. 1943. A logical calculus of the ideas immanent in nervous activity. *Bulletin of Mathematical Biophysics* 5: 115–133.

Mehta, Z., Newcombe, F., and De Haan, E. 1992. Selective loss of imagery in a case of visual agnosia. *Neuropsychologia* 30: 645–655.

Merzenich, M. M., Collwell, S. A., and Andersen, R. A. 1982. Auditory forebrain organization. Thalamocortical and corticocortical connections in the cat. In Woolsey, C. N., ed. *Cortical Sensory Organization*, vol. 3, *Multiple Auditory Areas*, pp. 43–57. Clifton, N.J.: Humana Press.

Merzenich, M. M., Jenkins, W. M., Johnston, P., Schreiner, C., Miller, S. L., and Tallal, P. 1996. Temporal processing deficits of language-learning impaired children ameliorated by training. *Science* 271: 77–81.

Merzenich, M. M., Kaas, J. H., Wall, J., Nelson, R. J., Sur, M., and Felleman, D. 1983. Topographic reorganization of somatosensory cortical areas 3b and 1 in adult monkeys following restricted deafferentation. *Neuroscience* 8: 33–55.

Merzenich, M. M., Recanzone, G., Jenkins, W. M., Allard, T. T., and Nudo, R. T. 1988. Cortical representational plasticity. In Rakic, P., and Singer, W., eds., *Neurobiology of Neocortex*, pp. 41–67. Chichester, Eng.: John Wiley.

Merzenich, M. M., and Sameshima, K. 1993. Cortical plasticity and memory. *Current Opinion in Neurology* 3: 187–196.

Merzenich, M. M., Jenkins, W. M., Johnston, P., Schreiner, C., Miller, S. L., and Tallal, P. 1996. Temporal processing deficits of language-learning impaired children ameliorated by training. *Science* 271: 77–81.

Mestel, R. 1995. Early start on signing vital for deaf children. *New Scientist* (25 February): 9.

Metzger, W. 1975. *Gesetze des Sehens*. Frankfurt am Main: Waldemar Kramer.

Miller, G. 1993. *Wörter: Streifzüge durch die Psycholinguistik*. Heidelberg: Spektrum Verlag.

Miller, G. A., and Glucksberg, S. 1988. Psycholinguistic aspects of pragmatics and semantics. In Atkinson, R. C., Herrnstein, R. J., Lindzey, G., and Luce, R. D., eds., *Steven's Handbook of Experimental Psychology*, pp. 417–472. New York: Wiley.

Minsky, M., and Papert, S. 1969/1988. Perceptions. In Anderson, J. A., and Rosenfeld, E., eds. *Neurocomputing*, pp. 157–169. Cambridge: MIT Press.

Mintz, S. 1969. Effect of actual stress on word associations. *Journal of Abnormal Psychology* 74: 293–295.

Mirenowicz, J., and Schultz, W. 1996. Preferential activation of midbrain dopamine neurons by appetitive rather than aversive stimuli. *Nature* 379: 449–451.

Modai, I., Stoler, M., Inbar-Saban, N., and Saban, N. 1993. Clinical decisions for psychiatric inpatients and their evaluation by a trained neural network. *Methods of Information in Medicine* 32: 396–399.

Mogliner, A., Grossman, J. A. I., Ribary, R., Joliot, M., Volkmann, J., Rapaport, D., Beasley, R. W., and Llinás, R. R. 1993. Somatosensory cortical plasticity in adult humans revealed by magnetoencephalography. *Proceedings of the National Academy of Science* 90: 3593–3597.

Morrison, J., and Hof, P. 1992. The organization of the cerebral cortex. *Discussions in Neuroscience* 11(2): 1–80.

Moss, F., and Wiesenfeld, K. 1995. The benefits of background noise. *Scientific American* (August): 50–53.

Mountcastle, V. B. 1957. Modality and topographic properties of single neurons of cat's somatic sensory cortex. *Journal of Neurophysiology* 30: 408–434.

Mountcastle, V. B., Alturi, P. P., and Romo, R. 1992. Selective output-discriminative signals in the motor cortex of waking monkeys. *Cerebral Cortex* 2: 277–294.

Mozer, M. C. 1993. Neural net architectures for temporal sequence processing. In Weigand, A., and Gershenfeld, N., eds., *Predicting the Future and Understanding the Past.* Reading, Mass.: Addison-Wesley.

Müller-Preuss, P., and Ploog, D. 1981. Inhibition of auditory cortical neurons during phonation. *Brain Research* 215: 61–76.

Mumford, M. 1992. On the computational architecture of the neocortex: II. The role of cortico-cortical loops. *Biological Cybernetics* 66: 241–251.

Mundt, D. 1984. Der Begriff der Intentionalität und die Defizienzlehre von den Schizophrenien *Nervenarzt* 55: 582–588.

Mundt, C. 1992. The history of psychiatry in Heidelberg. In Spitzer, M., Uehlein, F. A., Schwartz, M. A., and Mundt, C., eds., *Phenomenology, Language, and Schizophrenia*, pp. 16–31. New York: Springer.

Nauta, W., and Feirtag, M. 1990. *Neuroanatomie.* Heidelberg: Spektrum Verlag.

Neely, J. H. 1977. Semantic priming and retrieval from lexical memory: Roles of inhibitionless spreading activation and limited capacity attention. *Journal of Experimental Psychology* 106: 226–254.

Neumann, J. V. 1960. *The Computer and the Brain.* New Haven: Yale University Press.

Nichols, J. G., Martin, A. R., and Wallace, B. G. 1995. *Vom Neuron zum Gehirn: Zum Verständnis der zellulären und molekularen Funktion des Nervensystems,* Niehaus-Osterloh, M., and Bibbig, A., transl. Stuttgart: Gustav Fischer Verlag.

Ojemann, G. 1994. Intraoperative investigations of the neurobiology of language. *Discussions in Neuroscience* 10: 51–57.

O'Leary, T. J., Mikel, U. V., and Becker, R. L. 1992. Computer-assisted image interpretation: Use of a neural network to differentiate tubular carcinoma from sclerosing adenosis. *Modern Pathology* 5 (4): 402–405.

Oliver, S. G. 1996. From DNA sequence to biological funtion. *Nature* 379: 597–600.

Palermo, D., and Jenkins, J. J. 1964. *Word Association Norms.* Minneapolis: University of Minnesota Press.

Park, S., and Holzman, P. S. 1992. Schizophrenics show spatial working memory deficits. *Archives of General Psychiatry* 49: 975–982.

Park, S. B. G., and Young, A. H. 1994. Connectionism and psychiatry: A brief review. *Philosophy, Psychiatry and Psychology* 1: 51–58.

Parkin, A. J. 1996. H.M.: The medial temporal lobes and memory. In Wallesch, C.-W., Joanette, Y., and Lecourse, A. R., eds., *Classic Cases in Neuropsychology*, pp. 337–347. London: Erlbaum.

Pascual-Leone, A., and Torres, F. 1993. Plasticity of the sensorimotor cortex representation of the reading finger in Braille readers. *Brain* 116: 39–52.

Pechura, C. M., and Martin, J. B., eds. 1991. *Mapping the Brain and Its Functions*. Washington, D.C.: National Academy Press.

Penfield, W., and Boldrey, E. 1937. Somatic motor and sensory representation in the cerebral cortex of man as studied by electrical stimulation. *Brain* 60: 389–443.

Penfield, W., and Rasmussen, T. 1950. *The Cerebral Cortex of Man: A Clinical Study of Localization and Function*. Macmillan, New York.

Petrides, M., Alivisatos, B., Meyer, E., and Evans, A. C. 1993. Functional activation of the human frontal cortex during the performance of verbal working memory tasks. *Procedings of the National Academy of Science* 90: 878–882.

Pietrini, V., Nertempi, P., Vaglia, A., Revello, M. G., Pinna, V., and Ferro-Milone, F. 1988. Recovery from herpes simplex encephalitis: Selective impairment of specific semantic categories with neuroradiological correlation. *Journal of Neurology, Neurosurgery and Psychiatry* 51: 1284–1293.

Pinker, S. 1989. *Learnability and Cognition: The Acquisition of Argument Structure*. Cambridge: MIT Press.

Pinker, S. 1994. *The Language Instinct: How the Mind Creates Language*. New York: William Morrow.

Pinker, S., and Prince, A. 1988. On language and connectionism: An analysis of a parallel distributed processing model of language acquisition. *Cognition* 28: 73–193.

Plunkett, K. 1995. Language acquisition. In Arbib, M., ed., *Handbook of Brain Theory and Neural Networks*, pp. 503–506. Cambridge: MIT Press.

Plunkett, K. 1995. Connectionist approaches to language acquisition. In Fletcher, P., and MacWhinney, B., eds., *Handbook of Child Language*, pp. 36–72. Oxford: Blackwell.

Plunkett, K., and Marchman, V. 1991. U-shaped learning and frequency effects in a multi-layered perceptron: Implications for child language acquisition. *Cognition* 38: 1–60.

Pons, T. P., Garraghty, P. E., Ommaya, A. K., Kaas, J. H., Taub, E., and Mishkin, M. 1991. Massive cortical reorganization after sensory deafferentation in adult macaques. *Science* 252: 1857–1860.

Posner, M. I., and Raichle, M. 1996. *Bilder des Geistes*. Heidelberg: Spektrum Verlag.

Posner, M. I., Abdullaev, Y. G., McCandliss, B. D., and Sereno, S. C. 1996. Anatomy, circuitry and plasticity of word reading. In Everett, J., ed., *Visual Attentional Processes in Reading and Dyslexia*.

Pribram, K. H., and Gill, M. 1976. *Freud's Project Reassessed: Preface to Contemporary Cognitive Theory and Neuropsychology*. New York: Basic Books.

Purves, D. 1994. *Neural Activity and the Growth of the Brain*. Cambridge: Cambridge University Press.

Rakic, P. 1991. Plasticity of cortical development. In Brauth, S. E, Hall, W. S., and Dooling, R. J., eds., *Plasticity of Development*, pp. 127–161. Cambridge: MIT Press.

Raichle, M. E., Fiez, J. A., Videen, T. O., MacLeod, A.-M. K., Pardo, J. V., Fox, P. T., and Petersen, S. E. 1994. Practice-related changes in human brain functional anatomy during nonmotor learning *Cerebral Cortex* 4: 8–26.

Raleigh, M. J., and McGuire, M. T. 1984. Social and environmental influences on blood serotonin concentrations in monkeys. *Archives of General Psychiatry* 41: 405–410.

Raleigh, M. J., McGuire, M. T., Brammer, G. L., Pollack, D. B., and Yuwiler, A. 1991. Serotonergic mechanisms promote dominance acquisition in adult male vervet monkeys. *Brain Research* 559: 181–190.

Rall, W. 1995. Perspective on neuron model complexity. In Arbib, M., ed., *Handbook of Brain Theory and Neural Networks*, pp. 728–732. Cambridge: MIT Press.

Ramachandran, V. S., Rogers-Ramachandran, D., and Steward, M. 1992. Perceptual correlates of massive cortical reorganization. *Science* 258: 1159–1160.

Ramón y Cajal, S. 1988. *See* DeFelipe and Jones 1988.

Rauschecker, J. P. 1995. Compensatory plasticity and sensory substitution in the cerebral cortex. *Trends in Neuroscience* 18: 36–43.

Ravdin, P. R., and Clark, G. M. 1992. A practical application of neural network anlysis for predicting outcome of individual breast cancer patients. *Breast Cancer Research and Treatment* 22: 285–293.

Recanzone, G. H., Merzenich, M. M., and Dinse, H. R. 1992a. Expansion of the cortical representation of a specific skin field in primary somatosensory cortex by intracortical microstimulation. *Cerebral Cortex* 2: 181–196.

Recanzone, G. H., Merzenich, M. M., and Jenkins, W. M. 1992b. Frequency discrimination training engaging a restricted skin surface results in an emergence of a cutaneous response zone in cortical area 3a. *Journal of Neurophysiology* 67: 1057–1070.

Recanzone, G. H., Merzenich, M. M., Jenkins, W. M, Grajski, K. A., and Dinse, H. R. 1992c. Topographic reorganization of the hand representation in cortical area 3b of owl monkeys trained in a frequency-discrimination task. *Journal of Neurophysiology* 67(5): 1031–1056.

Recanzone, G. H., Merzenich, M. M., and Schreiner, C. E. 1992d. Changes in the distributed temporal response properties of SI cortical neurons reflect improvements in performance on a temporally based tactile discrimination task. *Journal of Neurophysiology* 67: 1071–1091.

Recanzone, G. H., Schreiner, C. E. , and Merzenich, M. M. 1993. Plasticity in the frequency representation of primary auditory cortex following discrimination training in adult owl monkeys. *Journal of Neuroscience* 13: 87–103.

Regan, D. 1989. *Human Electrophysiology*. New York: Elsevier.

Ritter, H. 1995. Self-organizing feature maps: Kohonen maps. In Arbib, M., ed., *Handbook of Brain Theory and Neural Networks*, pp. 846–851. Cambridge: MIT Press.

Ritter, H., and Kohonen, T. 1989. Self-organizing semantic maps. *Biological Cybernetics* 61: 241–254.

Ritter, H., Martinetz, T., and Schulten, K. 1991. *Neuronale Netze: Eine Einführung in die Neuroinformatik selbstorganisierender Netzwerke*. Bonn: Addison-Wesley.

Rock, I. 1984. *Wahrnehmung: Vom visuellen Reiz zum Sehen und Erkennen*. Heidelberg: Spektrum Verlag.

Rockel, A. J., Hiorns, R. W., and Powell, T. P. S. 1980. The basic uniformity in structure of the neocortex. *Brain* 103: 221–244.

Roland, P. 1994. *Brain Activation*. New York: Wiley-Liss.

Rose, S. 1992. *The Making of Memory*. New York: Anchor Books.

Rosenberg, R. N., and Rowland, L. P. 1990. The 1990s—Decade of the brain: The need for a national priority. *Neurology* 40: 322.

Roth, G. 1994. *Das Gehirn und seine Wirklichkeit*. Frankfurt: Suhrkamp.

Rueckl, J., Cave, K., and Kosslyn, S. 1989. Why are "what" and "where" processed by separate cortical systems? A computational investigation. *Journal of Cognitive Neuroscience* 1: 171–186.

Rumelhart, D. 1989. The architecture of mind: A connectionist approach. In Posner, M., ed., *Foundations of Cognitive Science*, pp. 133–159. Cambridge: MIT Press.

Rumelhart, D., and McClelland, J. L. 1986. On learning the past tense of English verbs. In Rumelhart, D., McClelland, J. L., *Parallel Distributed Processing: Explorations in the Microstructure of Cognition*, vol. 2, pp. 216–271. Cambridge: MIT Press.

Rumelhart, D., and McClelland, J. L., and PDP Research Group, eds. *Parallel Distributed Processing: Explorations in the Microstructure of Cognition*, 2 vols. Cambridge: MIT Press.

Rutledge, R. 1995. Injury severity and probability of survival assessment in trauma patients using a predictive hierarchical network model derived from ICD-9 codes. *Journal of Trauma* 38: 590–597, discussion, 597–601.

Rymer, R. 1992. Annals of science. A silent childhood. *The New Yorker* (13 April): 41–81, (20 April): 43–77.

Sacchett, C., and Humphreys, G. W. 1992. Calling a squirrel a squirrel but a canoe a wigwam: A category-specific deficit for artefactual objects and body parts. *Cognitive Neuropsychology* 9: 73–86.

Sahgal, A., ed. 1993. *Behavioural Neuroscience: A Practical Approach*, 2 vols. Oxford: Oxford University Press.

Sanchez-Sinecio, E., and Lau, C. 1992. *Artificial Neural Networks: Paradigms, Applications, and Hardware Implementations*. New York: IEEE Press.

Sano, I. 1956. Über chronische Weckaminsucht in Japan. *Fortschritte der Neurologie und Psychiatrie* 24: 391–394.

Sartori, G., and Job, R. 1988. The oyster with four legs: A neuropsychological study on the interaction of visual and semantic information. *Cognitive Neuropsychology* 5(1): 105–132.

Saß, H. 1989. The historical evolution of the concept of negative symptoms in schizophrenia. *British Journal of Psychiatry* 155 (suppl. 7): 26–31.

Schieber, M. H., and Hibbard, L. S. 1993. How somatotopic is the motor cortex hand area? *Science* 261: 489–492.

Schilder, P. 1923. Über elementate Halluzinationen des Bewegungssehens. *Zeitschrift für Neurologie und Psychiatrie* 80: 424–431.

Schlaggar, B. L., and O'Leary, .D. D. M 1991. Potential of visual cortex to develop an array of functional units unique to somatosensory cortex. *Science* 252: 1556–1560.

Schlicht, H. J. 1995. Anwendung und professionelle Nutzung der Kodak Photo CD. Bonn: Addison-Wesley.

Schmajuk, N. A. 1995. Conditioning. In Arbib, M., ed., *Handbook of Brain Theory and Neural Networks*, pp. 238–243. Cambridge: MIT Press.

Schmidt, R. F., and Thews, G. 1995. *Physiologie des Menschen*, 26th ed. Berlin: Springer.

Schöneburg, E. 1993. Industrielle Anwendung neuronaler Netze. Addison-Wesley, Bonn

Schwartz, E. L., ed. 1990. *Computational Neuroscience*. Cambridge: MIT Press.

Scoville, W. B., and Milner, B. 1957. Loss of recent memory after bilateral hippocampal lesions. *Journal of Neurology, Neurosurgery and Psychiatry* 20: 11–21.

Segal, Z. V., Williams, J. M., Teasdale, J. D., and Gemar, M. 1996. A cognitive science perspective on kindling and episode sensitization in recurrent affective disorder. *Psychological Medicine* 26: 371–380.

Segev, I. 1995. Dendritic processing. In Arbib, M., ed., *Handbook of Brain Theory and Neural Networks*, pp. 282–289. Cambridge: MIT Press.

Seidenberg, M. S. 1995. Linguistic morphology. In Arbib, M., ed., *Handbook of Brain Theory and Neural Networks*, pp. 546–549. Cambridge: MIT Press.

Semenza, C. 1988. Impairment in localization of body parts following brain damage. *Cortex* 24: 443–449.

Sereno, M. I., Dale, A. M., Reppas, J. B., Kwong, K. K., Belliveau, J. W., Brady, T. J., Rosen, B. R., and Tootel, R. B. H. 1995. Borders of multiple visual areas in humans revealed by functional magnetic resonance imaging. *Science* 268: 889–893.

Servan-Schreiber, D., Cohen, J. D., and Steingard, S. 1995. Schizophrenic deficits in the processing of context: A test of neural network simulations of cognitive functioning in schizophrenia. *Archives of General Psychiatry* XXX: XXX–XXX.

Servan-Schreiber, D., Printz, H., and Cohen, J. D. 1990. A network model of catecholamine effects: Gain, signal-to-noise ratio, and behavior. *Science* 249: 892–895.

Shallice, T. 1988. *From Neuropsychology to Mental Structure*. Cambridge: Cambridge University Press.

Shaywitz, B. A., Shaywitz, S. E., Pugh, K. R., Constable, R. T., Skudlarki, P., Fulbright, R. K., Bronen, R. A., Fletcher, J. M., Shankweiler, D. P., Katz, L., and Gore, J. C. 1995. Sex differences in the functional organization of the brain for language. *Nature* 373: 607–609.

Shepard, R. N., and Cooper, L. A. 1982. *Mental Images and Their Transformations*. Cambridge: MIT Press.

Shepherd, G. M. 1994. *Neurobiology*. Oxford: Oxford University Press.

Shepherd, G. M., and Brayton, R. K. 1987. Logic operations are properties of computer-simulated interactions between excitable dendritic spines. *Neuroscience* 21: 151–165.

Siebler, M., Rose, G., Sitzer, M., Bender, A, and Steinmetz, H. 1994. Real-time identification of cerebral microemboli with US feature detection by a neural network. *Radiology* 192: 739–742.

Siegle, G., Ingram, R, and Matt, G. 1995. A connectionist model of the emotional Stroop task (paper submitted).

Silbersweig, D. A., Stern, E., Frith, C., Cahill, C., Holmes, A., Grootoonk, S., Seaward, J., McKenna, P., Chua, S. E., Schnorr, L., Jones, T., and Frackowiak, R. S. J. 1995. A functional neuroanatomy of hallucinations in schizophrenia. *Nature* 378: 176–179.

Silveri, M. C., Daniele, A., Giustolisi, L., and Gainotti, G. 1988. Dissociation between knowledge of living and nonliving things in dementia of the Alzheimer type. *Neurology* 41: 545–546.

Sirigu, A., Duhamel, J. R., and Poncet, M. 1991. The role of sensorimotor experience in object recognition: A case of multimodal agnosia. *Brain* 114: 2555–2573.

Sklar, A. D., and Harris, R. F. 1985. Effects of parent loss: Interaction with family size and sibling order. *American Journal of Psychiatry* 142: 708–714.

Small, S. L., Hart, J., Nguyen, T., and Gordon, B. 1995. Distributed representations of semantic knowledge in the brain. *Brain* 118: 441–453.

Smyrnis, N., Taira, M., Ashe, J., and Georgopoulos, A. P. 1992. Motor cortical activity in a memorized delay task. *Experimental Brain Research* 92: 139–151.

Somoza, E., and Somoza, J. R. 1993. A neural network approach to predicting admission decisions in a psychiatric emergency room. *Medical Decision Making* 13: 273–280.

Spies, M. 1993. *Unsicheres Wissen: Wahrscheinlichkeit, Fuzzy-Logik, neuronale Netze und menschliches Denken.* Heidelberg: Spektrum Verlag.

Spillmann, L., and Werner, J. S. 1990. *Visual Perception: The Neurophysiological Foundations.* San Diego: Academic Press.

Spitzer, M. 1988. *Halluzinationen.* Berlin: Springer.

Spitzer, M. 1989a. *Wahn.* Berlin: Springer.

Spitzer, M. 1989b. What Are Thoughts Made of? Associations, Bits, Rules, and Neural Networks in the Light of Some Pathological Phenomena. In Klein, P., ed., *Praktische Logik: Traditionen und Tendenzen; 350 Jahre Joachimi JungII "Logica Hamburgensis,"* pp. 287–314. Proceedings of a seminar for the 13th International Wittgenstein Symposium, Kirchberg am Wechsel. 1988. Göttingen: Vandenhoeck und Ruprecht.

Spitzer, M. 1992. Word-Associations in experimental psychiatry: A historical perspective. In Spitzer, M., Uehlein, F. A., Schwartz, M. A., and Mundt, C., eds., *Phenomenology, Language and Schizophrenia,* pp. 160–196. New York: Springer.

Spitzer, M. 1993. Assoziative Netzwerke, formale Denkstörungen und Schizophrenie: Zur experimentellen Psychopathologie sprachabhängiger Denkprozesse. *Der Nervenarzt* 64: 147–159.

Spitzer, M. 1994. Neuronale Netzwerke. *Medizinische Monatsschrift für Pharmazeuten* 11: 329–341.

Spitzer, M. 1995a. A neurocomputational approach to delusions. *Comprehensive Psychiatry* 36: 83–105.

Spitzer, M. 1995b. Neural networks and the psychopathology of delusions: The importance of neuroplasticity and neuromodulation. *Neurology, Psychiatry and Brain Research* 3: 47–58.

Spitzer, M. 1995c. Conceptual developments in psychiatry and the neurosciences. *Current Opinion in Psychiatry* 8: 317–329.

Spitzer, M. 1996. History of neural networks. In Stein, D., ed., *Neural Networks and Psychopathology* (in press).

Spitzer, M. 1997. A cognitive neuroscience view of schizophrenic thought disorder. *Schizophrenia Bulletin* 23: 29–50.

Spitzer, M. 1999. *Psychiatry and Cognitive Neuroscience*. Cambridge: Harvard University Press

Spitzer, M., Braun, U., Maier, S., Hermle, L., and Maher, B. A. 1993a. Indirect semantic priming in schizophrenic patients. *Schizophrenia Research* 11: 71–80.

Spitzer, M., Braun, U., Hermle, L., and Maier, S. 1993b. Associative semantic network dysfunction in thought-disordered schizophrenic patients: Direct evidence from indirect semantic priming. *Biological Psychiatry* 34: 864–877.

Spitzer, M., Weisker, I., Winter, M., and Maier, S. 1993c. Semantische Aktivierungsphänomene bei gesunden Probanden und schizophrenen Patienten: Analyse auf Wortpaarebene. *Zeitschrift für Klinische Psychologie, Psychopathologie und Psychotherapie* 41: 343–357.

Spitzer, M., and Mundt, C. 1994. Interchanges between philosophy and psychiatry: The continental tradition. *Current Opinion in Psychiatry* 7: 417–422.

Spitzer, M., Lukas, M., and Maier, S. 1994a. Experimentelle Untersuchungen zum Verstehen metaphorischer Rede bei gesunden Probanden und schizophrenen Patienten. *Der Nervenarzt* 65: 282–292.

Spitzer, M., Weisker, I., Maier, S., Hermle, L, and Maher, B. A. 1994b. Semantic and phonological priming in schizophrenia. *Journal of Abnormal Psychology* 103: 485–494.

Spitzer, M., Beuckers, J., Maier, S., and Hermle, L. 1994c. Contextual insensitivity in schizophrenic patients is due to semantic network pathology: Evidence from pauses in spontaneous speech. *Language and Speech* 37: 171–185.

Spitzer, M., Böhler, P., Kischka, U., Weisbrod, M. 1995a. A neural network model of phantom limbs. *Biological Cybernetics* 72: 197–206.

Spitzer, M., Kwong, K. K., Kennedy, W., Rosen, B. R., Belliveau, J. W. 1995b. Category-specific brain activation in fMRI during picture naming. *Neuroreport* 6: 2109–2112.

Spitzer, M., Kammer, T., Bellemann, M. E., Gückel, F., Georgi, M., Gass, A., Brix, G. 1996. Funktionelle Magnetresonanztomographie bei Aktivierung des Arbeitsgedächtnisses. *Fortschritte auf dem Gebiet der Röntgenstrahlen und der neuen bildgebenden Verfahren* 65: 52–58.

Steinmetz, H., and Seitz, R. J. 1991. Functional anatomy of language processing: Neuroimaging and the problem of individual variability. *Neuropsychologia* 29: 1149–1161.

Strozer, J. R. 1994. *Language Acquisition After Puberty*. Washington, D.C.: Georgetown University Press.

Suga, N., and Jen, P. S. 1976. Disproportionate tonotopic representation for processing CF-FM sonar signals in the mustache bat auditory cortex. *Science* 194: 542–544.

Sulloway, F. J. 1982. *Freud: Biologie der Seele: Jenseits der psychoanalytischen Legende.* Köln-Lövenich: Hohenheim Verlag.

Suomi, S. J. 1991a. Primate separation models of affective disorder. In Madden, J., ed., *Neurobiology of Learning, Emotion, and Affect*, pp. 195–214. New York: Raven Press.

Suomi, S. J. 1991b. Early stress and adult emotional reactivity in rhesus monkeys. In *Papers of the Ciba Foundation Symposium* 156: 171–188. Chichester, Eng.: Wiley.

Suomi, S. J. 1991c. Uptight and laid-back monkeys: Individual differences in the response to social challenges. In Brauth, S. E., Hall, W. S., and Dooling, R. J., eds., *Plasticity of Development*, pp. 27–56. Cambridge: MIT Press.

Tallal, P., Stark, R. E., and Mellitis, . 1985. The relationship between auditory temporal analysis and receptive language development: Evidence from studies of developmental language disorder. *Neuropsychologia* 23: 537–544.

Tallal, P., Miller, S. L., Bedi, G., Byma, G., Wang, X., Nagarajan, S. S., Schreiner, C., Jenkins, W. M., and Merzenich, M. M. 1996. Language comprehension in language-learning impaired children improved with acoustically modified speech. *Science* 271: 81–84.

Teasdale, J. 1988. Cognitive vulnerability to persistent depression. *Cognition and Emotion* 2: 247–274.

Thomson, A. M., and Deuchars, J. 1994. Temporal and spatial properties of local circuits in neocortex. *Trends in Neuroscience* 17(3): 119–126.

Todd, L. 1900. *Pidgins and Creoles*, 2nd ed. London: Routledge.

Toga, A. W., and Mazziotta, J. C. 1996. *Brain Mapping: The Methods.* San Diego: Academic Press.

Trepel, M. 1995. *Neuroanatomie: Struktur und Funktion.* Munich: Urban und Schwarzenberg.

Tu, J., and Guerriere, M. 1993. Use of a neural network as a predictive instrument for length of stay in the intensive care unit following cardiac surgery. *Computation in Biomedical Research* 26(3): 220–229.

Tucker, D. M. 1993. Spatial sampling of head electrical fields: The geodesic sensor net. *Electroencephalography and Clinical Neurophysiology* 87: 154–163.

Tucker, D. M., Liotti, M., Potts, G. F., Russell, G. S., and Posner, M. I. 1994. Spatiotemporal analysis of brain electrical fields. *Human Brain Mapping* 1: 134–152.

Uexküll, J. v, and Kriszat, G. 1940/1970. *Streifzüge durch die Umwelten von Tieren und Menschen: Bedeutungslehre.* Frankfurt am Main: S. Fischer.

Ungerleider, L. G., and Mishkin, M. 1982. Two cortical visual systems. In Ingle, D. J., Goodale, M. A., and Mansfield, R. J. W., eds., *Analysis of Visual Behavior*, pp. 549–586. Cambridge: MIT Press.

Vines, G. 1996. Death of a mother tongue. *New Scientist* (6 January): 24–27.

Warrington, E. K., and McCarthy, R. 1983. Category specific access dysphasia. *Brain* 106: 859–878.

Warrington, E., and McCarthy, R. 1987. Categories of knowledge. *Brain* 110: 1273–1296.

Warrington, E. K., and Shallice, T. 1984. Category specific semantic impairments. *Brain* 107: 829–854.

Weinberger, D. R., Faith Berman, K., Suddath, R., and Fuller Torrey, E. 1992. Evidence of dysfunction of a prefrontal-limbic network in schizophrenia: A magnetic resonance imaging and regional cerebral blood flow study of discordant monozygotic twins. *American Journal of Psychiatry* 149(7): 890–897.

Welk, E., Leah, J. D., and Zimmermann, M. 1990. Characteristics of A- and C-fibers ending in a sensory nerve neuroma in the rat. *Journal of Neurophysiology* 63: 759–766.

White, H.1989. Learning in artificial neural networks: A statistical perspective. *Neural Computation* 1: 425–464.

White, L. E., Lucas, G., Richards, A., and Purves, D. 1994. Cerebral asymmetry and handedness (letter). *Nature* 368: 197–198.

White, M. W., Ochs, M. T., Merzenich, M. M., and Schubert, E. D. 1990. Speech recognition in analog multichannel cochlear prostheses: Initial experiments in controlling classifications. *IEEE Transactions on Biomedical Engineering* 37: 1002–1010.

Wiedling, J. U., and Schönle, P. W. 1991. Neuronale Netze. *Nervenarzt* 62: 415–422.

Wiesenfeld, K., and Moss, F. 1995. Stochastic resonance and the benefits of noise: From ice ages to crayfish and squids. *Nature* 373: 33–36.

Wilding, P., Morgan, M. A., Grygotis, A. E., Shoffner, M. A., and Rosato, E. F. 1994. Application of backpropagation neural networks to diagnosis of breast and ovarian cancer. *Cancer Letters* 77: 145–153.

Wilkins, E. G. 1917/1979. *"Know Thyself" in Greek and Latin Literature.* New York: Garland Publishing.

Williams, J., and Oaksford, M. 1992. Cognitive science, anxiety and depression: From experiments to connectionism. In Stein, D., and Young, A., eds., *Cognitive Science and the Clinical Disorders.* San Diego: Academic Press.

Wilson, F. A. W., Scalaidhe, S. P. O., and Goldman-Rakic, P. S. 1993. Dissociation of object and spatial processing domains in primate prefrontal cortex. *Science* 260: 1955–1957.

Wilson, M. A., and McNaughton, B. L. 1993. Dynamics of the hippocampal ensemble code for space. *Science* 261: 1055–1058.

Wilson, M. A., and McNaughton, B. L. 1994. Reactivation of hippocampal ensemble memories during sleep. *Science* 265: 676–679.

Wing, J. K. 1986. Der Einfluß psychosozialer Faktoren auf den Langzeitverlauf der Schizophrenie. In Böker, W., and Brenner, H. D., eds., *Bewältigung der Schizophrenie*, pp. 11–28. Bern: Huber.

Wise, R., Chollet, F., Hadar, U., Friston, K., Hoffner, E., and Frackowiak, R. 1991. Distribution of cortical neural networks involved in word comprehension and word retrieval. *Brain* 114: 1803–1817.

Wittgenstein, L. 1969. Schriften 1: *Tractatus logico-philosophicus; Tagebücher; Philosophische Untersuchungen.* Frankfurt: Suhrkamp.

Woolsey, C. N. 1982. Multiple auditory maps. In *Cortical Sensory Organization*, vol. 3. Clifton, N.J.: Humana Press.

Wu, Y., Giger, M. L., Doi, K., Vyborny, C. J., Schmidt, R. A., and Metz, C. E. 1993. Artificial neural networks in mammography: Application to decision making in the diagnosis of breast cancer. *Radiology* 187: 81–87.

Yamadori, A., and Albert, M. L. 1973. Word category aphasia. *Cortex* 9: 112–125.

Yang, T. T., Gallen, C., Schwartz, B., Bloom, F. E., Ramachandran, V. S., and Cobb, S. 1994. Sensory maps in the human brain. *Nature* 368: 592–593.

Yates, J., and Nasby, W. 1993. Dissociation, affect, and network models of memory: An integrative proposal. *Journal of Traumatic Stress* 6: 305–326.

Yeh, S. R., Fricke, R. A., and Edwards, D. H. 1996. The effects of social experience on serotonergic modulation of the escape circuit of crayfish. *Science* 271: 366–369.

Young, K. A., Brady, M. D., and Hicks, P. B. 1995. Psychophysiological evidence for neuroleptic-induced depolarization block in schizophrenics [abstract]. *Schizophrenia Research* 15: 170–171.

Zeki, S. 1993. *A Vision of the Brain.* Oxford: Blackwell Scientific Publications.

Zell, A. 1994. *Simulation neuronaler Netze.* Bonn: Addison-Wesley.

Zipser, D, 1990. Modeling cortical computation with backpropagation. In Gluck, M. A., and Rumelhart, D. E., eds. *Neuroscience and Connectionist Theory*, pp. 355–383. Hillsdale, N.J.: Erlbaum.

Zipser, D, and Andersen, R. A. 1988. A back propagation network that simulates the spatial tuning properties of posterior parietal neurons. *Nature* 331: 679–684.

Zipser, D, and Rumelhart, D. E. 1990. The neurobiological significance of the new learning models. In Schwartz, E. L., ed., *Computational Neuroscience*, pp. 192–200. Cambridge: MIT Press.

Zubin, J. 1986. Mögliche Implikationen der Vulnerabilitätshypothese für das psychosoziale Management der Schizophrenie. In Böker, W., and Brenner, H. D., eds., *Bewältigung der Schizophrenie*, pp. 29–41. Bern: Huber.

Zuk, G. H. 1956. The phantom limb: A proposed theory of unconscious origins. *Journal of Nervous and Mental Disease* 124: 510–513.

Index